Global Bioethics

Conflicts and Trends™ Studies in Values and Policies

Global Bioethics
The Collapse of Consensus

Edited by

H. Tristram Engelhardt, Jr.
Rice University, Houston

M&M Scrivener Press

Published by M & M Scrivener Press
72 Endicott Street, Salem, MA 01970

http://www.mmscrivenerpress.com

First published 2006

10 9 8 7 6 5 4 3 2 1

Library of Congress Control Number: 2006922383

ISBN - 13: 978-0-9764041-3-2
ISBN - 10: 0-9764041-3-3

Dust jacket: Hannus Design

Printed in United States of America on acid-free paper.

Contents

Foreword

Stephen A. Erickson

The volume before you stands as a threshold, for unavoidable questions arise regarding where we must go after absorbing its content. It is to these that I will speak. Such questions do assume that substantial agreement has been reached regarding where we currently stand. Such a consensus is in place, and the various and complementary arguments undergirding it are insurmountable: the conditions for the possibility of constructing a viable global bioethics do not exist. To the extent that they ever did they have been undermined. I will not survey and classify the various political, philosophical, cultural, and religious factors involved in this undermining. Rather, I will pause amidst the ruins of attempts at global bioethics to bring into further focus what must be addressed and what might be salvaged and carried forward as we move further into the twenty-first century. This amounts to a set of fundamental, critical and in some instances quite immediate issues and some ineradicable questions that accompany them.

For centuries it had been taken for granted that human beings have a nature. Also assumed was that though *in,* we humans are not altogether *of* this world, that we have a directedness or intentionality that point us toward a beyond. To be sure, the preposition 'of'—as in *not* of (*this* world)—has been required to shoulder a heavy metaphorical load by some, but whether its burden was construed as more literal or metaphorical, not being of this world was assumed to be an essential component of the human.

Is it time for a more open and engaged revisiting of this understanding of our human nature? Altogether certainly this should take place, precisely because of what has occurred in the interim. Enlightenment thinking, of which the discredited project of global bioethics is a contemporary variant, has attempted to rationalize and naturalize the human in a manner that rejects any transcendent dimension, as if human beings were *only* in this world. But no criteria other than internal, question-begging ones exist for justifying such a project, and, over the course of recent time, a set of conflicting secular agendas has arisen along these lines that at best sow confusion and at worst undermine all such undertakings. No, it is decidedly time to reconsider what it means to be human. Only on this basis might progress be made regarding those crucial issues to which bioethics must speak. To cast an eye over the globe is to see that its clustered, yet also dispersed inhabitants are both diverse and diversely religious. The religious dimension to human existence is no severable sideshow, neither to the historical nor to the contemporary human scene.

Also needing renewed consideration are questions regarding the meaning of history and possible configurations of our pending future. For many this might seem a strange statement. In the aftermath of large-scale nineteenth century philosophies of history we have been living within a pervasively secular set of assumptions, the core of which involve beliefs that the future can be successfully managed and that the goal of this management is a biotechnologically enhanced quantity and quality of worldly life. Might our human history have a different, complementary if not conflicting significance than this? A number of the world's major religions have believed this, and the manner in which the twenty-first century was dramatically and devastatingly launched tells us that there are those who are cruelly exploiting this belief today. Can our imminently pending historical future be construed solely as a battleground between the supposed superstitions of the varyingly religious and the allegedly enlightened resolves of those committed to advancing medical technologies? It is most doubtful. Philosophy of history has been decidedly out of fashion for over a hundred years. That it should rightly join company with alchemy and astronomy is by no means a foregone conclusion. If questions remain to be asked regarding our human nature, they must surely extend to a consideration of how and to what degree our nature is an historical one. Once begun, this consideration cannot avoid sustained reflections on History itself.

The aftermath of failed projects such as that of global bioethics is never easy to predict, though steps can be taken to ameliorate, if not altogether to prevent the most destructive consequences that such failures often engender. Some claim that the Enlightenment project's hope for secularly grounded universal values remained alive less because it was realistic than because it helped ameliorate some of the most rebarbative dimensions of those romantic reactions that it spawned. Enlightenment came to mean for many a concern for communication, the finding of common ground, and sometimes even the partial resolution of open conflict. In this sense, philosophers are often called upon to "enlighten," and there are at least four core issues needing to be addressed in this manner as we move further into the twenty-first century. Each, of course, opens up many other issues, and each will need to be taken up and be carefully pursued, both in context-specific and in more pervasive ways.

(1) With reference to particular writings and discussion, does 'global' truly mean global, as in reasonable and, once promulgated, minimally acceptable in most parts of the "educated" world? Or is the use of the term 'global,' whether intentionally or not, essentially a tactical means of forwarding a particular and in important respects exclusive and therefore polarizing agenda?

(2) What are the likely implications and trajectories for specific brands of bioethics, whether purportedly global or regional, in an age that is dramatically advancing scientifically, but that we also find almost bewilderingly diverse and fractious in its moral customs and practices?

(3) How is one to map and assign responsibility for resolving ethical quandaries in bioethics in terms of the overlapping, yet often conflicting *loci* of decision making suggested by the notions of individual, family, physician, community and state, especially when states are not only national but in some instances trans- or international in presumption?

(4) Why should it be that in our time medical practice has come so far toward the center not only of philosophical ethics, but of political and religious concern as well?

How might philosophical reflection of the sort needed take place? Here I must first offer an account of the generation of this volume. It is meant as a means of encouraging reflections on ways of structuring future philosophical venues. My concern is with open and ongoing discussion in a world that itself truly *is* global in the sense of being both international and multi-cultural, even if it is not amenable to a unifying set of global doctrines.

Compilations of papers, subsequently anthologized, typically involve authors who neither meet together nor even receive the benefit of studying each other's contributions in advance of publication. Such was decidedly not the case in this present undertaking. The volume before you grew up under unusually favorable interactive circumstances. Critical, yet integrative discussion was at a premium. The twelve contributors had three sustained opportunities over roughly a three-year period to come together to discuss their submissions in draft form. Not only did this make constructive revision more feasible, but it also fostered a measure of integration of effort and outcome more substantial than is usually found among a diverse set of writers. And, residing and working in Canada, Hong Kong, Germany, Italy and the United States, these writers are decidedly diverse, even in geography.

Each gathering took place over a two and one-half day period in a relatively secluded environment and involved six ninety-minute formal sessions devoted to the writers' drafts of their material. In the course of these days there were numerous informal discussions among the participants as well. Meals were taken together, and a hospitality suite was provided. These circumstances and their attendant opportunities were made possible through the extraordinary generosity of Liberty Fund, Inc. of Indianapolis, Indiana, a tax exempt, private operating foundation established to encourage the study of the ideal of a society of free and responsible individuals and those institutions that might be thought to support such an ideal. The Liberty Fund itself asked nothing of the participants except open, informed, diligent and civil discussion and exchange of views regarding the topic at hand.

My role at these meetings—held in Houston, Texas (October 2001), Palermo, Sicily (January 2003) and near Dublin, Ireland (June 2004)—merits a brief description, for it bears on this foreword. I served as moderator or, somewhat misleadingly, as the discussion leader. Not a direct contributor to the discussions except in the service of reformulations or clarifications of issues, my task was to direct very brisk and intellectually vigorous conversational traffic among the very engaged participants. It fell to me to make sure that only one conferee spoke at a time and that the themes that emerged received sustained consideration. Given six formal sessions per gathering and twelve contributing participants, it was possible to foreground and emphasize each participant's work for roughly one half of one session, thus for forty-five minutes. Since in each case the papers had been circulated well in advance of the meetings, however, and the formal discussions were directly preceded by and carried over into rich, informal conversations, each paper received more than this limited amount of attention. Whether this sort of environment, conducive as it is to probing and sustained exchange can be secured with any regularity in the future is of course doubtful. But it provided nearly an ideal environment for serious communication, and offered me an extraordinary vantage point for reflecting on future philosophical needs and possibilities.

The preparatory environment fostering this particular volume aside, how is further dialogue possible, what forms might it take, and what sorts of barriers might stand in its way? Let me begin with something recognized less helpfully than it should be. T.S. Eliot may well be right: the relation of culture to religion may be so intimate as to suggest that cultures are in important respects the incarnations of religions. Viewed anthropologically and epistemologically it is equally, if not more plausible that methods, even of spiritual/intellectual reflection have a cultural dimension to them. I have deliberately conjoined "spiritual" and "intellectual" in an ambiguous and indeterminate way, in order to leave open various, themselves possibly culturally bound possibilities of their integration or segregation. Much remains to be meditated upon and determined with respect to these matters.

From these two, admittedly unwieldy claims—regarding the intimacy of religion with culture and culture with methods of reflection and inquiry—it follows that at least in some settings intellectual investigation itself will have a religious dimension to it as well, whether unwitting, more cognizantly devotional, or in the service of some other dynamic or end. Obviously this circumstance might thwart, but possesses equally the potential to enrich the possibilities and dimensions of exchange, and hopefully of wisdom as well. And exchange will be increasingly needed, for, as this volume helps us realize, a plurality of increasingly overt religious perspectives as well as differing secular ones is likely to be, at a minimum, a major part of our twenty-first century dispensation.

Since the ascendancy of Enlightenment thinking in an increasingly rationalized West, secular in its aspirations, the conditions for human receptivity have been given a correspondingly decreasing degree of attention. On the one hand, receptivity had been understood for centuries as the capacity through which various forms of encounter were made possible. Of particular prominence had been divine revelation, mystically or straightforwardly construed. Receptivity, thereby, lived off what the Enlightenment took to be discredited capital. On the other hand, receptivity has been limited to what is available to the senses and, thus, to the confines of the physical world—the materials made available through inner sense providing a problematic, though largely unexplored and even unexamined exception to this exclusivist doctrine. Surely, this circumstance will need to change, for as Hegel could ask how a weighing machine (reason) could weigh itself, so we must ask how receptivity might also be receptive to its own nature and potential configurations, or whether it might actually with respect to itself be a glass only darkly seen, but not itself reliably seen through to its underlying foundations. In a world that is religious not just in action and doctrines, but also in ritual and in perception itself, such questions are not only disarming, but also disarmingly unavoidable.

Part of the problem we face going forward is surely bound up with the unraveling of the self-sustaining integrity of reason itself. Fashionably we might say that reason has undergone its own self-deconstruction, thereby losing purchase on any unaided claims it had to universality in any more than the most abstract and content-bereft sense. More directly, we can say that reason has become increasingly technological, and this is because it has needed to draw from human desires and purposes in order to achieve operational content. But what knowledge do we have of human purpose itself? Is it more generated or received, and in what proportions? Only through sustained reflection on matters such as these can any bioethics hope to speak foundationally and appropriately, insightfully and with transformative conviction.

The burgeoning technologies of our contemporary world, some even necessary, are nonetheless insufficient to our cultural, historical, and often pervasively religious embeddedness. But even the seeming innocence of the word "embedded" may too easily mislead us. It suggests an inner something lodged in an outer something else. Perhaps some form of duality is necessary to illumine our lives *in* (though not necessarily *of*) this world. But are words such as inner and outer the best means of conveying this? If they are, are our various "inners," as our corresponding "outers," themselves not complex pluralities, and how are varying inner-outer distinctions to be sorted out? If something (or perhaps everything) is said to be left or to reside in the hand of God, for example, how is inner and outer to be understood in terms of this very striking, though common perception?

Medicine and, with it, bioethics are already coming in our time to occupy that most central position once reserved for religion and theology, and later for science and conceptually oriented naturalistic philosophy. For bioethics to thrive it must not only take up this assignment, but do so in a way that is transparent to itself. Such transparency requires that bioethics not flinch from confronting those most fundamental questions which our age puts before it. These questions concern nothing less, but in fact much more than the meaning and purpose of human life. They equally concern the ground of human life. It is toward a reopening of these issues with courage, integrity, and humble confidence that my short foreword is directed.

Global Bioethics: An Introduction to the Collapse of Consensus

H. Tristram Engelhardt, Jr.

I. Passionately Seeking an Ever-Elusive Consensus

Although the title of this volume is *Global Bioethics,* this is not a book just about bioethics. It is a disturbing study of the contemporary moral predicament. More than that, it is an analysis of the human moral condition. The volume brings us to confront the circumstance that the culture wars that fragment bioethical reflections into contending partisan camps are grounded in intractable moral diversity. It is not just that there is a failure of consensus on all the major issues of human life, ranging from the significance of human sexuality, human reproduction, early human life, the allocation of scarce resources, and the nature of governmental authority, to the significance of suffering, dying, and death, but that no resolution of our controversies appears in sight. This state of affairs brings into question the ways in which Western Europeans have regarded morality for more than a millennium. In so doing, the essays in this collection, drawn from contributors from the United States, Canada, Western Europe, and the Pacific Rim, invite us to revise settled understandings of moral reflection, especially of moral philosophy. The cultural diagnosis offered requires us to determine how we can understand free and responsible action when there is disagreement about the nature of the good, the right, the virtuous, and the nature of human flourishing.

This volume acknowledges four striking features of contemporary morality. First, moral reflection is marked by prominent, indeed passionate disagreement. Moral philosophers support different moralities framed within incompatible settled moral judgments. One might think of the contrast

H.T. Engelhardt, Jr. (ed), *Global Bioethics* (pp. 1–17).

between a typically Singaporean and Texian understanding of a rightly-ordered polis, proper governance, and true human flourishing. There are competing moralities. There are competing bioethics. There are those who support and those who condemn homosexual activities and marriages. There are those who support and those who condemn abortion. There are those who support and those who condemn social democratic approaches to the allocation of resources. There are those who support and those who condemn physician-assisted suicide, euthanasia, and capital punishment. There is public debate and sustained disagreement about the significance of human sexuality, reproduction, property rights, the limits of governmental authority, the allocation of scarce resources, suffering, dying, and death, as well as about the nature of the good and human flourishing. The disagreements do not simply concern particular issues, but involve divergent worldviews. These disagreements are expressed in incompatible moral life-styles embedded in disparate moral life-worlds. The moral controversies involved give issue to cultural wars within societies, and indeed are manifested in clashes between societies shaped by different dominant moral perspectives. The disagreements are deep and at times they even issue in bloody conflict. Moral controversy defines the human condition.

Second, moral dispute is not just salient but persistent. The disagreements regarding the morality of abortion, homosexual liaisons, physician-assisted suicide, and euthanasia have histories that reach back over at least two and a half millennia. The disagreements are perennial; they characterize both ancient and contemporary moral reflections, though they may become muted in the face of a forcefully established orthodoxy.

Third, there are good grounds for holding that moral controversy is not just contingently persistent. Rather, it is impossible through sound, rational, secular argument to resolve the controversies dividing moralities along with their bioethics. This is the case because those in dispute frequently disagree regarding basic premises, as well as rules of moral and metaphysical evidence. This is to say that people are not just in disagreement regarding particular moral matters, but often about the foundational character of morality itself. It may be the case that all moralities have concerns regarding sexual relations, reproduction, the distribution of property, the significance of suffering, and the death of humans. These concerns, after all, reflect the character of human embodiment. Nevertheless, moralities differ in terms of the circumstances under which it is licit, forbidden, or obligatory to have sexual intercourse, to reproduce, to distribute property, or to kill humans. Different orderings of basic human goods and of cardinal right- and wrong-making conditions lie at the root of the differences separating disparate moralities and the settled judgments they sustain. Even if it were the case (as these essays show to be counter-factual) that all moralities were assembled from the same building blocks (in fact, moralities appear to use different building blocks; Christian concerns with the holy and Confucian concerns with ritual are not reducible to concerns of secular liberal morality), these basic moral building blocks are put together in quite different fashions. Moralities are also distinguished as to whether they acknowledge right-making conditions that cannot be reduced to interests in the good (i.e., as claimed by Kantian moralities), as well as to whether and how preferences should be corrected. As a consequence of the disparity of foundational moral premises and rules of evidence, attempts through sound, rational argument to secure a particular moral vision inevitably beg the question, argue in a circle, or engage in infinite regress. Most moral debates are as a result intractable.

Fourth, in the face of perennial disagreements, indeed despite such disagreement and its intractability, there are proclamations, at times passionately, of moral consensus. Confronted by bitter and persistent disputes, there is the studied pretense that the disputes do not exist or that they at least have no intellectual significance. Instead, there is the affirmation of the existence of a moral consensus supporting a common morality that is held to sustain a common understanding of a canonical bioethics and the health care policy it supports. One might think, for example, of the June 24, 2005, Declaration on Bioethics and Human Rights issued by the United Nations Educational, Scientific, and Cultural Organization. The Declaration is marked by a general vacuity of its principles, as well as a failure to take seriously the moral difference characterizing the contemporary age. There is, as it were, a desire to deny moral diversity's challenge to governance and political stability: there can be no substantive moral consensus. For instance, Article 10 states, "The fundamental equality of all human beings in dignity and rights is to be respected so that they are treated justly and equitably." However, the Declaration is silent as to the status of human embryos and fetuses, who are in a very important sense human beings, not to mention the nature of justice and equality. The Declaration thus ignores the major bioethical debates regarding the morality of abortion.

Indeed, no defense is offered of claims of human equality in the face of manifest human inequality. Such equality is advanced as a metaphysical truth despite empirical evidence to the contrary. Moral diversity for its part is recognized in a backhanded way. Though the Declaration acknowledges cultural diversity, it fails to appreciate the depth of moral diversity, for this would bring the very possibility of the Declaration into question. For example, Article 12 states that

> The importance of cultural diversity and pluralism should be given due regard. However, such considerations are not to be invoked to infringe upon human dignity, human rights and fundamental freedoms, nor upon the principles set out in this Declaration, nor to limit their scope.

In short, Article 12 announces without sufficient supporting considerations a vaguely articulated moral view of human equality, not to mention of human dignity, in terms of which all other views must be brought into conformity. Other articles, such as Article 13, are remarkably vacuous. "Solidarity among human beings and international cooperation towards that end are to be encouraged." The Declaration leaves undefined the nature and proper scope of claims on behalf of solidarity. In short, the claims are either platitudinous, ambiguous, or ungrounded.

At the beginning of the 21st century, moral reflection has a somewhat paradoxical character. Serious reflection regarding morality, moral controversies, bioethics, public policy, and health care policy in particular is characterized by the circumstance that moral debate is constant, perennial, often passionate, and frequently intractable, while at the same time many moralists deny the depth and significance of their manifest disagreements. It is not difficult to understand why in the face of persistent disagreement it is attractive nevertheless to assert the presence of moral consensus despite its absence. Those who would like to establish at law a particular health care policy will in general be advantaged if they can convince others that the policy they embrace reflects a consensus regarding basic human rights, claims grounded in human dignity, or the requirements of justice. This rhetorical move can disadvantage opposing positions by characterizing those who do not agree as obstinate, if not immoral, opponents of basic human rights, human dignity, and the claims of justice. Once the discourse is so structured, opponents of particular health care policies grounded in bioethical arguments that deny the regnant consensus will appear to be supporting an anti-moral vision. The rhetorical move to claims of basic human rights, human dignity, and the requirements of justice can in this fashion circumvent a democratic political discussion through which different parties with opposing moral visions hammer out compromise solutions for law and public policy. About such issues as human rights and dignity, it can almost seem indecent to be critical. In short, the invocation of a global ethics, a global bioethics, human rights, human dignity, and the claims of a universal understanding of justice plays an important part in a *Realpolitik* in the service of establishing particular laws and policies.

The attractiveness of invoking the presence of a consensus in the face of real, persistent, and intractable moral controversy and disagreement is augmented by the apparent ability of ethics commissions and ethics committees to create a consensus. This achievement of agreement is grounded in the dynamics guiding the appointment of ethics committees and ethics commissions. Those who appoint members would do a political disservice to their political and moral agendas if they impaneled individuals who fully reflected contemporary moral diversity. An ethics committee or commission that mirrors a society's actual range of moral views will reproduce within that committee or commission the passionate and intractable debates of the society at large, so that among other things no conclusions or recommendation will be reached. One might imagine, for instance, a bioethics commission composed of communists, socialists, free-market advocates, and libertarians examining the issue of the public allocation of resources. The result will be that debates will continue, but no resolution will be reached. Worse yet, from the political perspective of those supporting a particular program, they may have brought into jeopardy the possibility of having their agenda appear to be grounded in common, fundamental, moral commitments. In short, a false consciousness or dominant ideology can advance a particular bioethics and its health care policy by supporting the appointment of like-minded persons, thus marginalizing opposing views as lying outside the so-called ideological mainstream. Through such strategies, competing moral views and their adherents can be discounted if not effectively removed from public discourse. In this light, one can understand why appeal is made to a moral or bioethical consensus, even though no such consensus exists.

II. Reflections on Moral Controversy: The Implications for a Global Bioethics

This volume speaks to the salience of moral diversity and its denial. Each essay and commentary from its own perspective explores the possibility or for that matter the impossibility of a global morality, using bioethics as its heuristic. The essays were framed in a conversation that recurringly responded to the tension between a consensus sought and its illusiveness. The goal was to appreciate better the geography of our contemporary moral context and of the human moral condition, so as then better to appreciate the character of free and responsible choice. The failure to achieve, much less justify, a substantive consensus or common background morality may explain the success by default of market mechanisms of collaboration, as well as why moral strangers can collaborate peaceably together through contracts and within limited democracies.

The essays forming this volume grew out of meetings held in Houston, Texas (October 4-7, 2001), Palermo, Italy (January 9-12, 2003), and Rathnew, Ireland (June 3-6, 2004), supported by Liberty Fund, Inc., Indianapolis, Indiana. Eight individuals were commissioned to author major papers and four persons were charged with the role of commentator. Each commentator was given primary responsibility for critically responding to two of the major essays. One person, Stephen Erickson, served as the discussion moderator. His position proved analogous to that of a very talented conductor overseeing the flow and the development of the conversation. The result was a sustained, critical, frank, and not only civil but congenial dialogue. After each meeting, the papers were rewritten in light of the commentary essays and the discussions during the meetings, as well as the suggestions of the editor. In addition, both before and after meetings relevant literature, including ethics declarations, were sent to the group of twelve essayists. Each of the essays in the volume, including the commentary essays, passed through at least four substantive revisions (with the exception of one commentary, where a new participant joined the working group after the initial Houston meeting). The result is that a rich and complex discussion is reflected in the essays in this volume. Again, despite sustained interchange, no substantive moral consensus was reached. Discussions were amiable and sustained, but marked by foundational disagreement.

The discussions even compassed a movement within Chinese thought to step away from European and North American moral assumptions, so as to frame a moral vision and bioethics undirected by the dominant, American/Western European standard account of morality and bioethics. This issue raised implicitly by Ruiping Fan is perhaps the most challenging. It brings into question Western European affirmations of justice, fairness, human dignity, and human rights that fail to attend to the difficulty of justifying one among the numerous competing accounts. Fan's examination recognizes the moral and cultural colonization of Asia, South America, and Africa by dominant European and North America secular moral traditions. His approach invites the reader to cease taking for granted the moral premises and rules of moral evidence that support social-democratic viewpoints, especially those that nest an individualistic, anti-familist culture. Even when one might disagree with his views, one must acknowledge the importance of the foundational questions he advances as China again asserts its cultural and political strength.

Though the robust moral diversity of the reflections was expressed in a moral pluralism of bioethical accounts and norms, a moral relativism was not endorsed. It was recognized that, even though our moral-epistemological condition warrants substantive skepticism regarding the project of identifying through sound rational argument a particular moral or bioethical account as canonical, this state of affairs does not justify a metaphysical-moral skepticism, a denial of the existence of moral truth. Instead, in different degrees in some of the papers there is a recognition of the possibility of special moral insight, albeit insufficient for the achievement of a secular moral consensus or the identification through sound rational argument of a particular morality as canonical. This collection of essays thus compasses a rich, multifaceted presentation and assessment of the character of moral controversy and the roots of its intractability. It offers as well a view of the foundations of the disputatious character of bioethics. It provides a frank, critical appraisal of our contemporary moral condition.

These essays bear in particular against the plausibility of justifying a universal declaration on bioethics and human rights, such as that recently (June 24, 2005) advanced by UNESCO. There is no basis in sound, rational argument for a substantive consensus regarding material human rights, human dignity, justice, or fairness. The very invocation of consensus raises the crucial question as to what should count as a consensus and with what normative force and why. After all, one can envisage at least four different senses of consensus.

1. Consensus as an authorizing agreement—when there is actual agreement among parties to a contract.
2. Consensus as a hypothetical agreement—when there is no actual agreement, partisans of a particular account of moral rationality may nevertheless contend that persons, insofar as they are rational (i.e., rational according to the partisan's view of rationality), implicitly agree to the account that the partisans affirm.
3. Consensus as the produce of a procedural mechanism—a process can commit the participants so that a procedural consensus can be said to have been achieved, though the outcome is justified in nothing beyond the procedure itself (e.g., the UNESCO Declaration is the result of a consensus [i.e., agreement] produced by the procedure that enabled its drafting).
4. Consensus as the outcome of a deliberation—the outcome is held to have a claim to truth, even in the face of disagreement, as when in the sciences a preponderance of investigators agree with regard to a particular interpretation of data, this may establish a bias in favor of that interpretation (however, in moral controversies, where the disputants do not share basic moral premises and rules of evidence, such is not the case).

The UNESCO Declaration likely trades on the false supposition that a consensus of experts regarding a moral issue should have a standing analogous to that of a consensus of scientists. The difficulty is that, when it comes to moral matters, one cannot compare the predictive success of different accounts, because in each case the outcome is described differently. As a consequence, one cannot choose among alternatives without begging the question, arguing in a circle, or engaging an infinite regress.

The failure through sound rational argument to establish a particular canonical moral vision, brings into question the moral authority of legal systems, such as the material-rights constitutional frameworks born of the French Revolution's focus on human rights, given their reliance on particular thick moral views. On the other hand, this state of affairs weighs in favor of Anglo-American constitutional frameworks that support formal-right constitutional understandings that eschew claims regarding positive human rights, human dignity, justice, and fairness and instead (1) focus on protecting against tyrannies of the majority motivated by particular views of the good and (2) allow cooperation through procedural means in the face of intractable moral diversity. The result is an account of and defense of limited political authority. Even if one may not agree regarding the nature of the good, one may agree regarding the evil of unconsented-to force against peaceable minorities and the peaceable collaboration of individuals (as in the market).

Claims of substantive human rights and human dignity turn out not to be universal, but very particular. They are partisan to a particular account of the human good and human flourishing. When such claims on behalf of positive human rights and human dignity are accepted as a foundation for governance and political structures, they involve a majoritarian imposition of a particular view of proper governance. As such, they deny space for the peaceable interaction of individuals and communities committed to diverse moral visions. It is for this reason that the American and the Texian republican constitutions (among many others) never mentioned justice, fairness, or human dignity in their body or their list of basic rights. Instead, out of a recognition of moral diversity, they set limits to majoritarian legislation and offer procedural defenses of the individual over against the power of government. They take moral pluralism seriously. These essays provide not only an exploration of particular moral issues, but of the moral authority that can plausibly undergird governance and political authority in the face of intractable moral diversity. As these essays show, there is no universal, rationally justifiable, moral perspective, or even common notion of the reasonable, that could provide the basis for deliberative democratic polities or their governance. Instead, there are at best procedural modes of collaboration that allow negotiation and limited agreement, as in the markets. The paradigm for political discussion becomes not that of the Socratic seminar, but that of a limited market in which there are peaceable exchanges of political agreement.

III. Twelve Accounts of Moral Diversity

The volume opens with Engelhardt's assessment of the human moral condition: moral reflection is characterized by persistent and intractable moral disagreement. He identifies both the substantive character of this moral disagreement, as well as why sound rational argument fails to set such disagreement aside: we are separated by incompatible basic moral and metaphysical premises, as well as by disparate rules of moral and metaphysical evidence. Though sound rational argument cannot establish the authority to set moral pluralism aside, the conceit of the day is to fashion extensive lists of human rights, which often serve to set limits to peaceable individual choice. They are often meant to impose constraints on how peaceable persons can live within thick consensual moral communities as, for example, within traditional Christian, Islamic, and Confucian communities.

Corinna Delkeskamp-Hayes addresses a similar cluster of issues by critically exploring the ties between Immanuel Kant and the proclivity, especially in Europe, to develop statements on human rights and endorsements of human dignity. As she shows, such affirmations of human rights and human dignity generally do not admit of a grounding in Kant's views, though a Kantian grounding is often invoked. She explores as well how human rights are enlisted to set limits to tolerable bioethical diversity. In so doing, she draws out a contrast between claim rights and forbearance rights, finding the latter to be more easily secured by Kant's arguments. Claim rights, as she shows, are often incompatible with forbearance rights, such as the right to act peaceably with consenting others in the pursuit of one's own understanding of the human good and human flourishing. In particular, the contemporary penchant to assert claim rights is often connected, as she points out, to the disestablishment of traditional Christian norms in favor of a new secularity. An example of this state of affairs is the concern on the one hand to prohibit profit from the sale of organs, while on the other hand generally to accept abortion: the emergence of new secular moral taboos.

In commentary on the papers of Engelhardt and Delkeskamp-Hayes, Mark J. Cherry introduces a distinction among three senses of liberty often conflated in accounts of human rights and human dignity: (1) liberty as the entitlement to realize one's abilities and choices, (2) liberty as ingredient in an ideal, rather than actual, free choice, (3) liberty as lived human flourishing, and (4) liberty through forbearance rights that protect the freedom to venture and to fail. The first sense of liberty corrects actual choices in favor of a putatively rational understanding of the good. Accounts such as this can frequently focus on the importance of fair equality of opportunity. The difficulty lies in the circumstance that the good is plural, and therefore this account of secular moral rationality is plural. The second sense of liberty is grounded in a hypothetical account of rational choice. However, again, despite claims of the existence of a moral consensus on particular issues, moral rationality fragments into a plurality of accounts of rational decision-making. The third sense of liberty is grounded in particular thick understandings of human flourishing, as exist in traditional Christian, Islamic, and Confucian communities. Liberty is not seen as reflecting an historical, rational account of the good or of proper choice, but rather a thick communal experience of human flourishing. The last account of liberty focuses on eliminating constraints to actual, peaceable choice. Often, this elimination is justified on the basis of the limits of the authority of those who would interfere. As Cherry shows, these various accounts of liberty mirror the moral controversies of contemporary society in general and of bioethics in particular.

As Nicholas Capaldi argues, moral-epistemological (not moral-metaphysical) relativism is inevitable because of the disparities of basic moral premises and rules of evidence. Moral diversity defines the human condition. The rationalist hope to justify through sound rational argument a single, canonical account of moral rationality collapses, leaving in its wake at most procedural modes for collaboration. As he puts it, giving a gloss to one of Agrippa's *tropoi,* the persistent philosophical failure to establish a substantive, universal moral view as canonical leaves humans with the challenge of finding modes for collaboration in the face of substantive and persistent disagreement. The result is that political order and governance must make do with procedural norms, which are driven by instrumentalist concerns rather than substantive understandings of the good and human flourishing. It is for this reason, among others, as Capaldi notes, that market mechanisms possess an unavoidable centrality.

In her exploration of Confucian approaches to family-centered health care decision-making, Julia Tao ably displays the tensions between traditional Confucian commitments and the conceits of social-democratic aspirations. On the one hand, traditional Confucian moral and ontological understandings give priority to the family as an entity over the individual. The family is recognized as having a reality and moral status independent of its constituent members: the good of the family cannot simply be reduced to the good of its members. On the other hand, the liberal secular account of the family reduces the good of the family to the good of its constituent members. Indeed, the family is recognized as having only that reality and moral status which its members convey to it: the good of the family is understood in terms of the good of its members. Tao is well aware that the Confucian view is at odds with much of liberal, social-democratic sentiments. Confronted with this tension, she ventures creatively in the pursuit of a moderating integration of Western liberal commitments with a foundationally Confucian perspective. What she accomplishes is provocative and ingenious. From an analysis of physician-centered, patient-centered, and family-centered decision-making, as well as from a consideration of two different understandings of autonomy in health care decisions (i.e., autonomy as the right to self-determination, and autonomy as the capacity for critical self-reflection), Tao proposes a family-centered model of shared decision-making, which proceeds from the perspective of the patient-in-the-family. Through this model, she brings into interaction the patient, the physician, and the family. Her proposal offers an insight into as well as a response to the contemporary challenge to Chinese culture, namely, critically to decolonize itself from the intellectual occupation of secular European moral and metaphysical assumptions.

In response to Capaldi and Tao, Kurt Schmidt gives an analysis grounded in a social-democratic perspective. For example, he criticizes Capaldi's endorsement of the role of markets in health care, raising the question whether such will degrade humans to the level of a *homo oeconomicus* (presuming that that is bad), as well as whether health should be considered a marketable good. In particular, he reviews the prohibition by the *European Convention on Human Rights and Biomedical* of 1997 of financial gains from the human body and its parts. All of this is set within an analysis of the free market and libertarian medical decision-making that critically questions the claims of individuals to collaborate peaceably as they wish (especially in the market). He places these reflections in a general analysis of what he characterizes as the contrast between the I-identity and the we-identity, showing how this difference bears on Tao's account of the Confucian role of the family in medical decision-making. This leads Schmidt to note the unclear boundaries of families in Germany, as well as to raise concerns about truth-telling medicine. He observes as well that there are differences in approaches to truth-telling between northern versus southern Europe, with the latter showing similarities with China. In southern Europe there is more of a disposition to inform the family and to deceive the patient. Schmidt concludes by noting that, in the clinical context, patients are often less autonomous than many moral-theoretical approaches acknowledge, so that engaging family communication can appropriately assist in medical decision-making.

Kurt Bayertz, Angelo Petroni, and Ruiping Fan bring different perspectives to assessing the moral diversity defining contemporary bioethics. Bayertz offers a detailed picture of the multi-form European pursuit of a common European moral and bioethical identity. As Bayertz and Petroni show, there is a European moral and bioethical passion to affirm a consensus. His sketch can at best be described as disclosing a powerful but unsatisfied hunger for a common moral vision. As he shows, such a consensus, such a unity, has proven illusive. Europe is defined by diversity. This diversity becomes quite pronounced, once one places the United Kingdom within the ambit of European culture. The utilitarian dispositions of the British collide with the Kantian deontological dispositions of the Germans and the French. Continental Europeans, especially Germans, have a fondness for affirming human dignity, though this term is traditionally absent from British philosophy and British constitutional theory. When one attempts to identify European culture as focused on freedom, the individual, and rationality, one discovers the tension between more libertarian British approaches versus social-democratic Continental approaches to each of these key concepts. All of this is complicated by the influence of Roman Catholic social and natural-law reflection on laws bearing on cloning and embryo research, as well as on social policy through appeals to solidarity. Yet, over and against these to various extent secularized residua of Roman Catholicism, one finds aggressive laicist viewpoints. From the European search for moral and bioethical consensus, a European version of the culture wars emerges.

Petroni critically assesses the European community's attempt to regulate markets so as to abolish national and regional diversity, as well as to limit individual choices, in favor of a thick legal and policy framework. As he shows, a political framework is emerging that, although it is only deficiently democratically endorsed, is nevertheless forwarded as the basis of a European democratic vision for the future. It is engaged as well as the basis for a European policy identity with a wide range of implications for health care and bioethics. Among the issues examined by Petroni is the commitment of certain European political factions to imposing their own special moral understandings through appeals to the "precautionary principle", human dignity, solidarity, and respect for the human embryo. Such impositions are occurring through centralization of governance and through a growing list of human rights. As Petroni notes, the result is a tension if not a collision between the often-vaunted European principle of subsidiarity and the European ideology of centralization, with the latter triumphing. Indeed, the

European Union provides a prime example of a post-modern centralization achieved neither by military force nor through the centralization of taxing power, but rather through a harmonization of laws, regulations, and national policies. In all of this, there are central conflicts between socialist affirmations of basic human claim rights and liberal (in the libertarian sense) affirmations of negative rights or forbearance rights. The search for a consensus in bioethics thus emerges as a weapon in the culture wars wedded by the centralist cause of achieving greater harmonization and by proponents of variously secularized remnants of Europe's Christian past against libertarian solutions. It pits the centralist cause of achieving greater harmonization and secularized remnants of Europe's Christian past, as against libertarian sentiments supporting individual freedom and responsibility.

Fan assesses Bayertz and Petroni through introducing a Confucian appreciation of the rite-bearing nature of humans in order to diagnose the culturally impoverished circumstance of the emerging new Europe. As he puts it, humans are ritualizing beings, so that Kantian and Rawlsian philosophies (and here he would include Jürgen Habermas) proceed from a mistaken anthropology that ignores the ritual-requiring, familist character of humans. From his account of properly ritualized relationships, Fan addresses moral diversity, the European hunger for consensus, and the various processes of globalization. These issues are assessed in terms of three competing frameworks, what he terms the liberal view of bioethical globalization, the libertarian view of bioethical communitization, and the Confucian insight into bioethical localization. In the process, Fan responds to the anomie that threatens individuals, families, and communities through showing how persons should be located in ritual behaviors that disclose the relation of persons to each other and to the transcendent. The reality of human decision-making must be properly ritually shaped. In particular, as Fan underscores, humans are familist in their nature. Only when rightly ritually situated in a family will one have, according to Fan's gloss on Confucius, a morality and bioethics that can meet the challenges we face. As he argues, both the liberal and libertarian strategies sketched by Bayertz and Petroni are each in its own way one-sided and incomplete.

The last trio of papers explores with particular attention the problem of bioethical globalization: the attempt to create a global moral understanding for health care and the biomedical sciences. Joseph Boyle explores the increasingly globalized character of modern medicine, and therefore the prospect of an increasingly globalized understanding of bioethics and health care policy, drawing on the resources of natural law. The latter he defines in very broad terms as "the set of basic principles of moral life", but nevertheless embeds his account in the tradition of natural-law theory that took form through the labor of Roman Catholic canonists, theologians, and philosophers in the press of the Western philosophical/theological synthesis of the 12th and 13th centuries. He shoulders his project so as (1) to outline the normative implications of a globalized medicine for those who live in this natural-law tradition, and (2) to evaluate the capacity of his understanding of natural-law theory to meet the challenges raised by globalization. He develops an engaging overview of the growing nexus of bioethical conventions and international understandings under the rubric of an emerging bioethical ius gentium. With this term, he identifies the interplay of the more universalist elements of natural law with the particular contributions of specific cultures and contexts. He then critically assesses particular contemporary secular bioethical norms of patient autonomy. Boyle not only shows the heuristic strengths of natural-law reflection, but also offers an insight into one of the important intellectual traditions defining the bioethical culture wars in Europe, as well as in the United States.

Confronting the plurality of bioethical perspectives, as well as the imperialist ambitions of certain genre of bioethics, David Solomon evaluates the bioethics that arose in America, that is still largely produced in the West, and that is now zealously exported to the world. The issue of bioethical imperialism or, to put matters less tendentiously, the cultural export of Western bioethics, is placed by Solomon under the ingenious rubric, the export problem. He distinguishes the issue of exporting moral and bioethical issues from one culture to another from three other versions of the export problem: the temporal export problem, the local export problem, and the personal export problem. The first involves exporting ethical insights from one historical period to another, a problem one encounters when one questions whether Aristotle's understandings of morality are in fact at all like ours (so that one might question whether Aristotle's moral reflections were successfully exported across history). The second involves the exporting of ethical insights among persons in the same culture. The personal export problem involves the challenge of translating ethical insights within all dimensions of a single person's viewpoint. Solomon's exploration of the issue of the temporal export problem raises questions about the origins of bioethics itself and the extent to which bioethics represents a break from traditional Western moral reflections. Bioethics took shape as Western culture was developing a cult of authenticity, a focus on individualism and autonomy, and a privatization of religious views. The ethics revolution of the 1960s that spawned the bioethics of the 1970s carried with it a very particular set of assumptions and commitments that, among other things, ran counter to both traditional Christian and Confucian understandings. Bioethics may also in important ways differ from previous secular Western views of morality and moral reflection.

In any event, the ethics revolution, as the other papers in this volume concede, failed to overcome salient and intractable moral controversy (1) at the meta-ethical level, at the level of reflection about the cognitive status of moral claims, (2) at the normative level, at the level of determining the content of moral norms themselves, and (3) at the level of applied ethics, at the level of solving particular problems. As Solomon notes, the responses to moral pluralism and the controversies it engenders have been diverse, including: (1) strategies of assimilation, which deny the depth of the disagreements; (2) minimalist strategies, which deny that the differences are significant at the practical level; (3) casuistic approaches, which attempt to ignore the problems of pluralism by proceeding to the analysis of cases, drawing on whatever viewpoints appear useful; (4) triumphalist approaches, which affirm faith in the ultimate vindication of one particular account; and (5) what Solomon terms "rising above the ruins" as through embracing a political account as a substitute for the failure to establish a particular moral account (as, for example, with the later Rawls). The only hope that Solomon offers, following Alasdair MacIntyre, is to consider moral philosophy as a tradition-constituted inquiry. But yet again, multiplicity plagues us with the question of which tradition, guided by whose rationality, should prevail and why and under what circumstances. We are left with a plurality of foundations and a plurality of bioethics.

In closing, Kevin Wildes provides an overview of the geography of disagreement. He lays out the texture of controversy in morality, moral theory, and bioethics in terms of eight levels of disagreement.

1. Object level agreement with agreement on justification and foundations
2. Object level agreement with agreement about justification and disagreement about foundations
3. Object level agreement with disagreement about justification
4. Object level agreement with agreement/disagreement in part on the levels of justification
5. Object level agreement with disagreement about both justification and foundations
6. Object level disagreement with agreement on justification and foundations
7. Object level disagreement with justificatory agreement/disagreement in part
8. Object level disagreement with disagreement about justification and foundations

Rather than a substantive conclusion regarding the content of a normative morality and a global bioethics, we are left with reflections on and accounts of our disagreements. As Wildes ably shows, we can appreciate why we do not agree about issues in bioethics, ranging from the killing of human embryos to the allocation of scarce resources to the use of physician-assisted suicide. At best, we can erect procedural approaches to create areas of collaboration (as through contracts, the market, and limited democracies), though we are unable together to discover a common moral truth.

IV. Life in the Ruins: What Does the Failure of Moral Consensus Have to Teach us?

Moral diversity has been with us as far back as history records. Now, however, the failure of moralists to provide a coherent account of how one ought to act with regard to human reproduction, sexuality, the allocation of scarce resources, suffering, dying, and death is underscored by the dramatic character of medicine. Life and death decisions need to be made, and the standards to guide are contested. Dramatic new technologies give us unparalleled power, and we cannot in principle agree about how to use that power. We stand on the threshold of possessing capacities that will allow humans to redesign human nature and direct human evolution. Yet, we cannot agree on the constraints to be placed on those powers, or the goals to be pursued through those powers. In the face of conflicting accounts of the good, the right, the virtuous, and human flourishing, the challenges of how to shape the human future brings not common collaboration and a common vision, but impassioned disagreement and controversy.

A faith in reason born of the 12th- and 13th-century Western European synthesis of philosophy and theology has largely been lost. The modern and Enlightenment attempts to reground the Western medieval rational project have now been radically and foundationally brought into question. How should we proceed? We urgently need moral guidance, but we find ourselves confronted by an intractable moral pluralism with its cacophony of competing answers. Seemingly in desperation, Solomon remarks, "There may perfectly well be a non-relativistic truth about ethics, and perhaps this truth is even known and savored by, say, an Orthodox monk living in a cave on the Holy Mountain [Mount Athos, Agios Oros]" (ms p. 19). One may wonder whether Solomon's remark is quite as flippant as it at first blush might appear. Perhaps the observation serves as an implicit surrender to St. Gregory Palamas (A.D. 1296-1359), who along with what was equivalent to the Ninth Ecumenical Council (Constantinople V, A.D. 1341, 1347, 1351) knew that the Western synthesis is intellectually flawed and that the project would in time collapse. The Council knew that the only way to the Truth is through an asceticism integral to Christian mysticism.

We are returned to a moral and intellectual position that existed in the West before its Middle Ages. These reflections on the failure to justify a global bioethics disclose a fundamental challenge. A major rupture has occurred at the heart of the Western, now-global, moral-philosophical project of providing a justification for a particular moral vision that can direct human powers, as well as provide a warrant for political authority and governance. This rupture under the rubric of post-modernity discloses not just the failure of the modern or Enlightenment moral and intellectual project of creating a universal moral community grounded in reason, but the collapse as well of those universalist moral understandings that took shape at the beginning of the second millennium. There is now a growing recognition of not just the salience and persistence, but the irresolvability of moral pluralism. It is not simply that post-modernity takes moral diversity seriously, but that it involves as well an abandonment of moral truth. It is the fruit of the recognition articulated by David Hume (1711-1776) and Immanuel Kant (1724-1804) that, unless humans possess a noetic capacity (here we must again recall David Solomon's monk on Mount Athos), we are irretrievably locked not just within the sphere of immanence and finitude, but within subjectivity, and therefore at best within intersubjectivity. We are left with our sense impressions, guided by the structure and coherence we impose on them. The result is that there is no longer truth in the sense of an independent reality to be known, or at least in independent moral reality, but instead all truths become interpretations within the hermeneutic of a particular moral narrative.

In these circumstances, the character of the human condition brings into question traditional secular morality and bioethics. We are left with first a diagnosis and then the possibility of at least two forms of response.

1. The diagnosis lies in the recognition that post-modernity is the final outcome of the Western medieval philosophical and theological synthesis, which turned to look for traces of God in nature (e.g., through natural-law reflections) and ceased to look noetically through nature as through an icon to the Truth, to God. This creative, intellectual venture of the Western Christian Middle Ages in the end culminated in the secularization of the West, focusing with increasing zeal on studying nature and the recognition that one cannot find traces of the infinite in the finite. In the end, it came to regard humans as confined in the circles of their own intersubjective moral construction. This approach affirms as the heuristic and exemplar model for moral investigation the image of a Socratic critical reflection and dialogue, which, following the Euthyphro, seeks to domesticate the divine within the secular commitments of the West.
2. The first treatment for this circumstance, the first strategy for collaboration when truth becomes intersubjectivity and therefore multiple, is to recognize procedural means for working together in the face of moral and metaphysical disagreement. This strategy binds those separated by different moral and metaphysical visions, who draw their authority from neither God nor Reason, but from common agreement. This immanent approach affirms as the heuristic and exemplar model for moral investigation and collaboration the image of the market, a moral space where free and responsible individuals can through agreement venture together in limited enterprises.
3. The second treatment, only alluded to by David Solomon, is the one that prevailed in Europe before the philosophical-theological synthesis of the Western High Middle Ages, but that nevertheless remains

> at the roots of Western thought, and is independently appreciated by Ruiping Fan in his reflections on the place of ritual. This approach affirms as the heuristic and exemplar model for moral investigation an ascetic struggle to mystical insight, to noetic union of the knower with the known.

A secular bioethics that is to transcend the battles of the culture wars an doffer a means for morally authoritative collaboration in the face of intractable moral diversity will need to take seriously the role of agreements, contracts, the market, and limited constitutional polities.

The conclusion is that there is no conclusion, or at least no conclusion regarding which moral claims are normative, the content of moral claims, or how to resolve particular cases of moral controversy. One is left only with a description of our state of affairs, of the tensions and conflicts that mark our fallen human condition. To put the matter in different terms, there is only a meta-conclusion, namely, that we do not and cannot in general secular terms come to substantive conclusions regarding matters moral and bioethical through sound rational argument. Moreover, it is clear as to why we lack this capacity. We disagree about basic moral premises and rules of evidence (i.e., one must remember the monk on Mount Athos). Nevertheless, other strategies still invite their consideration. At the very least, we can by default find procedures, strategies to live together as moral strangers in the face of irresolvable moral diversity.

The Search for a Global Morality: Bioethics, the Culture Wars, and Moral Diversity

H. Tristram Engelhardt, Jr.

I. Moral Pluralism and the Post-Modern Crisis of Morality

Can morality be more than a dominant mores? Is morality as a set of universally binding norms possible? The some two thousand five hundred-year history of philosophical reflections on morality and moral diversity gives little empirical basis for holding that it is possible to establish a universally binding morality, at least in terms justifiable to all. As a conceptual matter, controversies regarding the normative content of morality do not appear resolvable by sound rational argument without begging the question, arguing in a circle, or engaging an infinite regress. This state of affairs brings the project of a global morality into question. Indeed, these considerations challenge the very project of morality as a set of universally binding norms regarding right and wrong, good and bad actions. Modernity's faith in a universal vision of right conduct has been brought into question (Heller, 1990).

Matters are no better in the field of bioethics. There is real bioethical diversity. The disagreements range from abortion and euthanasia to the reallocation of private resources to support health care. This diversity is often denied or strategically overlooked in the service of making plausible embracing a common morality and common bioethics to guide health care policy

H.T. Engelhardt, Jr. (ed), *Global Bioethics* (pp. 18–49).

across the globe. For some, it may have taken the events of September 11, 2001, to remind them of what should have been obvious: the world is not united in a common understanding of the good, the right, and human flourishing. People do not share a common set of settled moral judgments. People really do disagree, often violently, about the significance of sexuality, reproduction, property rights, suffering, dying, and death. Moreover, the public policies both formal and informal of numerous polities disclose deep disagreements regarding the substance of bioethics (Alora, 2001; Cherry and Engelhardt, 2004; Fan, 2002; Fan and Li, 2004; Hoshino, 1997). These disagreements merit careful study and attention. As important as the disagreements, if not more important, is an understanding of the possible conditions for peaceable collaboration[1] in the face of substantive moral disagreement. At stake are fundamental issues regarding the unity and diversity of morality.

Despite obvious moral diversity, there are substantial interests in elaborating and justifying a global ethics, bioethics, and health care jurisprudence.[2] The current pursuit of a global bioethics (Council of Europe, 1997; International Bioethics Committee, 2003) has grown out of the ascendancy of a particular moral view associated with the emergence in 1971 of this field of applied ethics under the term bioethics (Beauchamp, 1997; Engelhardt, 2002; Jonsen, 1998; Potter, 1970a, 1970b, 1971; Reich, 1994). Bioethics was largely a movement to establish a liberal, social democratic morality with its health care policies. Critical voices have come to recognize this particular genre of bioethics as constituting only one among a number of possible understandings of bioethics (Engelhardt, 1986; Alora and Lumitao, 2001; Hoshino, 1997). This essay assesses the possibility of establishing a single, content-full, canonical bioethics that can justify a global approach to health care policy and law. The conclusion is that there is a range of moralities having at best a family relationship with each other, among which one cannot choose the canonical morality in a principled fashion through sound rational argument. Moreover, these moralities carry with them starkly different understandings of freedom and responsibility. By default, the only global or universal secular morality that can be justified is secured at the cost of forgoing content. This state of affairs requires a fundamental reconsideration of the nature of morality and the proper character of biolaw.

This paper begins by contrasting the dominant view of bioethics (a view born of the Enlightenment) with a view of morality that recognizes that secular moral reflection must compass through procedural mechanisms a plurality of moral perspectives. Fukuyama's recent defense of the global regulation of genetic engineering is critically examined as a case example of the failed aspirations to global health care policy and law (Fukuyama, 2002). This essay then explores the axes of moral difference along which moral controversies are constituted, such as the contrast between traditional versus post-traditional, family-oriented versus individual-oriented approaches to health care morality and decision-making. Attention is also directed to the grounds for the ineradicable pluralism of moral views we confront. In conclusion, a brief reflection is advanced regarding health care policy and biolaw, in light of the moral pluralism that defines the contemporary human condition. This reflection underscores the watershed implications of moral pluralism for a secular morality and its radical consequences for a secular account of liberty and responsibility.

II. How Could a Global Morality and Bioethics Be Problematic?

At first blush, it would seem wrong to oppose a global morality along with a global bioethics and biolaw. After all, moral claims should be universal. All humans should be united in a common pursuit of the good, the right, and the just. Morality by its very nature calls out for universal recognition. If killing persons is wrong in some particular circumstances, killing persons should be wrong in relatively similar circumstances everywhere in the universe. The same should be true for all the moral issues addressed by bioethics, from third-party-assisted reproduction, human reproductive cloning, the production of embryos for research, and prenatal diagnosis with selective abortion, to physician-assisted suicide and euthanasia. So, too, for matters of the allocation of health care resources: whatever the requirements of morality are, the requirements should be universal (although one might recognize local excusing and modifying circumstances). At least insofar as this can be accomplished without greater collateral moral harms, all law and public policy should be brought into harmony with the universal requirements of morality, so as to protect the human rights of all. There should be no moral room for off-shore islands and miscreant sovereignties within which morally divergent approaches to health care or economic policy can be pursued to the injury of justice and human rights. The matter appears resolved at the outset in favor of a content-rich global morality and its bioethics[3] so that morality's universality should be reflected in a global consensus regarding the foundations of health care policy and the general lineaments of health care law. Aside from differences in local circumstance, there should be no particularly American, European, Japanese, Roman Catholic, Mohammedan, or Texan bioethics or health care policy.

Bioethics should liberate from unjustified customs and constraints, those contrary to the demands of universal moral reason. As such, bioethics should support the Enlightenment's and the French Revolution's aspiration to the realization of a universal moral community.[4] In this light, who could in good faith be opposed to this global commitment to liberation other than those recalcitrantly and misguidedly committed to the immoral peculiarities of their traditions, religions, superstitions, and cultures? Those opposed to a global bioethics would appear to be the party of reactionaries, partisans of the unjustifiably particular over against the universal claims of reason. From this point of view, defenses on behalf of regional moralities and moral pluralism can be opposed as hidden ways of seeking exemption from the universal demands of morality.

One might envisage a bioethics framed under a United-Nations-sponsored global health care policy and legislation, which, when necessary, could be enforced by the United Nations and the International Court of Justice. Such an international biomedical juridical framework would likely eventually include:

1. the harmonization of health care globally in order to justly redistribute resources so as to guarantee a universal, global standard of health care;
2. the prohibition of forced pregnancy through requiring physicians as a part of their licensure to provide abortion services;
3. the requirement that all hospitals, regardless of their historical religious roots (e.g., as Roman Catholic or Orthodox Jewish), provide euthanasia services.

In this fashion, a global bioethics could be elaborated and then achieved through a network of internationally enforceable health care policies and law.

This essay is written in opposition to such a content-full bioethics as well as to the national, not merely the international, pursuit in law of a content-rich view of the good, the right, and the just. At issue are radically different understandings of the possibilities for a global morality and the bioethics it could ground. On the one hand, there is a vision with roots in Greek philosophy, crucially reshaped in the Western Middle Ages that endorses a centrally enforced uniformity of moral understanding and deportment. This vision combines the Western medieval faith in reason's capacity to disclose a proper account of deportment with the Western Middle Ages' commitment to a unique central authority able to guarantee uniformity of practice, even when this requires inquisitorial interventions.[5] It is this vision that is the remote historical source of a global bioethics developed by UNESCO and affirmed by the United Nations (International Bioethics Committee, 2003). On the other hand, there is a view of morality that by default accepts the ineradicable plurality of human moral viewpoints.

The acceptance of eradicable moral pluralism is more congenially nested in pagan Anglo-Saxon jurisprudence, which resisted grounding the law in a universally binding appreciation of justice, as occurred in legal systems grounded in Roman law. This acceptance of moral pluralism has as well important roots in the Reformation and its consequences. As Hegel in *The*

Philosophy of Right (1830) observes, the disunion of the Western church "is the best piece of good fortune which could have befallen either the church or thought so far as the freedom and rationality of either is concerned" (Hegel, 1952, §270, p. 174). The result is that contemporary civil societies and states fashioned in the light of common law and the Protestant Reformation can no longer be understood as single moral communities. They must instead be appreciated as a framework that embraces a plurality of communities separated by a diversity of moralities (Engelhardt, 1994). Common law, the Protestant Reformation, the Thirty Years' War, the British Civil War, the American Revolution, the French Revolution, and Napoleon's impact on jurisprudence on the Continent, along with the subsequent 19th-century secularization of Western Europe, produced societies variously opened or closed to acquiescing in individuals and groups pursuing their own morally incompatible projects. The United States, more than any other polity of its size, were established so as to encompass robust moral difference.[6]

Two major foundationally different secular moral-political understandings have emerged in response to this state of affairs. They conflict with respect to the possibilities for, and the character of, a global ethics and bioethics, and the law and health care policy that they would warrant, as well as their appreciation of free and responsible action. The first is committed to the establishment of a universal social democratic framework defined by a single thoroughgoing vision of justice within which an acceptable moral pluralism must fit. The other is committed to securing a libertarian framework that can unite persons and communities who at the same time are divided by diverse concrete views of the moral life and of justice, but who are nevertheless associated through the market and protected by the state against unconsented-to force. The first envisages a rationally discoverable vision of morality, justice, and proper conduct, which authorizes state or international governmental authority to constrain and direct citizens, groups, and communities. This is the normative perspective of the universal legislator of Kant's categorical imperative (grown beyond the actual aspirations of Kant's rational impartial observer[7]), or of the privileged utilitarian calculator of benefits and harms, who assumes that, out of an already available account of moral rationality, rational volition, or human preference satisfactions, a concrete understanding of responsible human choice can be derived.[8]

In this first vision of morality, one finds one of the roots of hypothetical choice accounts, including hypothetical contractor accounts of moral rationality and justice: an ahistorical, content-rich, moral viewpoint.[9] In this account, to act freely and responsibly is to act informed by a rationally disclosable universal moral vision, or at least a common view of the reasonable (Rawls, 1993), that can provide the basis for a universal or global public policy cum legislation. To act freely, to act autonomously is not to act in accordance with one's own wishes and desires, but in accord with the dictates of right reason, often disclosed via an image of hypothetical free choice specifiable at least in general outline by reference to an ideal of choice as it would occur in Kant's kingdom of ends or the original position of John Rawls (1971) or a more limited view of the reasonable (Rawls, 1993) or decent (Rawls, 1999).[10] In consequentialist accounts, the focus is on a supposed privileged standpoint for the comparison of the likely results of different choices issuing in pleasures and pains, as well as preference satisfactions. A bioethics created in this image and likeness is committed to a thick notion of mutual respectful affirmation (e.g., forbidding as hate speech statements such as "abortionists are murderers"), to a robust realization of equality (e.g., forbidding as in Canada the purchase of better basic health care), and to the elimination of "exploitative" health care policies (e.g., prohibiting organ sales, family's consent on behalf of competent members and enforced pregnancy through the non-availability of abortion). A bioethics is affirmed that can be characterized as falling generally within what can be termed a social democratic ethos (Rawls, 1993; Daniels and Sabin, 2002). In this account, governmental power assures that people will in general act according to a thick understanding of liberty, as well as according to an ideal, not actual, account of appropriate free choice.

The second vision in contrast affirms secular morality as a framework, as a marketplace of moral ideas and moral understandings within which each person peaceably can pursue his own ends without sharing a common, content-full moral vision or concrete view of justice. In this case, the image is not that of a universal legislator, but of a moral trading floor: a space within which peaceable, consenting moral agents can frame joint projects with willing others. Instead of envisaging the content of the moral life as discoverable through the heuristic of such expository devices as a kingdom of ends, a disinterested observer, an original contractual position, or a privileged calculator of benefits and harms, the expository device is that of peaceable participants engaged in a complex of free collaborations creating outcomes they could not in advance have been envisaged.[11] Free and responsible individual choice is realized through actual choices by actual individuals allowing them peaceably to pursue their own wishes, desires, and views of the good with consenting others. Through the market and within limited state structures, moral competition can produce a higher good: an economically and culturally enriched society which none of the individuals and communities explicitly affirmed or sought. Thus (slightly recasting Mandeville), much can be "full of Vice, Yet the whole Mass [can be] a Paradise" (Mandeville, 1988, vol. 1, p. 24).

This essay criticizes the global aspirations of a concrete, social democratic bioethics, along with the harmonization of health care policy and law it endorses. It does so through recognizing the irreducibility of moral diversity, and how it renders the claims of a secular, content-rich bioethics unjustifiable. The view of secular morality as a procedural framework is defended as a default understanding of moral probity for a global ethics, because

1. There is widespread disagreement regarding the existence of God and about His requirements (i.e., there is significant and apparently irreducible religious pluralism).
2. There is widespread disagreement regarding the content of a secular morality and the settled moral judgments (e.g., the ranking of such cardinal human goods as liberty, equality, prosperity, and security) that should guide human choice (i.e., there is significant moral pluralism).
3. These theological and moral disagreements cannot be resolved by sound rational argument without begging the question, arguing in a circle, or engaging an infinite regress, because many of those in disagreement are separated by divergent foundational moral premises and rules of moral evidence (Engelhardt, 1996, ch. 2 and 3).[12]
4. The establishment through state coercion (i.e., by law) of a comprehensive view of morality and justice, even though one knows that one cannot in general secular terms know that the morality imposed is the canonical secular morality is an illegitimate use of force; the level of certainty in secular moral theory delegitimates any all-encompassing, coercive imposition of a particular view of morality and justice, in that it becomes an unjustified use of force against the innocent.
5. Therefore, a secular morality must be a framework for peaceable moral diversity and collaboration based on permission, not a concrete ethos to be imposed coercively.

This critical account of the possibility of a common or global morality is embraced by default through recognizing the moral inescapability of attempting to resolve moral controversies by agreement rather than by the common discovery of a canonical normative moral vision.

In short, humans do not share one common morality, if by that one means sharing a common understanding of the good and the right. For example, if one considers only the ordering of such cardinal human moral concerns as liberty, equality, prosperity, and security, different rankings will lead to quite different moralities grounding divergent settled moral judgments (e.g., regarding the propriety of surrogate mothers for hire). So, too, depending on whether one holds that consent cures the wrong-making prohibition never to use persons as means merely, one will also hold substantively different settled moral judgments. As a result, different substantive visions of the good and the right will undergird different moralities in the sense of different clusters or systems of settled judgment as to right and wrong, good and bad behavior.

It may be the case that all human moralities are concerned with liberty, equality, prosperity, and security, but depending on how these concerns are ordered and articulated, a quite different morality is constituted. So, too, human moralities may in general hold that it is wrong, all things being equal, to kill humans and to lie. But human moralities differ precisely regarding when (if ever) it is held to be good or indeed obligatory intentionally to kill humans or to lie. Human moralities may share a large number of common moral concerns (e.g., they may recognize there is a moral significance to liberty, security, prosperity, the killing of humans, and lying). The differences lie at least in how these concerns are ordered in a particular morality with its particular settled moral judgments affirming particular proscriptions and prohibitions (e.g., it is always wrong to take human life even in self-defense; it is good to kill humans when an issue of honor is at stake), etc. These differences among moralities are not reducible to differences among philosophical accounts of morality (e.g., act-utilitarian, natural law, or Kantian theories), although some philosophical accounts may fail to reconstruct cardinal elements of particular moralities (e.g., that there are forbearance rights that hold, independently of consequences). The libertarian global moral framework explored in this essay offers a morality at a meta-level (not the same as a meta-ethics) within which a wide plurality of moralities can be placed, although this meta-morality does not affirm any particular content-rich morality (i.e., it does not involve a particular ranking of human goods or values), though it does possess moral implications (in that it derives authority from the permission of peaceable collaborators). It is a moral space within which persons can peaceably exchange opportunities to realize a range of interests, including moral interests. It is this circumstance that recommends as a moral exemplar the image of the market as the place for the secular moral self-understanding of free and responsible individuals.

Because this latter account acknowledges that individuals and communities are separated by divergent understandings of God's requirements, moral rationality, and reasonableness, moral authority is derived from the permission of those who choose peaceably to collaborate in acting morally, thus establishing only two cardinal moral constraints:

1. actual persons (i.e., actual moral agents) may only be used (a) with their actual permission (this requirement is a right-making condition grounded in the possibility of a morality transcending the diversity of moral-theological and moral-philosophical perspectives) or at least (b) in terms of the practice of resolving controversies in the light of the recognition of persons as in authority over themselves;
2. moral agents are never to act malevolently, for this is to act against the project of morality itself, the pursuit of the good (this requirement is empty of moral content until specified within a particular moral understanding, which can supply content to the *bonum* and the *malum*).

It will be argued that the defenders of a content-full secular global morality and bioethics, along with the global enforcement of health care law and policy, have radically misunderstood the human condition and the character of secular morality.

III. Two Conflicting Moral, Bioethical and Political Understandings

Social democratic universalist and libertarian pluralist approaches disagree foundationally regarding the nature of the secular moral project. This disagreement demarcates a cleft between a moral vision that presupposes robust capacities for moral rationality and a moral vision that acknowledges the finitude of secular moral knowledge and authority.

1. On the one hand, the possibility of a global bioethics is understood by liberal cosmopolitans in terms of morality as a framework of concrete obligations and claim rights, which can be disclosed by or justified through right reason, and which morality should be brought effectively to direct the conduct of all persons. Morality is taken to be grounded in a universal, content-rich, moral perspective available through discursive rational reflection and investigation, or at least available by reference to a particular understanding of reasonable discourse, which can inform moral agents who should then act

a. informed by moral premises or commitments garnered from
   i. rational analysis and/or
   ii. discursive reflection on the human condition, combined with
   iii. scientific investigation of the character of human proclivities
b. This view is not skeptical regarding the existence of moral truth or at least concerning a common sense of the politically reasonable
c. that will allow one to endorse
   i. inalienable liberty rights (therefore condemning consensual illiberal social relations, e.g., traditional Confucian and Mohammedan social arrangements, even when all participants consent to be bound by them),
   ii. inalienable equality rights (therefore condemning market outcomes that lead to significant differences in wealth and social power, or which undermine equality of opportunity),
   iii. inalienable rights to mutual affirmation and respect (e.g., therefore excluding the condemnation of abortionists as murder ers).

2. On the other hand, the possibility of a global bioethics is understood by libertarian cosmopolitans in terms of morality as a framework within which persons can peaceably agree to collaborate, despite their being separated by incompatible views of the good, the right, the just, and the nature of

human flourishing. Global morality in this account is understood as grounded in the peaceable agreement of persons authorizing collaboration. The image of this collaboration is not that of a legislator, a participant in a rational discourse, or persons bound by a shared sense of the reasonable, but that of participants in a marketplace of moral interests, making various agreements in the face of unavoidable moral diversity so as to pursue particular joint projects set within the moral constraints of:

a. never using persons without their permission (as long as persons conform to this practice; e.g., one may defend against murder) and
b. never acting with malevolent intent, while
c. attempting (as a further elaboration of ii. above) to act prudently in the sense of pursuing the realization of more benefit than harm (although there will not be agreement across moral communities regarding the nature of harms and benefits, or of how they should be compared).

This view is skeptical regarding either the existence of a content-full moral truth or a sense of the rational (or reasonable) independent of the conventions of particular communities (i.e., it involves a metaphysical skepticism) or regarding the possibility of knowing that truth (or the fabric of the reasonable) through discursive rational means (i.e., it involves an epistemological, but not a metaphysical skepticism). This view of the possibility of a global morality is thus in accord with moral viewpoints that could hold, for example, either of the following positions:

a. The moral life is realized within the particular traditions of particular communities and their moral conventions framed through the thick experience of communal and/or individual histories, such that, given the plurality of human goods, there is a plurality of moralities.
b. The moral life is only fully realized within the veridical understanding of virtue, character, moral obligations, and moral probity, which understanding cannot be secured through discursive rational reflection, the deliverances of history, or any other merely immanent access to moral knowledge and experience (Engelhardt, 2000), but only through a unique experience of God and His requirements; this understanding of proper action requires individuals to be converted freely and not by coercion, such that advocates of other understandings of the moral life will be tolerated (but their beliefs and actions not approved), even when they are seriously misguided (e.g., one has a right to do X but it is wrong), as long as they are peaceable, by default acquiescing (however reluctantly) in the presence of a plurality of moral visions due to human moral blindness and willfulness.

The recognition of the ineradicable character of moral pluralism gives substantive grounds for rejecting arguments in favor of a single content-full universal morality and bioethics to be realized through international law and public policy.

IV. An Ill-Directed Hunger for a Content-Rich Global Morality: Francis Fukayama as a Case Example[13]

In the face of intractable moral-theological and moral-philosophical diversity, there is the aspiration, nevertheless, to justify a content-rich bioethics that can authorize a global approach to bioethics, health care policy, and health care law. A heuristic example of this drive to a universal, content-full bioethics (along with its biolaw) and its attendant difficulties is provided by Francis Fukuyama. In *Our Posthuman Future: Consequences of the Biotechnological Revolution,* Fukuyama is rightly uneasy at the prospect that a better understanding of human genetics and genetic engineering may lead, if not within this century, then surely within this millennium, to humans guiding their own evolution (Fukuyama, 2002). The challenge is to determine which among the numerous alternative futures to choose and why. Fukuyama recognizes that important moral and policy questions are at stake. The puzzles raised by the book are fourfold: first, why are answers to these important questions so difficult to secure? Why are they in particular difficult for Fukuyama? Why are such questions so irresistible? Finally, how is one to proceed in the face of intractable moral difference?

As to the difficulty of supplying a normative foundation or consensus within which to anchor a global bioethics, as has already been observed both in this essay and in Alasdair MacIntyre's *After Virtue,* a characteristic of our contemporary culture is that debates go on and on about matters of great moral importance with no end in sight (MacIntyre, 1981, p. 6; Engelhardt, 1986). It is not just that such debates are interminable. Worse yet, generally acceptable grounds for their resolution are not apparent. The parties are separated by incompatible metaphysical commitments (e.g., embryos do or do not have an immortal soul), religious moral beliefs (e.g., euthanasia does or does not involve the sin of murder), and by divergent rankings of cardinal moral concerns (e.g., the claims of security do or do not trump concerns for prosperity). As a consequence of these differences, we disagree and will continue to disagree about the moral issues at stake in abortion, euthanasia, and health care reform. Fukuyama's recent book further illustrates this state of affairs by focusing on germline genetic engineering and the human control of human evolution, thus despite himself showing that no content-full secular moral constraints can in principle be established by discursive rationality alone.

Fukuyama finds himself in the troubling circumstances of contemporary culture: mankind possesses more power than ever before but with no common vision of how to use it. There is a legitimate sense of urgency about matters that require answers in the very near future. Wringing his hands, Fukuyama calls for appropriate regulations to control these new technologies: we should act prudently, rightly, and with restraint so as to preserve human nature as we find it.[14] However, he fails to provide a substantive account of why restraints should be absolute, rather than prudential, uniform, rather than pluralist. This is particularly the case where there is no direct threat to human liberty (e.g., as there is with governmentally augmented psychiatric interventions in the service of state power coercing the innocent without their permission), but where instead the choice is one among a number of alternative, genetically-designed futures. His fear is that genetic technologies will increase the biological and mental inequalities separating humans, leading to untoward legal and moral consequences. Yet, the genetic technologies may diminish such inequalities as well as increase them.

The challenge is doubly difficult for Fukuyama. After his 1989 article in *The National Interest* (Fukuyama, 1989), as well as in his book that followed (Fukuyama, 1992) in which he prophesies a consumer, social democratic capitalist world culture, Fukuyama is in principle barred from the moral content needed for the substantive guidance he now seeks so as to justify the global regulation of genetic engineering, which he takes to be required to avoid humans taking command of their own evolution. We, and in particular he, lack the secular moral resources to give substantive answers to the questions that *Our Posthuman Future* raises. The reason is this: Fukuyama has been largely right concerning the emergence of a dominant, Western liberal cosmopolitan culture focused on self-determination, self-satisfaction, and mutual recognition. The morality of his last man,[15] the person at home in this culture, can affirm self-determination, self-fulfillment, and mutual recognition, but cannot specify how one ought to pursue self-determination so as consensually and peaceably to seek self-fulfillment. The mutual recognition required by the last man provides no grounds for condemning mutually respectful consensual lifestyles, including the consensual redirection of human evolution.

Once upon a time, Western culture recognized human biological nature as created by God and then taken on by Christ in the Incarnation. What Fukuyama termed "the murky depths of religious faith" (Fukuyama, 1992, p. 202) cannot within the horizon of the immanent secure canonical content for the morality of Fukuyama's last man. Nevertheless, Fukuyama in *Our Posthuman Future* argues that "religion provides the clearest grounds for objecting to the genetic engineering of human beings" (Fukuyama, 2002, p. 88). As Fukuyama once stressed, "liberalism [has] vanquished religion in Europe [and] [r]eligion has thus been relegated to the sphere of private life…" (Fukuyama, 1992, p. 271). The best moral advice that the last man can offer for the project of directing human evolution is (1) to proceed prudently so as to achieve more benefit than harm, and (2) to seek a future that enhances self-determination and self-fulfillment, while not (3) significantly increasing current biological and psychological inequalities among humans in order not to endanger mutual moral recognition. Numerous different directions for human evolution fall within these constraints.

This problem cuts even deeper for Fukuyama. Substantive categorical guidance regarding the uses of genetic engineering requires a comprehensive, moral-metaphysical viewpoint. Such viewpoints, however, divide. In *The End of History and the Last Man,* Fukuyama argued that mankind was entering an age of perpetual peace grounded in the abatement of ideological struggles. Rather than battles over ideas, there is to be an anesthetizing, pacific pursuit of individual satisfaction within the embrace of social democratic guarantees of self-determination, self-fulfillment, and mutual respect. Respect is found through mutual recognition in the pursuit of self-satisfaction rather than in transcendent ideals, norms, or concerns. It is precisely the sunset of transcendent ideals that promised the peace of a social democratic consumerist market future. Or as Fukuyama put it, paraphrasing Alexandre Kojève,

> The end of history would mean the end of wars and bloody revolutions. Agreeing on ends, men would have no large causes for which to fight. They would satisfy their needs through economic activity, but they would no longer have to risk their lives in battle. They would, in other words, become animals again.... A dog is content to sleep in the sun all day provided he is fed... (Fukuyama, 1992, p. 311).

But in this circumstance, one is no longer able to give canonical moral content to notions of human dignity or discover an ultimate purpose for human existence. As Fukuyama observed, "modern thought has arrived at an impasse, unable to come to a consensus on what constitutes man and his specific dignity, and consequently unable to define the rights of man" (Fukuyama, 1992, p. 337).

It is remarkable that Fukuyama is disappointed that ethicists, embedded in the morality of his last man, acknowledge few limits in principle to the new biomedical technologies. "In any discussion of cloning, stem cell research, germ-line engineering, and the like, it is usually the professional bioethicist who can be relied on to take the most permissive position of anyone in the room. But if the ethicist isn't going to tell you that you can't do something, who will?" (Fukuyama, 2002, p. 204). The morality of Fukuyama's last man cannot provide direction for the human control of human evolution. In *The End of History,* Fukuyama correctly saw the force of the cultural changes framing our contemporary moral context. As Hegel (in *Glauben und Wissen* in 1802) and later Nietzsche recognized, God and metaphysics, the foundations for ultimate goals, are now dead for the dominant liberal culture, thus producing the consequent loss of ultimate points of direction.

In the dominant secular culture, all lies within the horizon of the finite. All is immanent to human narratives, including narratives about absolute spirit. In a moral context bereft of ultimate or transcendent points of anchorage, humans find themselves in a seemingly ultimately senseless universe. The point of *The End of History* is that this loss of metaphysical depth and ultimate orientation should no longer matter to those integrated within the satisfactions of a consumerist, post-metaphysical culture. Peace is promised precisely because humans cease to worry about making ultimate sense of it all. At the supposed end of history, the concerns for ultimate meaning and purpose that once drove history and its struggles are dead—or at least dead in the dominant culture. All this Fukuyama once seemed to accept in a positive light. The end of ideological wars was to be insured because people sought immanent satisfactions, not ultimate truths that can divide and engender conflict (*pace* September 11, 2001). Now as Fukuyama only partially realizes, quoting Nietzsche's castigation of John Stuart Mill, one cannot have a semblance of Christian morality in the absence of belief in a Christian God (Fukuyama, 2002, p. 155).

Fukuyama notices as well that, unlike in Europe and North America, in the Pacific Rim where bioethics and health care policy are relatively untouched by residual Christian concerns, there is not the same moral interest in setting limits to the development and use of genetic technologies (Fukuyama, 2002, p. 192). In this circumstance, is there less moral hesitation about transforming "the stable human essence" (Fukuyama, 2002, p. 217)? After all, there is a considerable list of human biological characteristics that suggest themselves as appropriate targets of human genetic engineering, ranging from auto-immune diseases, presbyopia, benign prostatic hyperplasia, and the various vexations of menopause, to predispositions to heart disease and cancer. The line between genetic treatment and genetic enhancement is difficult, if not largely impossible to make out (e.g., if one could do away with presbyopia via genetic engineering, would that involve curing a disease or instead enhancing humans?). Moreover, aside from practical concerns (e.g., when treating a disease, one can balance possible harms from the treatment against known harms from the disease), why as a matter of principle should one care about the distinction between treatment and enhancement? In a post-metaphysical, post-religious age, there may still be moral remembrances from a past that suggest that limits should be set to the biotechnological reshaping of human nature. Yet, there is no common sense of where limits should be placed: moral narratives are doggedly plural and the dominant social democratic moral vision lacks ultimate goals. How, then, can one decide what particular direction to give to human evolution, or whether one should prohibit such an undertaking, as Fukuyama now wants?[16]

One is brought to ask why, despite the presence of intractable moral-theological and moral-philosophical diversity and the inability to resolve disputes through sound rational argument, would there still be partisans of a content-rich global bioethics such as Fukuyama? This state of affairs can be explained in terms of two phenomena defining the character of secular morality, at least in the West.

1. The immanent displacement of theological commitments. Moral concerns drawn from the theological background culture of the West still provoke questions regarding the proper biological character of humans and the appropriate direction of human evolution; however, in a secular context, these questions are not answerable.
2. The de-orientation of cosmic and human history. Once human moral concerns are placed fully within the horizon of the finite and immanent, then the cosmos in general, and human evolution in particular cannot be appreciated as aiming towards any ultimate purpose. In this context, humans are left with the task of attempting to make sense of a seemingly senseless universe within various finite moral narratives, none of which can be definitive.

The result is that questions that appear to concern important matters are posed in a secular moral context with the expectation that definitive answers will be forthcoming although, given the character of secular morality, this is impossible. A transcendental illusion is generated within the context of secular morality, fed by a human hunger for meaning, leading to the hope for moral insights that secular morality can never produce. It is for this reason that the aspiration to a content-rich global secular morality and its bioethics is both intense and misguiding.

V. Taking Pluralism Seriously: Axes of Moral Difference and Disagreement

Morality and bioethics are plural. Any account of bioethics, and in particular any reflections on the possibility of a global bioethics, must take into account the remarkable moral pluralism at the roots of bioethics, as well as the breadth of its diversity. Many of the disagreements can be identified along five intersecting axes or dimensions of disagreement.

A. Traditional Versus Post-Traditional Accounts of Bioethical Issues

In the West, traditional moral understandings are in great measure rooted in Western Christian assumptions, though the particular arguments may often be framed in a secular idiom, as is illustrated by Fukuyama's attempt to defend the preservation of the contemporary, general characteristics of human biological nature. In other cultures, arguments for traditional approaches to moral issues in medicine may have roots in Confucian or Islamic commitments. Controversies thus emerge between partisans of Christian versus post-Christian (or post-traditional Christian), Islamic versus post-Islamic (or post-traditional Islamic), Confucian versus post-Confucian (or post-traditional Confucian) moral perspectives. The debates concerning traditional versus post-traditional accounts of bioethical issues address the role of third parties in reproduction (e.g., the traditional Christian judgment is that the use of donor gametes involves a form of adultery), the propriety of abortion (traditionally forbidden by Christianity), the propriety of cloning (Christianity traditionally requires all sexual activity and reproduction to occur within the marriage of one man and one woman), the acceptability of genetic engineering (opposition being expressed, particularly in Europe and especially in Germany (Bayertz, 1997), against alterations of the human genome as it currently exists), and the appropriateness of using animals in research (post-traditional rejection of humans as the masters of creation), as well as the licitness of physician-assisted suicide and euthanasia (traditionally, Christianity rejects such interventions). Though much of the defense of traditional moral prohibitions historically has Judeo-Christian roots, many traditionalist arguments lack a religious grounding (Kass, 1985, 2002).

B. Family- or Community-Oriented Authority Versus Individual-Oriented Authority in Health Care Decision-Making

Views contrast as to who is in authority to make decisions on behalf of patients. In China, for instance, the dominant assumption is that decisions will be made by family members, unless patients explicitly take steps to the contrary (Fan and Li, 2004), as opposed to North America and northwestern Europe, where currently the dominant assumption is that decisions will be made by the individual patient, unless the patient has explicitly empowered someone to act as an agent of the patient. At stake are contrasting positions regarding the initial taken-for-granted decision-makers for health care choices. These differences are expressed as well in assumptions at law as to whether, in the absence of medical powers-of-attorney, members of the family will be considered as authorized to act on behalf of the patient. At issue are even deeper moral-political views regarding the sovereignty of families and communities over against society and the state. Insofar as families and particular communities possess sovereignty over themselves, others will bear the burden of proof of justifying their intrusion into these exclaves.

In the full development of this latter position, communities will bear the responsibility for articulating their own understandings of bioethics and for framing their own health care policy and biolaw within the protection afforded by a society and state that guarantee the right of individuals peaceably to pursue their own views of human flourishing within the communities they choose and/or fashion.[17] On the other hand, insofar as such sovereignty is denied, families and communities must bear the burden of proof in establishing their authority to act contrary to general societal norms, not to mention public policy and law. They become subject to state invasion, given any suspicion of child, spouse, or elder abuse. Differences will also be reflected in whether health care savings plans are individual or family specific. For example, communities with a familialist commitment will encourage health savings plans for families as self-directing wholes, so as to encourage family-based responsibility and choice.

C. North American and European Versus Non-Western Culturally Framed Approaches to Bioethics

At stake are contrasting assumptions regarding the ranking of values and right-making conditions. On the one hand, one finds accounts of justice in health care framed in terms of hypothetical decision-makers or understandings of the reasonable that affirm a social democratic ranking of interests in liberty, equality, security, and prosperity, such as in Rawls (Rawls, 1971, 1993). On the other hand, one finds health care policies, grounded in rankings such as Singapore's, which focus primarily on family, security, prosperity, and responsibility (Healthcare Research Group, 1999). To put matters more broadly, one can envisage policy makers in China, after the chaos following the fall of the Soviet Union, concluding that a more orderly transition to the future can be achieved by giving priority to market rights (e.g., rights to amass wealth) over civil liberty rights (e.g., the right critically to assess the government in the press). The Chinese might also conclude that only in such circumstances could a developing country such as China peaceably compass areas with radically different levels in the availability of modern high-technology health care. Indeed, they may affirm in principle that market rights have a priority over other liberty rights. In different cultural contexts, different assumptions will govern regarding the appropriate ordering of human moral concerns, leading to quite different portrayals of the appropriate content for bioethics, health care policy, and health care law.

D. Market Freedoms Versus Special Claims to Respect or Dignity

A cluster of concerns are at issue, including the commodification of health care services, the sale of gametes, the availability of services held by the larger society to demean those involved in their provision (e.g., surrogate motherhood for hire), as well as the patenting of sequences from the human genome. Those supporting the priority of market freedoms will hold that no secularly cognizable harm has been done, if all parties to a peaceable transaction consent. Those who defend certain accounts of an inalienable respect or dignity due humans will hold that some market transactions are exploitative and/or are wrong in inducing persons to use themselves or others in ways that are improper, even if all directly involved consent. Although there is an overlap of issues under this rubric with those surfacing in disputes between partisans of traditional versus anti-traditional understandings of bioethics, the matter here also turns on contrasting secular moral visions regarding the relationship between the market and human dignity (although

Western philosophical appeals to human respect and dignity have generally had Judeo-Christian roots).

E. Visions of Equality Versus Freedom

Debates regarding health care allocation policies are often rooted in foundational conflicts between freedom of choice and equality. As long as individuals have a morally prior right to act peaceably and consensually with each other, differences in resources and other opportunities, as well as differences in access to health care, will inevitably occur. Only if equality interests trump actual free choice may uniform, all-encompassing health care systems legitimately be imposed contrary to the wishes of particular individuals and groups. Family loyalties, for example, undermine claims on behalf of equality of opportunity (Fishkin, 1983). In addition, there are numerous and incompatible visions of equality and its demands. There are egalitarianisms of envy that regard equality as in itself worth pursuing, versus egalitarianisms of altruism that have a concern with inequality only if it results in the significant suffering of particular individuals.[18] The latter often involve accounts of how needs generate claims or rights against others for resources. Contemporary controversies regarding health care allocation policies are sustained by fundamentally contrasting (to differing degrees) libertarian versus egalitarian understandings of polity and human flourishing.

F. A Summary: Bioethics as a Field of Controversy

Bioethics has failed to produce a generally accepted account of appropriate deportment so as uncontroversially to justify a single account of health care policy and biolaw. The disputes are substantive: the pluralism of moral understandings supports the view that all do not recognize a similar background morality. The depth of the differences is reflected in a starkly hostile rhetoric separating many of the opponents in these debates. On the one hand, abortionists and physicians assisting suicide are characterized as murderers or assistors in self-murder. On the other hand, such physicians are described as liberators from unjust, enforced pregnancy and terminal suffering. Those who impose all-encompassing, single-payment, egalitarian health care systems such as exist in Canada are characterized as violators of basic human freedoms and market rights. On the other hand, those who support access to different levels of basic health care are characterized as violating basic rights to equality. As a matter of descriptive ethics, one finds widely divergent understandings of moral probity. Moral pluralism is substantial.

VI. Why Are There Moral Pluralism and a Diversity of Bioethics?

Not only are there significant moral disagreements about substantive issues in bioethics and health care policy, many if not most of those controversies are not resolvable through sound rational argument. On the one hand, as already noted, many of the controversies depend on different foundational metaphysical commitments, as with respect to the significance of abortion, the production of embryos for research, and infanticide (i.e., whether the entities involved should be considered persons on a par with competent adult humans). As with most metaphysical controversies, resolution is possible only through granting particular initial premises and rules of evidence. On the other hand, even when foundational metaphysical issues are not at stake, the debates turn on different rankings of the good.

Again, resolution is not feasible without conceding what is at issue. As far as the issue is metaphysical, the claims at stake involve matters that lie beyond the horizon of common experience, as Immanuel Kant has amply shown. Insofar as the issue turns on a correct ranking of values, then in the background one must already have conceded what is at issue to resolve such a controversy. Which is again to say, such controversies cannot be resolved without begging the question, arguing in a circle, or engaging in infinite regress. One cannot appeal to consequences without knowing how to rank the impact of different approaches with regard to different moral interests (e.g., with respect to liberty, equality, prosperity, and security interests). Nor can one uncontroversially appeal to preference satisfaction unless one already grants how one should correct preferences and compare rational versus impassioned preferences, as well as calculate the discount rate for preference satisfaction over time. Appeals to disinterested observers, hypothetical choosers, or hypothetical contractors will not avail either. If such decision-makers are truly disinterested, they will choose nothing. To choose in a particular way, they must be fitted out with a particular moral sense or thin theory of the good. Intuitions can be met with contrary intuitions. Any particular balancing of claims can be countered with a different approach to achieving a balance. In order to appeal for guidance to any account of moral rationality, one must already have secured normative content for that moral rationality.[19]

Bioethics as we find it is plagued by the torments of post-modernity. Strident moral diversity defines the debates regarding all substantive issues in health care. Moreover, in principle there is no good reason to hold that these debates can in a principled fashion be brought to closure through sound rational argument. The partisans of each position find themselves embedded within their own discourse with its own fundamental presuppositions: they are unable to step outside of their position's hermeneutic circle without embracing new and divergent premises and rules of evidence. This is not to say that the parties cannot understand each other's positions. Indeed, in understanding the other's position, they can appreciate why, given their initial commitments, the commitments of the other are wrong, if not deeply evil. The contemporary character of bioethics is thus defined not just by controversies, but by the absence of a basis for principled resolution of the controversies through analysis and discursive argument.

There are six possible grounds for this intractable moral pluralism or diversity. Given the truth of any one of these, by default at least some health care policy and legal diversity ought to be tolerated over against an aspiration to establish a single morally authoritative, content-specific, global bioethics carrying with its own biolaw.

A. Moral Pluralism Due to Primary Moral Relativism

This account of the inevitability of moral pluralism rests on a deep metaphysical skepticism regarding the availability of an objective canonical moral truth, a canonical normative account of a subjective truth, or a common normative sense of the reasonable. In such circumstances, morality becomes community-relative: there is no moral truth that transcends communities with their specific commitments and conventions. This position is compatible with different states, communities, and groups acting on quite contrary moral understandings regarding bioethical issues such as physician-assisted suicide and the sale of human organs. There are strong grounds, given this moral skepticism against a state coercively establishing a particular, content-full moral vision, much less a particular moral account globally.

B. Moral Pluralism Due to a Secondary Moral Relativism Grounded in a Moral Epistemic Skepticism

This position by default accepts moral pluralism as inevitable because of a moral epistemic skepticism regarding the possibility of knowing in generally available discursive terms that one knows the morality that is in fact canonical. The possibility of moral truth is not denied. What is recognized is the impossibility of resolving moral controversies by sound rational argument based on generally justifiable secular moral premises. This position is compatible with different states, communities, and groups acting on contrary moral understandings of physician-assisted suicide and the sale of human organs. There are strong grounds (e.g., based on not using unjustified coercive force against peaceable, innocent, unconsenting persons), given this moral skepticism against a state coercively establishing a particular, content-full moral vision, much less a particular moral account globally.

C. Moral Pluralism Due to Secondary Moral Relativism Grounded in the Special Conditions Necessary for Moral Knowledge

This position in favor of accepting a moral pluralism as inevitable rests on the understanding that true moral knowledge presupposes a personal transformation of the knower, which is unlikely on the part of persons generally. Such accounts of the acquisition of true moral knowledge are often tied to particular religious understandings, such as that of Orthodox Christianity, which continues the tradition of Christianity's first millennium (Engelhardt, 2000, chap. 4). When this view of the difficulty in acquiring rightly-ordered moral knowledge is combined with a toleration of those who are morally wrongly directed but peaceable, moral diversity will be accepted by default. For example, force would not be used against a peaceable pagan polity in order to interdict physician-assisted suicide and the sale of human organs; one might recall that one of the grounds advanced for the Spanish subjection of Mexico was to stop sodomy (Vitoria, 1991, pp. 205-292).

D. Limited Moral Pluralism Due to the Application of General Moral Principles in Divergent Local Circumstances

This position accepts a moral pluralism as inevitable based on an acknowledgement that general moral principles must be applied in particular circumstances, often leading to divergent moral approaches, even in the absence of a true moral pluralism. In part, the acceptance of local variations is grounded in a principle of subsidiarity that recognizes that many elements of governance can only be successfully accomplished when undertaken at a local level. For example, one can hold that standards of medical care should ideally be uniform, while yet recognizing that there must be acquiescence in a more limited standard of care being developed for remote resource-poor areas.

E. Limited Moral Pluralism Accepted Because of Respect for Individual and Community Choice

This position favors moral diversity because of the importance of individuals through their communities and with peaceable consenting others making choices for themselves as well as learning responsibility through bearing the consequences of their own choices. Even if one held that allowing (or forbidding) physician-assisted suicide is improper, yet one might acquiesce in communities choosing wrongly. A communal variation on this approach to moral pluralism is found in federal polities that within constitutional constraints accept a diversity of regional approaches to matters of criminal and civil law recognizing the benefits from local governance and from competition among moral and juridical models.

F. Limited Moral Pluralism Accepted Out of Concerns for Prudence: Recognizing the Inability to Assure Full Uniformity

This position in favor of limited moral diversity is justified in terms of the moral, political, and other costs involved in imposing a uniform moral standard. Thus, a polity may take the position that surrogate motherhood and prostitution violate important moral norms, while nevertheless not criminalizing such activities, on the ground that this would produce more moral harms than benefits. There will often be good moral reasons for not making all that is immoral illegal (e.g., the moral danger to the development of individual responsibility, given all-pervasive police oversight).

G. A Critical Summary

Given the inability in the face of divergent foundational understandings of metaphysics and morality to resolve most substantive moral controversies by sound rational argument, moral pluralism will need to be accepted. Positions 1-3, which acknowledge the full depth of moral diversity, provide the strongest considerations in favor of politically and legally recognizing a robust space for moral diversity. In addition, the strength of the acceptance of moral pluralism will be enhanced if, in the face of moral diversity, one also recognizes that one cannot in general secular terms draw common authority from a common understanding of God, moral rationality, or the reasonable, so that by default one is left with deriving secular moral authority from the consent of those who collaborate.[20] The plurality of moral visions will then be set within a procedural framework that establishes the possibility for secular moral collaboration on a basis (e.g., permission of the collaborators) that all the collaborators can affirm (i.e., insofar as they wish to share a commonly recognized source of authority), with the result that persons may not be used without their permission, including those who in a peaceable fashion act immorally with willing others. Once these limits on secular moral authority are recognized, regional diversity will be most salient at the community level, which community need not be geographically located (e.g., Roman Catholics). States, and the societies they represent, will lose the secular moral warrant to impose one community's moral vision on all, under the color of the authority of societal norms and state policy, much les a content-rich global morality.

Living in freedom with human diversity requires taking seriously the limits of discursive moral epistemology and the possibilities nevertheless to draw limited common authority from the consent of willing collaborators. Political space must be made not just for a diversity of communities within particular states, but for the emergence of worldwide networks of non-geographically based communities with their own particular understandings of moral probity, including bioethics, health care policy, and law. In such a framework, members of particular moral communities will be at liberty to carry with them and their property their own special criminal and civil legal constraints. In particular, a particular non-geographically based community's morality and bioethics could be established so that its own criminal and civil law could be enforced on its own health care facilities (e.g., Vaticare International, were Roman Catholics to establish such). Thus, on Vaticare premises throughout the world the death penalty could be visited against those who perform abortions in such facilities, while physicians could be severely punished in Atheistcare facilities, were they not to provide euthanasia as agreed to under previously established contracts requiring them to do so. Insofar as states compass a preponderance of particular communities with common moral traditions and cultural understandings, "national" differences would remain. The bearers of substantive moral difference would be the communities of collaborating individuals who organize themselves around particular content-rich understandings of morality and human flourishing.

The implications of moral diversity, the limits of moral knowledge, and the possibility for drawing moral authority from the consent of collaborators demands a radical restructuring not only of the state, but also of the ways in which the contrast between regional and global bioethics will be understood. With respect to the possibility of a justified global bioethics, a global bioethics can at best provide a thin moral framework, a space within which individuals and moral communities can peaceably pursue divergent understandings of morality and bioethics within limited democracies and within a global market. Such a global bioethics cannot provide a content-full understanding of the right, the good, virtue, or human flourishing. Content will have to be found within particular moral communities and the moralities and bioethics they sustain.

VII. Two Images of Public Conversation and Collaboration: Reason vs. Free choice

How one comes to terms with moral and bioethical diversity is a function of fundamentally different images of moral collaboration tied to quite different views of liberty and responsibility. Two in particular have been contrasted under the rubrics of a libertarian versus a liberal cosmopolitan ethos. These moral views involve divergent understandings of appropriate governance, one endorsing a limited polity spanning persons and communities divided by their concrete views of justice but united by the market and the state as the protector against unconsented-to force, and the other endorsing a social democratic polity bound in a single totalizing vision of justice. These engage two divergent understandings of how the moral behavior of free and responsible individuals should be understood, overseen, and then directed by state authority.

At stake are contrasting understandings of what it is to choose as free and responsible individuals. In the liberal, social-democratic account, to act freely and responsibly is to act informed by a rationally disclosable universal moral vision that can guide all and that can provide a uniform basis for a universal or global public policy and legislation. To act freely, to act autonomously is not necessarily to act in accordance with one's own wishes and desires, but in accord with the dictates of right reason, which are legitimately to be imposed through public policy and law. In this account, the state in the service of responsibility assures that people will act freely according to a particular thick understanding of liberty, according to an ideal, not actual, account of free choice, discoverable independently of particular free choices by individuals. As has been shown, this approach cannot be justified in general secular terms.

In the libertarian account, to act freely and responsibly is peaceably to act on one's wishes, desires, or vision of the good, collaborating with others insofar as they are willing in the pursuit of common undertakings. The liberal, social-democratic vision of the free and responsible individual's choice is often disclosed via an image of hypothetical free choice specifiable at least in general outline by reference to ideal free choice as would occur in Kant's kingdom of ends or the original position of John Rawls (1971).[21] The first vision of free and responsible individual choice is disclosed in terms of the image of the market within which actual choices by actual individuals allow them both to pursue their own wishes and desires while in unanticipated fashions enriching themselves as well as others. The cardinal image of the public forum is in this case not one of rational deliberation, but one of free trade. Rather than construing individuals as bound together in rational deliberation about proper common action, one recognizes them as engaged in limited peaceable exchanges of opportunities to realize particular interests. It is the image of the market as the exemplar of peaceable collaboration that discloses a possibility to take seriously peaceable collaboration in the face of robust moral pluralism.

This last account of global morality and governance confronts the collapse of excessive expectations rooted in the Western High Middle Ages with respect to the powers of secular discursive rationality. As post-modernity discloses, discursive rationality cannot discover a way to a canonical secular moral rationality. By default, one is left with the freedom of individuals as the source of the authority for peaceably collaborating on a global scale through the market and limited contracts. Free and responsible individuals are also left at liberty to pursue robust understandings of moral obligations with consenting others. In this circumstance, peaceable secularists and religious fundamentalists of various sorts can co-exist within a limited global framework nested within a libertarian cosmopolitan ethos, as long as they eschew unconsented-to force against non-aggressors. Rather than attempting to make the world safe through the global spread of social democracy, one is left only with the general moral authority to seek space within which communities of starkly incompatible moral commitments may peaceably pursue their particular visions of the good and human flourishing with willing collaborators. After September 11, 2001, one should more than ever cease to take moral diversity seriously.

Notes

1. In this account, peaceable collaboration is understood to involve the eschewal of coercion against the unconsenting innocent. The notion of peaceable interaction does not preclude employing justified punitive or defensive force.
2. The last few years have seen a groundswell of interest in international declarations on bioethics and on global ethics generally. For a study of the April 4, 1997, European Convention on Bioethics, see Schmidt, 2000. See also Draft Report on Human Rights Aspects of Traffic in Body Pats and Human Fetuses for Research and/or Therapeutic Purposes, UNESCO, 1989. In addition, there is a wide range of statements on global governance and ethics. See, for example, Commission on

Global Governance, 1995; Shafer, 1998; Parliament of the World's Religions. Some of these statements endorse limits on freedom of the press ("Sensational reporting that degrades the human person or dignity must at all times be avoided" [InterAction Council, May 1996, Article 14]), as well as world-wide indoctrination in the new global values ("Education, at all levels, has a crucial role to play in inculcating global ethical values in the minds of the younger generation. From the primary school to the university, curricula and syllabi should be restructured to include common global values and to promote understanding of religions other than one's own. Education programmes should inform values like 'affirmative tolerance' and curricular materials should be produced accordingly. The development of the aspirations of youth should be a major emphasis. UNESCO and the United Nations University and other international bodies should work together to achieve this objective. The electronic media should be enlisted" [InterAction Council, March 1996, § 17]).

3. The terms "content-rich" and "content-full" are used to identify moral accounts that are committed to particular rankings of cardinal human values (e.g., liberty, equality, prosperity, and security).
4. Immanuel Kant provides an example of the project of a common moral vision for all humanity. Toward the end of "The Metaphysical Elements of Justice" in *Metaphysics of Morals* (1797), as well as in *Perpetual Peace* (1795), Kant endorses a universal league of nations constituting a world community under international law. "The rational Idea of a peaceful, even if not friendly, universal community of all nations on earth that can come into mutual active relations with one another is not a philanthropic (ethical) principle, but a juridical one" (Kant, 1965, § 62, p. 125). It is to be noted that Kant's international community is one marked by free trade bound within an international legal framework. "The kind of community that they hold is that of possible physical interaction (*commercium*), that is, a community that involves a universal relationship of each to all the others such that they can offer to trade with one another; consequently, they have a right to attempt to trade with a foreigner without his being justified in regarding anyone who attempts it as an enemy. These rights and duties, insofar as they involve a possible unification of all nations for the purpose of establishing certain universal laws regarding their intercourse with one another, may be called *world Law (jus cosmopoliticum)*" (Kant, 1965, § 62, p. 125). Kant did not presume that individual states or a league of nations would enforce a particular, content-full morality in all its detail. Given Kant's opposition to revolutionary change and his faith in the progressive force of the Enlightenment, he expected that the forces of reason would gradually reform polities world-wide. Out of these considerations, he would have tolerated a limited diversity of bioethics, albeit in the expectation that through the Enlightenment's advance there would be a final emergence of a global bioethics with its international public policy and law.
5. The development of the Western Christian moral and theological synthesis is contemporaneous with the establishment of the Inquisition as a means of securing through force and threat of torture a universally accepted understanding of appropriate belief and conduct. Although the Inquisition has roots in Augustine of Hippo's notion of righteous persecution (Wakefield, 1974, p. 82), the institution did not emerge until the 13th century, after the Fourth Lateran Council (1215) in Canon III offered the same indulgences for the elimination of heretics as were pro-

vided for engaging in a Crusade to the Holy Land. In 1232 Conrad of Marburg was appointed as the first *Inquisitor haereticae pravitatis.* The Inquisition received enhanced support after a mob on April 6, 1252, killed Peter of Verona, leading to the issuance of the bull Ad extirpanda by Pope Innocent IV on May 15 of that year, followed by the canonization of Peter as the patron of inquisitors in 1253 (in 1586 Pope Sixtus V honored Peter of Verona as the second head of the Inquisition, following Dominic). One must recognize as well the important contributions of Thomas Aquinas (1225-1274) in providing theological justification for the Inquisition's use of the death penalty against unrepentant heretics. For a critical brief overview of the Inquisition, see Burman, 1984. For two sympathetic accounts, see Vacandard, 1908, and Walsh, 1940. For an example of the Western Christian unification of theological and governmental power, see the bull *Unam Sanctam* of 18 November 1302. There the claim is advanced that both the spiritual and the material swords of power are under church authority, in particular that of the papacy. "In hac eiusque potestate duos esse gladios, spiritualem videlicet et temporalem, evangelicis dictis instruimur.... Uterque ergo est in potestate Ecclesiae, spiritualis scilicet gladius et materialis" (Denzinger, 1965, 873:469, p. 280). From this basis the Spanish were able to develop the famous Requirement, a manifesto that was to be read as of June 14, 1514, to the Indians of America prior to their subjugation by the Spaniards. This manifesto declared that the Indians should capitulate, since Pope Alexander VI had given the offshore isles of America and Tierra Firma to the Spanish. The title of the Spanish to this territory, so it was claimed, came from "the Church as the Ruler and Superior of the whole world and the high priest called the Pope, and in his name the King and Queen Juana in his stead as superiors, lords, and kings of these islands and this Tierra Firme by virtue of said donation" (Hanke, 1949, p. 33).

6. The United States, when they fashioned their second constitution in 1787, needed to compass sovereign states, some of which allowed slavery and others which did not. The result was the creation of a robust moral space for difference generally unavailable on the Continent.
7. See, for example, Immanuel Kant, *The Foundations of the Metaphysics of Morals,* AK IV 393.
8. Kant identifies appropriate moral deportment through conceiving of human moral community in terms of a concurrence of volition, ideally understood so that the particular wishes and concerns of moral agents become irrelevant. This account of autonomy versus heteronomy, as well as of appropriate moral deportment, is grounded in the "concept of each rational being as a being that must regard itself as giving universal law through all the maxims of its will, so that it may judge itself and its actions from this standpoint…" (Kant, 1959, AK IV.433, p. 51). The third formulation of the categorical imperative captures the idea of each individual willing for all "in the idea of the will of every rational being as a will giving universal law" (Kant, 1959, AK IV.432, p. 50). The first and last formulation of the categorical imperative presupposes the universal standpoint of a global law and lawgiver.
9. Kant grounds in his supposedly general secular rational arguments all of his particular commitments as a sometime pietist Christian. For an account of Kant's actual beliefs, see Kuehn, 2001. Kant argues not only against suicide, but also against masturbation as worse than suicide. See Kant, 1964, AK VI.424-425. He

supplies in addition arguments against inoculation in order to protect against smallpox (AK VI.423-424), as well as against the sale of one's tooth (AK VI.423).

10. Rawls employs the heuristic of the original position (a fictive rational contract) in order to feed into its moral rationality all of the choices his hypothetical contractors are to make. "One way to look at the idea of the original position, therefore, is to see it as an expository device which sums up the meaning of these conditions and helps us to extract their consequences" (Rawls, 1971, p. 21). Like Kant's kingdom of ends, all members of the original position are to be in accord in their understanding of morality. "The original position is so characterized that unanimity is possible; the deliberations of any one person are typical of all" (Rawls, 1971, p. 263). Much is packed into his view of the reasonable, though the later Rawls abandons any strong Kantian claim to a universally normative moral rationality. Instead, he moves to a notion of the politically reasonable by endorsing "a reasonable comprehensive doctrine [that] does not reject the essentials of a democratic regime" (Rawls, 1993, p. xvi). Rawls then places substantial social democratic commitments into his answer to the crucial question, "What are the fair terms of social cooperation between citizens characterized as free and equal yet divided by profound doctrinal conflict?" (Rawls, 1993, p. xxv). In this way, Rawls establishes robust welfare rights so as to ensure "all citizens adequate all-purpose means to make effective use of their freedoms" (Rawls, 1993, p. 6). The claims made by the later Rawls are, in short, substantial, even after he has traded moral rationality for the seemingly less robust notion of the politically reasonable. Though Rawls may at first blush seem sympathetic to a moral pluralism, he radically restricts what is acceptable, as when he requires the reform of traditional families in order to achieve equality between the sexes. "[T]he principles of justice enjoining a reasonable constitutional democratic society can plainly be invoked to reform the family" (Rawls, 1997, p. 791). The Amish, the Hassidim, supporters of limited democracies, and libertarians fall beyond the pale of the reasonable.
11. Hegel, through his notion of *die List der Vernunft,* the cunning of reason, introduces a higher-level moral rationality through which collaborators such as traders in the market achieve goods unanticipated by any of the participants. "Reason is as cunning as it is powerful. Cunning may be said to lie in the intermediative action which, while it permits the objects to follow their own bent and act upon one another till they waste away, and does not itself directly interfere in the process, is nevertheless only working out its own aims" (Hegel, 1892, § 209 Zusatz, p. 350).
12. For over two thousand years, the difficulty of providing a foundation for moral or general philosophical accounts has been well recognized. One might think of the view attributed to Protagoras, "that there are two sides to every question, opposed to each other" (Diogenes, 2000, p. 463). Given different initial premises, one can derive contradictory conclusions. This state of affairs was recognized not just by Sophists, but by early Christians as well. For example, Clement of Alexandria observes, "Should one say that Knowledge is founded on demonstration by a process of reasoning let him hear that first principles are incapable of demonstration; for they are known neither by art nor sagacity" (Clement, 1994, vol. 2, p. 350). Such appreciation of the limits of discursive rationality led to the recognition of the impossibility of establishing through sound rational argument a particular moral account without begging the question, arguing in a circle, or

engaging an infinite regress. A third-century articulation of this circumstance for moral (and indeed other) epistemological skepticism (but not for moral metaphysical skepticism) is found in the *pente tropoi* or five modes of the later Skeptics and the late Academy, which Diogenes Laertius (3rd century A.D.) attributes to a Greek Skeptic, Agrippa. "But Agrippa and his school [affirm five] modes, resulting respectively from disagreement, extension *ad infinitum,* relativity, hypothesis and reciprocal inference" (Diogenes Laertius, 1931, vol. 2, IX.88, p. 501). Sextus Empiricus (probably third century) gives the following summary of the five modes: "the first based on discrepancy, the second on regress *ad infinitum,* the third on relativity, the fourth on hypothesis, the fifth on circular reasoning" (Sextus Empiricus, 1976, vol. 1, p. 95).

13. Francis Fukuyama was appointed in 2001 by President George W. Bush to the President's Council on Bioethics.
14. "An international consensus on the control of new biomedical technologies will not simply spring into being without a great deal of work on the part of the international community and the leading countries within it. There is no magic bullet for creating such a consensus. It will require the traditional tools of diplomacy: rhetoric, persuasion, negotiation, economic and political leverage. But in this respect the problem is not different from the creation of any other international regime, whether in air traffic, telecommunications, nuclear or ballistic missile proliferation, and the like." Fukuyama, 2002, pp. 193-194.
15. Fukuyama's last man stands at the end of ideological or conceptual struggles, so that he looks to the end of history where man disappears and becomes culturally an animal. Fukuyama takes this notion in part from Kojève's very particular reinterpretation of Hegel, where "the disappearance of Man [is] at the end of history," where then "Man remains alive [only] as animal" (Kojève, 1969, p. 158), as well as from Nietzsche, who saw in the transformation of the slave ideology of Christianity into democracy the emergence of the last men who are more beast than man (*Also sprach Zarathustra,* IV.1).
16. Fukuyama hopes to justify restraints that can set strong limits to a human-directed evolution by appealing to human rights grounded in human nature as the sum of the behavioral characteristics typical of the human species.

> What is it that we want to protect from any future advances in biotechnology? The answer is, we want to protect the full range of our complex, evolved natures against attempts at self-modification. We do not want to disrupt either the unity or the continuity of human nature, and thereby the human rights that are based on it. ... That aspect of our complex natures most under threat has to do with our emotional gamut (Fukuyama, 1992, p. 172).

For Fukuyama, human dignity is grounded in the emotions that flow from human nature. In developing this point, Fukuyama makes the astonishing claim that we should feel no guilt for actions taken against a Star Trek Spock-like person devoid of feelings, such as anger or betrayal. Fukuyama never acknowledges that such an emotionless moral agent could act with a Kantian good will and not simply on the basis of a utilitarian calculus (Fukuyama, 2002, p. 169). One should also note that Fukuyama reduces utilitarian concerns to economic considerations (Fukuyama, 2002, p. 91). Fukuyama also conflates moral emotions with grounds for moral judgment and action. For example, Christian theology has regarded the Persons of the Trinity, not to mention angels, as acting without passion, but nevertheless with a moral will, and as such being worthy of respect. Because of this approach, Fukuyama dismisses the view that the rights, dignity, and equality of humans lie in their standing as moral agents. Fukuyama's quick try at the development of moral theory is crucially underdeveloped. Nevertheless, Fukuyama's volume is important in providing an example of the desire in intellectual circles for global regulation, especially concerning human germline genetic engineering, in order to forbid humans from refashioning the character of their human biological nature.

Our Post-human Future gives the impression of an author who up until the writing of this work, perhaps with some sympathy, reflected on the marginalization of traditional religiously- and metaphysically-rooted morality. Fukuyama, like Hegel, recognized in Napoleon's victory at the Battle of Jena (August 6, 1806) the emergence of a new age, bringing with it not only the abolishment of the Western empire and the liberal recasting of European culture, but also wide-ranging deconstruction of traditional Christian morality. These cultural changes, as Fukuyama argues, are tied to the end of history and the emergence of his last man: a person who, satisfied with immanent goods, has abandoned disputes about ultimate concerns. Having seen the abyss, Fukuyama in *Our Postmodern Future* seems to step back, seeking to secure a way to avoid the collapse of traditional moral constraints and loss of metaphysical orientation. He has recognized that in a post-metaphysical context there are no ultimate directions for guiding human evolution as it comes under human control. Unlike Nietzsche's superman, Fukuyama is uneasy at the loss of ultimate meaning and direction. Against this backdrop, Fukuyama attempts to confront the startling, long-range promises of new technologies, especially human genetic engineering.

17. If one takes communities seriously as well as the limited character of the authority of the secular state, then one can imagine the emergence of world-wide, non-geographically located, quasi-sovereign communities, such as the Roman Catholic church, Islam, Orthodox Jewry, Orthodox Christianity, and the International Texan League providing their own health care through their own health care institutions. There would thus be international networks of Vaticare, Islamicare, Jewishcare, and Texicare (Engelhardt, 2000, pp. 379-383).
18. To distinguish egalitarianisms of envy from egalitarianisms of altruism, consider the different moral claims involved in morally characterizing the following three possible worlds. The first is the original reference world in which there are ten individuals, each possessing six units of the good. In the second world, there are again ten individuals, but one individual possesses ten units of the good, while the other nine still have six. If one considers this world worse than the reference world, even though the total amount of good has been increased, and would prefer this first world, one embraces an egalitarianism of envy. In the third world, there are again ten individuals, nine with six units of the good and one with one. If one is concerned as cheaply as possible to bring the person with less to the standard of those with more, one is not concerned with inequalities for their own sake, but only insofar as they are associated with harm to such individuals.
19. I have explored these arguments in greater detail in Engelhardt, 1996, chs. 1-3, and Engelhardt, 2000, chs. 1-2.
20. For an account of this sparse moral fabric grounded in the permission of collaborators as the one framework to ground a general secular approach to health care policy, see Engelhardt, 1991, chap. 5.

21. Rawls employs the heuristic of an original position to feed into his moral rationality all of the choices his hypothetical contractors are to make. "One way to look at the idea of the original position, therefore, is to see it as an expository device which sums up the meaning of these conditions and helps us to extract their consequences" (1971, p. 21). Like Kant's kingdom of ends, all members of the original position are to act in accord with their content-full understanding of morality. "The original position is so characterized that unanimity is possible; the deliberations of any one person are typical of all" (1971, p. 263).

References

Alora, A., & Lumitao, J.M. (Eds.). (2001). *Beyond a Western Bioethics: Voices from the Developing World.* Washington, DC: Georgetown University Press.

Anderson, G. R., & Poullier, J.P. (1999). Health Spending, Access, and Outcomes: Trends in Industrialized Countries. *Health Affairs,* 18 (May/June), 178-192.

Bayertz, K. (1997). 'The normative status of the human genome: a European perspective,' in K. Hoshino (Ed.), *Japanese and Western Bioethics* (pp. 167-180). Dordrecht: Kluwer.

Beauchamp, T.L. (1997). 'Comparative studies: Japan and America,' Iin K. Hoshino (Ed.), *Japanese and Western Bioethics,* (pp. 25-47). Dordrecht: Kluwer.

Burman, E. (1984). *The Inquisition: Hammer of Heresy.* New York: Dorset.

Cherry, M. J., & Engelhardt, H.T., Jr. (2004). 'Informed consent in Texas: theory and practice,' *Journal of Medicine and Philosophy,* 29(2), 237-252.

Clement of Alexandria. (1994). 'The Stromata,' in A. Roberts and J. Donaldson (Eds.), *Ante-Nicene Fathers.* Peabody, MA: Hendrickson Publishers.

Commission on Global Governance. (1995). *Our Global Neighbourhood.* [On-line]. Available: http://www.cgg.ch/index.html.

Council of Europe. (1997). *Convention for the protection of human rights and dignity of the human being with regard to the application of biology and medicine: convention on human rights and biomedicine.* Oviedo [On-line]. Available: http://conventions.coe.int/Treaty/en/Treaties/Html/164.htm.

Daniels, N., & Sabin, J.E. (2002). *Setting Limits Fairly.* New York: Oxford University Press.

Denzinger, H. (Ed.) (1965). *Enchiridion Symbolorum* (33rd ed). Freiburg/Breisgau: Herder.

Diogenes L. (1931). *Lives of Eminent Philosophers.* (Trans., R.D. Hicks). Cambridge, MA: Harvard University Press.

Engelhardt, H. T., Jr. (2002). 'Secular priests, moral consensus, and ethical experts,' *Social Philosophy and Policy,* 19(1), 59-82.

Engelhardt, H. T., Jr. (2000). *The Foundations of Christian Bioethics.* Lisse, Netherlands: Swets & Zeitlinger.

Engelhardt, H. T., Jr. (1996). *The Foundations of Bioethics* (2nd ed). New York: Oxford University Press.

Engelhardt, H. T., Jr. (1994) 'Sittlichkeit and post-modernity: an Hegelian reconsideration of the state,' in H. T. Engelhardt, Jr., & T. Pinkard (Eds.), *Hegel Reconsidered* (pp. 211-224). Dordrecht: Kluwer.

Engelhardt, H. T., Jr. (1991). *Bioethics and Secular Humanism.* Philadelphia: Trinity Press International.

Engelhardt, H. T., Jr. (1986). *The Foundations of Bioethics.* New York: Oxford University Press.
Fan, R. (2002). 'Reconstructionist Confucianism in health care: an Asian moral account of health care resource allocation,' *Journal of Medicine and Philosophy,* 27(6), 675-682.
Fan, R., & Li, B. (2004). 'Truthtelling in medicine: the Confucian view,' *Journal of Medicine and Philosophy,* 29(2), 179-193.
Fishkin, J. S. (1983). *Justice, Equal Opportunity, and the Family.* New Haven, NJ: Yale University Press.
Fukuyama, F. (2002). *Our Posthuman Future.* New York: Farrar, Straus and Giroux.
Fukuyama, F. (1992). *The End of History and the Last Man.* New York: Free Press.
Fukuyama, F. (1989). The End of History? *The National Interest,* 16 (Summer), 3-18.
Hanke, L. (1949). *The Spanish Struggle for Justice in the Conquest of America.* Philadelphia: University of Pennsylvania Press.
Hayek, F.A. (1976). *Law, Legislation, and Liberty.* Chicago: University of Chicago Press.
Healthcare Research Group. (1999). *Health Care Services in Singapore: A Strategic Entry Report, 1999.* San Diego, CA: Icon Group International.
Hegel, G.W.F. (1952). *Hegel's Philosophy of Right.* (Trans., T.M. Knox). Oxford: Clarendon Press.
Hegel, G.W.F. (1892). *The Logic of Hegel* (2nd ed). (Trans., W. Wallace). Oxford: Oxford University Press.
Heller, A. (1990). *Can Modernity Survive?* Berkeley: University of California Press.
Hoshino, K. (Ed.) (1997). *Japanese and Western Bioethics.* Dordrecht: Kluwer.
InterAction Council. (1996, March 22-24). *In search of global ethical standards.* [Online]. Available: http://asiawide.or.jp/iac/meetings/Eng96ethics.htm.
InterAction Council (1996, May 19-22). *Communiqué of the InterAction Council.* [Online]. Available: http://asiawide.or.jp/iac/sessions/communiq14.htm.
International Bioethics Committee (2003). Report of the IBC on the Possibility of Elaborating a Universal Instrument on Bioethics. Paris: UNESCO.
Jonsen, A. (1998). *The Birth of Bioethics.* New York: Oxford University Press.
Kant, I. (1959). *Foundations of the Metaphysics of Morals.* (Trans., L.W. Beck). Indianapolis: Bobbs-Merrill.
Kant, I. (1957). *Perpetual Peace.* (Trans., L.W. Beck). New York: Macmillan Publishing Co.
Kant, I. (1965). *The Metaphysical Elements of Justice.* (Trans., J. Ladd). Indianapolis: Bobbs-Merrill.
Kant, I. (1964). *The Metaphysical Principles of Virtue.* (Trans., J. Ellington). Indianapolis: Bobbs-Merrill.
Kass, L. R. (2002). *Life, Liberty and the Defense of Dignity.* San Francisco: Encounter Books.
Kass, L.R. (1985). *Toward a More Natural Science.* New York: Free Press.
Kojève, A. (1969). *Introduction to the Reading of Hegel.* (Trans., J. H. Nichols, Jr.). New York: Basic Books.
Kuehn, M. (2001). *Kant: A Biography.* Cambridge: Cambridge University Press.
MacIntyre, A. (1981). *After Virtue.* Notre Dame, IN: University of Notre Dame Press.
Mandeville, B. (1988). *The Fable of the Bees.* Indianapolis: Liberty Classics.

Parliament of the World's Religions. (1993). *Declaration toward a global ethic.* [On-line]. Available: http://www.uni.tuebingen.de/stiftung weltethos/dat_eng/ st_3_e.htm.
Potter, V. R. (1970a). Bioethics, the Science of 'Survival'. *Perspectives in Biology and Medicine,* 14, 127-53.
Potter, V.R. (1970b). Biocybernetics and Survival. *Zygon,* 5, 229-46.
Potter, V.R. (1971). *Bioethics, Bridge to the Future.* Englewood Cliffs, NJ: Prentice-Hall.
Rawls, J. (1999). *The Law of Peoples.* Cambridge, MA: Harvard University Press.
Rawls, J. (1993). *Political Liberalism.* New York: Columbia University Press.
Rawls, J. (1971). *A Theory of Justice.* Cambridge, MA: Harvard University Press.
Reich, W. (1994). 'The word 'bioethics': its birth and the legacies of those who shaped its meaning,' *Kennedy Institute of Ethics Journal,* 4(4), 319-335.
Schmidt, K. (Ed.) (2000). *Journal of Medicine and Philosophy,* 25(2), 123-266.
Sextus Empiricus. (1976). Outlines of Pyrrhonism. I.164. In: *Sextus Empiricus.* (Trans., R.G. Bury). Cambridge, MA: Harvard University Press.
Shafer, I. (Ed.) (1998). *Envisioning a global ethic.* [On-line]. Available: http://astro.temple.edu/~dialogue/anthocon.htm.
Vacandard, E. (1908). *The Inquisition* (2nd ed). (Trans., B. L. Conway). Green, NY: Longmans.
Vitoria, F. (1991). *Political Writings.* New York: Cambridge University Press.
Wakefield, W.L. (1974). *Heresy, Crusade and Inquisition in Southern France 1100-1250.* London: George Allen and Unwin.
Walsh, W. T. (1940). *Characters of the Inquisition.* New York: P.J. Kennedy & Sons.

Implementing Health Care Rights Versus Imposing Health Care Cultures: The Limits of Tolerance, Kant's Rationality, and the Moral Pitfalls of International Bioethics Standardization

Corinna Delkeskamp-Hayes

Cultures, understood as collectively lived particularities, rest on normative identities. Such identities also extend to the moral sphere. A diversity of cultures may therefore imply a diversity of moralities. How different may these moralities be and still deserve the name? What separates a culture from a un-culture (or anti-culture)? The Western theory of human rights claims to have the answer: On the one hand, cultural diversity is affirmed as globally (as well as societally) enriching and as an outgrowth of individuals' right to cultural self-determination. On the other hand, such diversity is accepted only to the extent that individual human rights are respected and protected within any given culture. Only under the constraints thus imposed can, and must, (and both, as a matter of right) cultural diversity be tolerated. Western-style human rights thus determine the master-moral limits to moral and cultural diversity tolerance.

H.T. Engelhardt, Jr. (ed), *Global Bioethics* (pp. 50–94).

On the political level, numerous documents have been prepared for international and even global recognition of this principle. These documents specify, for the areas of economics, labor law, education, social relationships, and health care, how the endorsement of such rights should translate into legislating and policy-making. "Transnational networks of human rights activists" (Hawkins and Humes, 2002, p. 233) use a number of "socializing" methods for implementing such rights globally. Among these methods are, as the authors quote from the literature,

> media attention and public accusations to raise the profile of norm-violating states at the international level in an effort to shame them into compliance...empower[ing] domestic opposition groups by mobilizing and strengthening them through funding and moral-political support... creat[ing]e transnational structures that pressure the state both from within and from without (Hawkins and Humes, 2002, p. 233).

For traditional cultures with strong emphasis on particular, family, and community-oriented values, such political pressure can be profoundly unsettling.[1] Understandably, therefore, the Western theory of human rights is not everywhere welcome.[2] Can that theory be defended in a way that could compel even non-Westerners (or traditionally minded Westerners) to accept the cultural integrity sacrifices it imposes on them? Such a defense would require appealing to an authority all humans acknowledge. The most promising candidate for such universality[3] is rationality:[4] mathematicians and even empirical scientists across the world agree about standards of coherence, explanatory power, verification and relevance. The technological advances reached on the basis of these disciplines are in worldwide demand, quite irrespective of differences in culture. Rationality as a criterion is applied not only for determining what is reliable and useful in theories and institutions; it also distinguishes what must be respected in claims advanced by individuals. In a more encompassing sense, rationality serves even as a criterion for respectability in individuals themselves. If the Western theory of human rights can establish its rationality, then it can be claimed to be valid for all humans who (self-respectingly) understand themselves as rational beings. Whoever would then contest that validity would disqualify himself in view of a universally respected standard. He would repudiate the respectability of his very contesting. On the political level, where such contesting translates into the refusal to grant human rights, this refusal would defeat a state's moral respectability. Just as an individual violating what rationality morally requires defeats his claim to have his autonomy respected, so a state using its power in a way that violates human rights defeats its own "natural law" claim to be left in peace. Such a refusal and violation would even establish a moral obligation on the part of other states to intervene, and to use force against such a state.[5]

This essay opposes Western human rights theorists' claim to rationality in the universally compelling sense just outlined. It offers as evidence an analysis of the most promising secular foundation for such rights: the practical philosophy of Immanuel Kant.[6] At the end of his *Rechtslehre in the Metaphysik der Sitten* (1797a, p.216f and p.235)[7], Kant envisages a moral ideal of eternal peace on earth, to be secured by a universal league of nations. His faith in the moral progress of humanity (1796, p. 86f) was nourished from the French Enlightenment's project of replacing the theological justification of political power by a secularly moral one.[8] Kant's rational morality has inspired[9] today's call for the universal acknowledgement of human dignity[10], understood as a specific and yet culture-transcending (Andorno, 2002, p. 960) value, and for the securing[11] of encompassing human rights which are derived from that dignity[12] The problem with this inspiration, so this essay argues, lays in the fact that Kant's definition of humans' specifically rational dignity endorses (at most) only a negative right to individual autonomy. It offers no support, either for the substantial positive rights[13] or the (implied as well as further stipulated) substantial moral standards limiting that autonomy, which contemporary human rights advocates affirm.[14]

A particularly prominent example of international human rights promotion concerns health care and bioethics.[15] Technological advances in these fields present allocation and risk management problems as well as challenges to the traditional ethos of medicine. Numerous proclamations from UNESCO, WHO and European as well as Asian intergovernmental councils have responded to what they perceived as a resulting need for international cooperation. These technological advances, moreover, in touching on issues of life and death, illness, procreation, body and species integrity, concern especially culture-sensitive areas, which in many ways resist Western-style human rights implementation. The diversity of moral cultures in this realm is therefore held to pose the problem of the extent and limits of a properly "moral" tolerance in a particular urgent manner. Yet as H. Tristram Engelhardt Jr. has shown (2005, p. 4 ff), it is also this realm, which exposes with particular clarity the contested nature of "Western-style" human rights even within the (post-traditional) West.[16] Whereas (most) Europeans (and along with them the international human rights policy players) follow Kant in taking the very notion of human rights to rest on a content-rich understanding of human dignity, which imposes, in addition to political respect for such rights, very specific bioethical norms, the Anglo-Saxon (or, to a certain extent, Lockean) tradition which exerted its formative influence on the political culture of the United States, (typically) refrains from asserting such further norms. Accordingly, Europeans, unlike (typical) representatives of that latter culture, affirm more encompassing social rights.[17] Moreover, they take failure to enforce non-discrimination for genetic reasons, failure to secure equity[18] in health care resource allocation, or take the permission of germ line interventions (Andorno, 2002, p. 960), genetic enhancement (Andorno, 2002, p. 961), organ sale, surrogate motherhood, sex choice and therapeutic cloning to be contrary to human dignity and therefore beyond the limits of what may be tolerated as cultural diversity in medicine. By contrast, human rights advocates who argue from the specific legal tradition of the United States restrict their commitment to securing a much wider scope for negative rights (as for example in informed consent requirements). They oppose non-Western practices only (and without much concern about reasons) when it comes to reproductive cloning and germ line enhancement.

In addition to such disagreements on the content-level of bioethical standards, even the (majority-enforced, post-traditional) European position suffers from divergent methodological interpretations concerning the question of how bioethical claims are to be grounded. Sometimes the texts suggest that bioethical issues can be exhaustively (even if in merely general terms) derived from what is implied in the notion of human dignity itself. (Most prominent among such issues are health care rights—sometimes even presented as "rights to health", cf. WHO in United Nations 2001, Add II.). Sometimes these same texts claim that their bioethical standards derive from agreement and compromise formation, as a result of which cultural differences were discounted for the sake of scientific, technological, or epidemiologic cooperation. This methodological difference is veiled through the invocation of a "common consensus". Such a consensus, however, can either be grounded in a regard to an objective reality (here of moral norms), which all agree to be valid, or it can be grounded in a discursive process, where the outcome is not a discovery of something objectively given but the production of something subjectively agreed upon. In the case of the first interpretation, global harmonization of laws and regulations in biomedicine (Andorno, 2002, p. 959) and biotechnology is understood as an endeavor that aims at hindering what is objectively unacceptable (hence intolerable). In the second case this endeavor is seen as resulting from negotiations between consenting partners, each of who pursues what they consider desirable.[20] To be sure, to some extent both interpretations are compatible: to consider negotiation between consenting partners as a validating procedure presupposes, after all, that one respects their autonomous right to enter such agreements. Endorsement of a formal concept of human dignity thus is common to both accounts. It is only the material aspects of that notion, and what they imply for bioethics, which are posited as inviolable by the first interpretation, but subject to bargaining by the second. Only the first understanding, of course, requires that the bioethical standards recommended for global implementation partake—via their content rich human-dignity foundation—of the rational credentials, which are also claimed for human rights (and for their tolerance limiting potential in view of justifying the use of force).

Only this (first) understanding, so it may seem, is therefore vulnerable to the criticism offered in this essay. A closer look however reveals that the same holds for the second as well: its vulnerability is merely less immediate. The consenting partners to the bioethical treaties, after all, are not individuals (using their respective autonomy rights) but governments. Through such treaties they establish an (ever more) extensive international recognition of their authority, through the processes of "harmonizing laws" which these treatises impose, to restrict their citizens' (individual and communal) bioethical autonomy rights (as well as border-crossing ability to secure these rights abroad)—and thus to act in an individual-human-rights violating manner.[21] Only if it could be shown that, as a matter of rationally compelling moral obligation, health care rights must be recognized and the corresponding services supplied by governments, only then could one restrict one's moral concerns to the human-rights-compatible (i.e. democratic) procedures by which the ethical standards that will guide that supply are determined. Only then would the arbitrary element implied in national bioethics enforcement as well as in international bioethical compromise formation, as it were, itself be covered by a rational necessity. Each partner state, after all, would have to somehow opt for some one (of the many possible, but from the standpoint of rationality equally arbitrary) way of normatively guiding public biomedicine. In this case the (obvious) lacking compelling-ness of some chosen guidance would not defeat a government's authority to enforce it. It remains only the fact that health care is publicly provided itself which would have to be defended as morally obligatory in a universally valid sense. As a result, both interpretations of Western human rights implementing in the field of health care and gene technology, whether by direct appeal to a content rich notion of human dignity, or by detour of scrutinizing governments' authority legislate bioethics and to negotiate about it, presuppose the rational necessity of health care rights. Both interpretations, thus, can be questioned in view of that rational necessity, and can be exposed to the "Kantian test".

And in fact, both interpretations are even advocated by reference to Kantian claims and insights. This somewhat surprising fact is reflected in the way in which—irrespective of their opposing presuppositions concerning the function of "human dignity"—both interpretations are so indiscriminatingly endorsed along one another in the human rights documents. There is a reason, so this essay will argue, for such conflating: Kant's own texts are ambiguous. His project of rationally reconstructing the specifically Christian moral culture of his social environment tempted him into overestimating what his purely secular and at the same time purely noumenon-oriented rationality can accomplish. His moral imperative (basically) addresses rational beings (1786, pp. 82, 84). It takes humans' embodiment merely as a contingent circumstance, to be considered only on the level of securing moral compliance. Kant's own pronouncements on bioethical subjects (such as children's right to life and adequate care, the in-permissibility of suicide and of self mutilation, his "consumptive" and sexuality) are therefore particularly vulnerable to bias in favor of rationally un-warranted cultural commitments.[22]

Not surprisingly, present day human rights advocating, as it endeavors to update Kant's concept of human dignity so as to promote it to the status of a bioethical guiding principle is hampered by inconsistencies. A good example is the most encompassing present day international bioethics declaration, the Council of Europe's (1997a) *Convention for the Protection of Human Rights and Dignity of the Human Being with regard to the Application of Biology and Medicine* (the *Oviedo Convention*). An analysis of this inconsistency will be the subject of the first part of this essay. As a result, it will become clear that any attempt to defend the rational compelling-ness and thus the bioethical tolerance-limiting function of human rights advocating in bioethics must take issue with the second, negotiation-based interpretation of bioethical standards. The question of rational compelling-ness must thus be restricted to governments' obligation to recognize (and fund) rights to health care, or more generally (positive) social rights, merely as such. This question will be the subject of the second, Kantian part of the essay.

I. Human Rights in Biomedicine: The Example of the *Oviedo Convention*

Cultivating human rights is claimed to be not merely a cultural thing. It is conceived as a criterion of moral legitimacy. This criterion can be depicted as a wicker fence weaved around rights-securing posts and enclosing a free space for the cultivation of permitted diversity. At the same time, cultivating human rights centrally implies respecting autonomy and cultural self-determination. It thus not only permits but even encourages normative diversity, both for individuals and their communities. It celebrates cultural diversity.[23] This welcome is generally taken to also include polities[24] as bearers of different cultures. The biomedicine implications of this commitment on both the individual and the political level are illustrated with particular clarity by the Oviedo convention. On each of these levels, the endorsement of human rights requires balancing the appeal to a common obligatory core-morality with acceptance of moral diversity within the confines of what is tolerated by that core morality. In the first case (A) this balancing concerns the relationship between the state and the individual; in the second case (B) between core-moral human dignity and individuals' own normative pursuits.

A. Moral Diversity Among Polities

As the essays by both Angelo Petroni (2005, p. 1) and Kurt Bayertz (2005, p. 15) affirm, Europe takes pride in the richness of cultural diversity among its member states. Legal harmonization therefore is to leave room for national differences in how to (a) implement public health care (Council, 1997a, Art.3), and (b) devise standards of rights-protection (Council, 1997a, Art. 27). The political cultivation of particular normative identities is thus encouraged.[25]

Yet on this inter-state level, the wicker fence model presents the problem already indicated in the introduction. Whereas for individuals this image represents the relationship between what is prohibited (by the law doing the fencing-in) and what is permitted in the fenced-in space, on the inter-state-level the permitted cultural autonomy (within the fenced-in space left for individual states' discretion) endorses their restricting their members' autonomy (thus further fencing in their free space). Individuals' human rights encompass normative (moral and religious) self-determination (General Assembly, 1948, Art. 18-20). Acknowledging such individual normative self-determination implies accepting that the days of homogenous nations with their presumed cultural "general will" has passed. It implies that one endorses normative pluralism even within a state. But then the act of also acknowledging polities' (cultural) "self-determination" in fact authorizes governments to disrespect individuals' self-determination.[26] How can one and the same human rights endorsement support such opposing principles? A solution is often sought in terms of "public debate".

The quest for public debate (General Assembly, 1948, Art. 28) affirms the need for societal agreement on social, economic, and ethical issues, as raised by medicine and biotechnology.[27] Not only is the democratic form of government itself supposed to secure (an at least procedure-mediated) general consent of voting members to their state's cultural identity. The discursive processes, which accompany the voting, are also supposed to symbolize some general participation in cross-societal developments of normative compromises. Does that mean that the political-culture problem is solved and the contradiction noted above removed? Let us consider the two issues the Convention addresses.

Varieties in implementing public health care

The first issue concerns health care rights. Different ways of implementing such rights reflect—among other things like different historical, geographic, social and economic circumstances—different value rankings. These rankings may respond to such external circumstances, but they cannot be exhaustively derived from them.[28] Any particular implementation of health care rights will thus enforce only one particular ranking among many possible ones. Such implementation forces even those individuals who rank differently. To be sure, public health care can be provided only if all (can be forced to) not only contribute, but also comply. As the provision of such care will always be normatively biased, some losses in moral diversity are unavoidable. Acknowledging a right to health care, and thus the necessity of such a provision, merely as such, implies accepting such losses.

These losses are not negligible, even already within the "West". In many developed countries with a high level of public health care, even those who object to such "care" publicly finance services like abortion, in-vitro-fertilization, and sex-change-operation.[29] As Petroni has pointed out, moreover, European Union subsidies of enormous dimensions are being devoted to stem cell research, which is forbidden in several countries (Petroni, 2005, p. 30). In Germany, the reform of home care for the elderly or helpless forced religious orders (which had long been integrated into a system of subsidiary cooperation) to discontinue their no-pay charity services. Because of the strong government involvement (through taxes) that comes with acknowledging health care rights, resources for financing private alternatives are drained away. In addition, chances of having such alternatives succeed in a subsidy-distorted market are reduced. In Belgium, Roman Catholic Hospitals contemplating a policy of not offering euthanasia and physician assisted suicide services were threatened with withdrawal of government funding. In both Belgium and Germany even religious hospitals are unable to hinder[30] their staff from responding to patient demands for euthanasia[31]: such hindering is interpreted as denying patients their right to end-of-life autonomy. Acknowledging health care rights (and to do so in the context of a liberal culture that is—as Mark Cherry has clearly pointed out (2005, p. 7ff)—inherently hostile to all non-secularized religion) thus severely compromises moral and cultural diversity, especially among minorities. The hope that "public debate" and the general consent to the democratic procedure could remedy the corresponding losses of autonomy among minorities is vain: ultimately, no discursive veneer can hide the fact that minorities must succumb to the decisions of the majority. The discursive model itself, while appropriate for voluntary cooperation (or the enterprise associations for which Nicholas Capaldi has invoked Oakeshott), fails when applied to a context in which no one is free to withdraw.

Combining negative rights (to autonomy and cultural diversity) and positive rights (to social services) in bioethics compromises the former in yet another sense: in constitutional democracies, human rights limit majority rule. It is precisely by withholding what these rights grant from what is publicly negotiable, that such democracies respect human rights. The very meticulous attention which documents proclaiming positive rights (for instance in economics and social affairs) devote to the detailed listing of the benefits to be secured through such rights (United Nations, 1997, Art.7, pp. 10-14, 15) reflects an effort to withdraw these issues from what can be decided by a voting public. The Convention, on the other hand, permits the extent to which health care rights are granted to be determined in view of signature states' "needs" and "available resources". In democracies, the perception of which health services answer "needs", which needs have priority, and what resources should be reserved for them, are settled (ultimately) through voting. Accordingly, the extent to which health care rights are honored in such states, and property rights earmarked for their financing, becomes an issue of public negotiation.[32] Since it is one of the decisive purposes of Western human rights advertising to de-emphasize any difference between negative and positive rights[33], the rock bottom non-negotiable character of "rights" is compromised.

Different levels of rights-protection

The second issue concerns the problem of moral reasons for restricting negative rights. Germany did not sign the *Convention* because it considered the restriction Article 17 imposes on medical research with subjects who are unable to consent too weak. Belgium did not sign because it considered that same protection too strong. Different protection levels imply different perceptions of how much social solidarity obligation is imposed not only onto property, but also—so one is led to conclude—onto the human body. While here the burden imposed on the few is small (*op.cit.* Art. 17.2ii) in comparison to the large benefit expected for the many, research on human embryos (*op.cit.* Art. 18.2, who are also bearers of human rights, see Council, 1997b #19) is qualified by a demand of "an adequate protection" that does not honor even their right of life. Even "existential earmarking" (or should we say: ear-chopping) of human beings' right to life is thus accepted. In permitting the imposition of such sacrifice of life and bodily integrity, and in subjecting the extent of such imposition to public negotiation, Western democracies renounce what was to distinguish them from a morally unacceptable mere majority rule. They have cancelled their presumed fundamental difference vis à vis traditional autocracies, or even plain despotism.

Obviously research imposed sacrifice has a benevolent motive: those unable to consent and those not yet born are to benefit from medical progress.[34] Germany's higher protection standards in medical research however to some extent deprive the protected individuals of their positive rights. Germany accepts this disadvantage in view of her National Socialist past, the repudiation of which still shapes her present-day cultural identity. The same holds for Germany's prohibition of euthanasia (a subject not covered by the Convention): on the basis of Germany's particular moral commitments (and concerns about the integrity of the medical profession) individuals' right to (terminal) self-determination (in the sense of being able to procure physicians' assistance in suicide or euthanasia) is denied. But if such *Sonderwege* are to be protected under the umbrella of Western individual rights endorsement, it becomes difficult to understand why moral toleration should be withheld from non-Western cultures, if they (benevolently) lower solidarity impositions with respect to (negative) property rights by abstaining from positive health care rights altogether. Why, to cite another example, should Germany's concern for her cultural identity be permitted to severely limit stem cell research, thus favoring in vitro fertilized eggs' right to life at the expense of her competent members' right to benefit from that research, whereas non-Western (or traditionally minded Westerners') concerns for cultural identity are not to be permitted (because convicted of sexual discrimination) to limit women's access to the work place, thus favoring infants' right to a health-promoting family environment at the expense of their mothers' right to professional self-determination?[35]

Let us summarize: The way in which the *Oviedo Bioethics Convention* makes space for cultural diversity on the political level compromises human rights in three respects: 1. the commitment to the protection of cultural minorities' moral self-determination could not be sustained, 2. the political significance of negative rights was repudiated, 3. the limits for the legitimate violation of negative rights, and thus the criteria which were to centrally distinguish tolerable (rights-granting) from intolerable (rights-denying) cultures, could not even be rendered intelligible.

B. Moral Diversity on the Individual Level

If commitment to human rights is to maintain its tolerance for and even celebration of cultural and moral diversity in a more consistent manner, that diversity must be restricted to individuals. Even if states are the primary[36] addressees of the human rights master-morality, diversity cultivating must be for individuals (and their voluntary associations) exclusively. The fact that politically (enforced) culture-cultivating still persists (and that the *Convention* accepts it even still in Europe) must be discounted as a relic of pre-Enlightenment periods that will be worn away by ever progressing global protection of all polity members' individual rights.

But precisely the (at least implied) opposition to the political implementation of cultural values thus endorsed, or precisely the commitment to individualism underlying that opposition, will be conceived as a threat to non-individualist political cultures.[37] Members of such polities often claim a right to have their culture protected politically. (Islam and Confucianism are just two prominent examples.)[38] Some tradition-oriented cultures tolerate or even welcome enforcing their culturally communal duties politically.[39] What is considered legitimate in such environments is usually perceived as overstepping the toleration limits endorsed by the Western (post-traditional) commitment to individual human rights.

Thus, (post-traditional) Western individualism is what is usually taken to be the cardinal bone of contention. This individualism is thought to undermine non-Westerners' ability to accept even that rationality-condition of human respectability, without which the effort to prove that human rights have rational foundations is pointless. Given this predicament, it seems to make sense that "human dignity" in the West is defined not merely in rational but also in moral terms. Such dignity then entitles humans to rights insofar as it rests on rationality not just *per se* but insofar as that rationality encompasses a moral conscience (General Assembly, 1948, Art.1) taking up the Kantian understanding (1786, p. 76 f; 1797a, p. 22). The Western appeal to human dignity implies individualism in a pointedly moral sense. Whereas the General Assembly considers humans' moral dignity in terms of mere moral accountability (and of responsibility as the ability to answer for oneself), in Europe that dignity also encompasses some altruistic concern (and responsibility "for others").[40] Dignity in the first sense addresses only the possibility of moral achievement (along with moral failure). It derives the right to have one's autonomy respected from mere ability to be called to account. Dignity in the second sense addresses realized achievement. It grants autonomy rights only under the condition of such (enforced) achievement: Here the sacrifices of individual autonomy that culture demands, or the solidarity burdens it imposes on (species-) human life and bodily integrity, personal property, spiritual integrity, and consensual contracting are all believed to deny merely negligible fringe areas of individual autonomy. They are believed to deny spaces for self-determination, which no decent individual (i.e. no individual properly socialized into the European human rights world view) would wish to claim anyway.

Usually, both one of these readings is thought to be sufficient to overcome non-Western reservations against Western individualism, and to invite agreement even from non-Enlightenment-transformed cultures: with regard to the first reading, this is indeed unproblematic. While linking moral responsibility for failures and achievements more strongly with individuals' home communities, these cultures still restrict societal reward and legal punishment to the responsible individual himself. With regard to the second reading, it is usually held that politically enforced moral achievement in the (European main stream) West is somewhat akin to such cultures' emphasis on communal cohesion, and compatible with politically enforcing what is culturally endorsed as normatively obligatory (as long as this does not overstep the master-morally fixed definition of "negligible autonomy fringes").[41]

Nevertheless both readings, whatever their virtues for overcoming non-individualistic cultures' hostility to the Western human rights theory, raise serious further problems for the consistency of the bioethics convention, and thus of that theory itself, insofar as it finds itself embodied in the convention: how can one reconcile granting human rights where no moral accountability can be attributed? And how can one reconcile endorsing individuals' culture diversity celebrating with legally imposing the very concrete moral norms connected with the (secular) European understanding of human dignity, as these determine where the "negligible fringe" part of one's autonomy is supposed to begin? Those two problems arise with particular urgency with regard to (a) medical treatment of humans unable to consent, and (b) commitment to autonomy resources protection.

The extension of rights-bearer-ship

The *Oviedo Convention*, its *Explanatory Report* (# 19), as well as all other bio-medical human rights documents, extend rights-bearer-ship beyond the realm of moral accountability, or beyond personhood in the narrow sense. Potential persons, to be sure, will later develop into real persons. One can grant them an anticipated "retrospective" right (that "matures" as their personhood unfolds) to protection of life and bodily integrity during their growing stages.[42] But such anticipation is valid only for potential persons who will in fact realize their potential. It does not cover any obligation to permit such realizing. If it is only on account of their later accomplished personhood that they are granted protection-rights beforehand, then, as long as one hinders the former, why should they enjoy the latter? Why, more specifically, and in the purely secular context addressed here, should real persons' rights be restricted with regard to those who will not be permitted to mature? The *Oviedo Convention* prohibits in vitro fertilization for the production of human research material (Art. 18.2). (By implication it also prohibits the breeding of cloned organ banks for therapeutic purposes.) It is unclear on what (secular, and thus potentially universally acceptable) grounds it can impose such restrictions.[43]

The protective measures the Convention institutes to "make up for" potential persons' inability to consent raise difficulties of their own. Forbidding genetic (germ line) therapy that affects future generations (Art. 13) gets justified in view (not of a precautionary principle, as in UNESSCO 2003b #81, but in view) of future generations' right to bodily integrity (which includes their genetic heritage). But future generations are also granted a right to benefit from medical research (*Oviedo Convention*, 1997, *Preamble*). The convention's prohibition deprives them of that right. Even their right to life is jeopardized if their genetic defects are to be left in principle un-tampered with: they might fall victim to pre-birth routine genetic screening. They are thus even existentially discriminated against on the basis of their genetic heritage (*Oviedo Convention*, 1997, Art. 11). Protecting potential persons' one right to genetic integrity thus violates three other of their acknowledged rights. In this area the human rights account even increases its inconsistency.

In what concerns, on the other hand, humans who are born but never will be moral persons in the full sense, these are, of course, also counted as bearers of human rights. The only secular, and thus potentially universally acknowledgeable, solution for the problem of their dignity consists in membership in the human species (which they also share with potential persons). The rights established for human non- (and not even potential) persons on the basis of that attributed dignity (again) restricts the rights of (potential as well as realized) persons. It remains unclear how a dignity that had been grounded for some classes of human species members in their moral personhood could be transferred to other (non moral-person) classes of human species members.[44] On what secular ground could "species membership" constitute an unconditional value so as to be able to ground norms in the first place?

With regard to therapeutic interventions on such "never moral person"-humans, the *Convention* recognizes proxy consent as valid only if it benefits (those non-person) patients themselves (1997, Art.6.1). But proxy consent for non- therapeutic research (offering no benefits) is permitted, even if it violates the research subjects' right to bodily integrity (1997, Art. 17.2). The burdens and risks must be "minimal" (1997, Art. 17.2ii), to be sure. But we do not force the minimal risk and burden of non- therapeutic research on those able to consent. Bodily integrity is not universally "earmarked" for (medical research-) solidarity reasons. Those unable to consent are thus not only instrumentalized, they are also discriminated against. Granted, that discrimination is unavoidable in order to avoid discriminating against other non-persons in their age-, disease- or condition-group (1997, Art. 17.2i), whose right to benefit from medical research had been acknowledged (Council, 1997a, Preamble).[45] Thus again, recognizing human rights in non-(moral) persons is not only incomprehensible with regard to those rights' foundation of moral dignity, it also introduces further inconsistencies.

Concern for autonomy resources

The *Oviedo Convention* prohibits deriving financial gain from bodily organs (Art. 21, UNESCO, 2003c # 54). It thereby limits persons' autonomy rights with respect to the integrity of their own bodies. The argument that persons do not own their bodies but are obligated to maintain those bodies' integrity cannot be rendered secularly comprehensible.[46] The argument that inducing others to sell their organ would be immoral is not helpful either: acknowledging moral accountability as basis of a moral dignity that entitles to autonomy rights means accepting the risk of moral failure in exchange of the chance of moral achievement. We do not prohibit prostitution, or selling alcohol to an alcoholic, or gambling away one's family assets. Wishing to avoid such risks in order to secure the achievements betrays a lack of faith in humans' ability to answer for themselves, which repudiates the very (minimal version) basis of rights-acknowledging. With regard to the second version of that basis (where moral dignity is linked with some basic moral achievement), inducing someone to sell his organs could indeed be classified as in principle immoral (and proscribed) only if all organ-sale could be shown to be morally irresponsible (in the sense of "objectionably egoistic"). The *Convention* seems to assume this. While it classifies donating bodily organs as dignified (because altruistic), it classifies selling them as undignified (because indicative of base motives). The possibility that selling an organ (just as selling sperms and ova or surrogate motherhood, which are implicitly also prohibited) may also be altruistically motivated[47] is disregarded.[48] Moreover, in restricting ("imputedly altruistic") organ donation from those unable to consent to the saving of siblings' lives (1997, Art. 20.2.ii), and proscribing it with regard to aunts or cousins (not to even speak of parents), who may be involved in caring for such donors, the *Convention* permits, on no rationally comprehensible grounds, weakening potential donors' often indispensable family support system.[49]

It is often argued that societal situations in which persons have to resort to medical self-mutilation (as well as, so we could add, sperm- or ova- selling and uterus-renting) are themselves "undignified". But even if we granted this, it would not justify—in a way that respects human rights—not permitting individuals to adjust their life plans to whatever social situations they find themselves in.[50]

A further motive[51] frequently adduced for human rights advocates' concern with organ sale is concern for autonomy: respecting dignity implies granting rights to life and bodily integrity, both of which are also resources of for autonomous action. It is concluded that granting such rights also means protecting these resources. (The Convention therefore empowers governments to protect a person's life and bodily integrity even against the embodied person himself.) But that conclusion has fallen prey to an ambiguity in the concept of "respecting": respecting someone's autonomy on the basis of his moral personhood (first reading: accountability) by itself merely implies respecting his autonomy as a principle. It means placing side constraints on others' actions. Respecting someone's autonomy as a value that must be protected, by contrast, authorizes and even obligates others to interfere with that person's autonomously disregarding that value in himself. Such interference (in the sense of the second reading: enforced moral achievement) again defeats humans' moral accountability.

Moreover, as there are different, and in each case particular, ways in which such a value (or any moral achievement in general) can be defined, any such enforced protection will imply a respectively particular understanding of human dignity. If some uses of autonomy which lead to the compromising of autonomy-resources are declared "undignified", it becomes hard to understand why other such uses (as when engaging in a marriage with non-Western, or traditionally-minded Western, husbands so as to restrict one's autonomy resources as a woman, or when renouncing the use of most of one's autonomy resources by joining a monastery) should not equally be prohibited. The invocation of human rights for limiting only some, but not other aspects individuals' normative autonomy cannot be rendered intelligible. (Of course, human rights advocates are usually not much taken by non-Western marriages or monasteries anyway.)

To summarize the results of our survey of the *Oviedo Convention* on Heath Care and Bioethics: even after discounting its troublesome commitment to polities as bearers of cultural autonomy rights, and attending only to the individual level, two central problems have remained unsolvable. The extension human rights to non-persons introduced inconsistencies, and the claimed dependence of human dignity on protected autonomy resources reduced the criterion of what is morally tolerable in bioethics, once again, to something merely particular, thus repudiating its claimed cross-cultural generality. The toleration limit defended by Western human rights advocating in biomedicine in this Convention cannot even be intelligibly drawn.

As the references to other bioethical documents made clear, moreover, there exists presently no alternative account of human rights in this field, the consistency and coherence of which could be tested. The question concerning the rational compelling-ness and corresponding universal validity of such an account can thus not even be posed. At least in the field of bioethical standards implementation, no global policing in the name of human-rights-securing can—at least so far—be defended. Since there is obviously nothing rationally compelling about the bioethical standards proposed in these documents, there remains no alternative but to accept their second interpretation: we shall assume that these standards, as they are recommended for global implementation, result from negotiation and political compromise. We shall assume, in other words, that these standards—in a more properly constraint-defying sense than that exemplified by national public debates (establishing what—regardless of the discursive efforts invested to accommodate minorities—in the end will be enforced as majority vote anyway) secures at least the participating political partners' consent. But that does still not solve the legitimacy question noted in the introduction. Since such compromise agreements between states determine limits to tolerance in bioethics, they still authorize the use of force against these states' own constituents. Both with respect to imposing such (from a rational standpoint arbitrary) norms on their own members, and with respect to un-avowed advantage taking (from the unequal bargaining power) in their negotiations with other states, the invoked moral commitment to human rights must be shown to justify the normative and cultural diversity losses incurred as a result of such imposing and advantage taking. As stipulated above, both parts of this justification require that granting social rights (as these can be argued to include health care) is, in fact, rationally compelling. If this could be shown, even the incompatibilities between positive and negative rights that had turned out to hamper the bioethical context could, as it were, be allotted to a philosophically irrelevant "level of phenomena", which, like a material cloak, envelops the hard and ideally consistent core of equally compelling positive and negative "human rights". The second part of this essay is devoted to the way in which Kant's moral theory addresses this task.

II. A Kantian Rational Check on Health Care Rights and Tolerate Limits

Looking for a rational ground for positive human rights seems a paradoxical undertaking. Suppose, as this is generally conceded, that the existence of a "natural human freedom right" can be rationally grounded in humans' both rational and moral dignity. Suppose that right imposes a moral ban on using force against anyone (without his consent). Suppose further that this negative right can even be proven to be compatible with the use of some political force against some (without their consent, in cases where they themselves have disrespected that right in others). Given all of that, the possibility of including positive rights to publicly subsidized goods and services will, from the very start, authorize the use of political force for limiting humans' rationally grounded (negative) freedom right. Such a limiting could be considered legitimate only if humans' moral dignity were interpreted as responsibility in the second sense, as implying (and hence imposing) some altruistic concern for others. Determining the extent to which such social rights ought to be granted would then amount to determining the extent of dignity-implied (and hence politically imposable) altruistic concern. But if social rights are to be rationally grounded in such a doubly oriented human dignity, that dignity must encompass a biological and psychological dimension, for the sake of which providing humans with social goods and services may be considered obligatory.[52] And in fact, textual evidence proves that Kant himself endorsed all of that. Not only did he explain the obligation to form a state with the goal of securing persons' survival (1797a, p.157) and thereby acknowledged the state's obligation to care for those in need (1797a, p. 186ff). He even specified certain allocative adjustments (1798, p. 178) for such care in a way that parallels the Oviedo Convention's lee-way for "available resources" and "perceived needs", when determining levels of public health care.[53]

Accordingly, if the search for Kantian rationality credentials for Western-style human rights is not from the very start to run aground on the obvious paradox of social rights granting, his unfortunate passion for accommodating moral norms derived from the Christian tradition must be discounted. The rational core of his theory must be reconstrued from carefully dissected texts. What can be proposed as universally valid grounds for limiting culture tolerance, both in bioethics and other areas for human rights, must be separated from what commands only the historian's interest.

In pursuing this dissection, I shall first consider what Kant's strictly noumenal approach accomplishes for founding human rights (A). It will turn out that a negative freedom right can be established in a way that includes even (phenomenal) property- and bodily integrity-considerations. In a second section (B) the question of positive rights will be addressed.

A. Negative Rights

Negative rights have (1) a moral and (2) a political dimension.

1. The moral obligation to respect

Only if persons are morally accountable (Kant, 1797a, p. 22) in a sense that presupposes (1797b, p. 33) "noumenal" (1797a, p. 48) freedom from causally operating motivations (and all humans consider themselves to be in that moral sense free (1786, p. 113), does imposing unconditional moral obligations make (secular) sense. On the other hand, only if such genuinely moral agency (or responsibility in the sense of accountability) exists can one even worry about devising a (master-) morality which grounds the obligations guiding that agency. In linking such moral agency with rationality (or the ability to govern one's actions by a regard for what practical reason legislates, 1786, p. 83), Kant further specifies those obligations: no one can claim to be (even just morally) entitled to freedom rights unless he pays the "entrance fee" of endorsing the rationally imposed respect for such rights in others. In view of this morally legislating rationality, after all, as it is shared by all persons, everyone must conceive himself "on a par" with all others (1786, p. 83). Everyone is obligated to respect (in the sense of not instrumentalizing 1786, p. 66f) that rational "nature" (1786, p. 84f) in himself just as in them. In positing such a "mystical brotherhood of all rational beings" (1787, p. 836), Kant has succeeded in introducing a normative element in humans' moral dignity, which does not involve the material value implications of responsibility-as-altruism. He has succeeded in keeping his account clear of any universality defying particularities.

Kant's acknowledgement of a freedom (1786, pp. 79, 101f) defies empirical verification (1786, p. 26) and even flies in the face of common experience and scientific evidence concerning the causal conditioned-ness of human behavior. This acknowledgement presupposes that one resolutely separates the different (and profoundly incompatible) ways of considering persons either noumenally or phenomenally (1786, p. 107ff; 1797b, p. 65).[54] This additional dimension is often regarded today as a metaphysical burden. But it accounts for precisely that dualism in individuals, between what explains any actual (or actually lacking) consent and what can be appealed to in terms of persons' own "higher nature", which (dualism) is in turn indispensable for the moral justification of political power. Without such power, on the other hand, the morally legitimate use of which even against those who do not actually consent is at least (and for the moment) conceivable, a morally legitimate (human rights respecting and protecting) state is inconceivable. (For both, respecting and protecting, require that even among its citizens such respect is—if this loose way of speaking is permitted—"enforced", and their freedom thus protected.) Kant's two-fold approach to human persons, in other words, permits to both acknowledge freedom in whatever way individuals may happen to use and value it (and thus permits to endorse freedom as a principle) and, at the same time, to impute to them (as moral persons) a commitment to their rationally self governing freedom (and thus to moral achievement), where the latter imposes moral constraints on the exercise of the former, some of which the state (once its own legitimacy has been established) may enforce.

2. *The Political Dimension of Respect*

Obviously, a state erected on the basis of such a morality, authorized to play some of the "oughts" governing those moral constraints against the "is" of actual consent, can be kept from engendering a rights-violating moral despotism only if its "play" is stringently limited. The use of power for forcing the actually non-consenting must be confined to what is rationally compelling: whoever would contest the legitimacy of such force must be proven to thereby contest his own moral personhood. How does Kant's accomplish this task?

The moral legitimacy of political power rests on what Kant called the "legal" necessity of forming a state (1797a, p. 43). If that necessity is to override the (human dignity-based) moral obligation never to use (institute, ratify, or authorize) force against a person without his (actual) consent, the former (legal necessity) must take priority over the latter (moral obligation). Being an author of many minds, Kant offered several accounts of that higher necessity. The most important ones invoke, (1) securing members' survival (1797a, p. 187), (2) securing universal obedience to the moral law (for property respect: 1797a, pp. 73, 157), and (3) securing for all the autonomy resources they are entitled to (1793, p. 233). But on the noumenal level of Kant's morality none of these accounts works: (1) Biological survival cannot function as normative ground in the context of a theory that reserves normative significance to humans' rational existence.[55] (2) The presupposition that the moral obligation to respect others comes into force only if all comply is (rightly) repudiated by Kant (1786, p. 84ff). (3) Since threats of penal force do not effectively prevent (and since applications of such force do not effectively undo) all criminal disrespect, and thus are not sufficient for securing everyone's rightful autonomy resources, prevention cannot justify the state's use of force. Accordingly, Kant himself dismisses all three accounts: the legal system instituted by the state does not derive its validity from any regard for consequences (1793, p. 234; 1796, p. 93f).

A better account of the legitimacy of political power, as used against citizens, can be derived from the very moral necessity to respect itself: in order to respect someone's autonomy, so Kant argues, one must know what worldly things (over and above his bodily integrity) he has a right to. Whereas in the state of nature, property lines are determined merely individually, the state represents a commonly acknowledged authority to resolve the unavoidable conflicts in this regard (1797a, p. 162 f). Offering respect presupposes generally known and recognized property (and property transference) laws. The obligation to form a state is therefore more properly not a legal obligation (which would be inconvenient anyway, since legal obligations are a function of the state), but a meta-moral one: the state is indispensable for the very possibility (in the sense of case-by-case conceivability) of moral respect, and thus quite generally, of morality.[56]

If thus the state's legitimacy is derived from its function for making morality possible, its authority to use force (and play the "ought" of imputable consent against the "is" of actual consent) must be limited by that meta-moral function. But how can the state's authority even be extended, beyond defining property lines, to the use of force? Kant offers two reasons: prevention (by deterrence), and retaliation (1797a, p. 196ff). Prevention, insofar as it effectively hinders what threatens to violate the obligatory respect, presents a morally innocuous negation of a negation (1797a, p. 35), and thus must be morally licit. When considering penal retribution, Kant seems to have presupposed a general agreement. He does not argue for its meta-moral indispensability. Such an argument can be supplied, however. Retaliative force solves a paradox that arises, when one tries to extend the morally obligatory respect to trespassers of the moral law: Infringing upon others' rights disrespects not only those others, but also the noumenon (or humanity) in oneself (1797a, p. 197).[57] But to respect someone (by refraining from interfering with his autonomy), who voluntarily renounced his own respectability, is to disrespect his voluntary renouncing. The only way in which one can respect someone who disrespected others (and thereby himself) is to join in with his disrespect of himself, and to do so in a way commensurable to his own disrespect. Since such commensurability, when determined individually, will always be contested, the state's authority is required. Its use of penal force institutionalises that disrespect of the trespasser's autonomy (1797a, p. 193), which, as it were, removes (1798, p. 170) his self-directed disrespect. Such force against (even the actually un-consenting) trespasser is therefore not only licit but even (once again) indispensable if the state is to fulfil its function for rendering morality possible.[58]

As a result, the moral legitimacy of a state as the addressee of claims to (negative) human rights has been established as rationally compelling (in the Kantian, i.e. transcendental sense of the term). The following section will discuss the possibility of also accommodating states' obligation to care for those in need. In spite of the fact that Kant explicitly acknowledges only one human freedom right (1797a, p. 45) and explicitly rejects needs-based rights (1797a, p. 33), his endorsement of such an obligation presents at least a chance of imputing to him an endorsement of social right as implied in that obligation.

B. Positive Rights

The three most important grounds, which can be invoked for reconciling such a beneficence obligation with Kant's moral account of the state, are (1) the relevance of basic needs for the meta-moral obligation to found such a state, (2) the inclusion of beneficence among what is required by the categorical imperative, and (3) the virtue duty to care for one's phenomenal needs.

1. Basic needs

The issue of basic needs raises the problem of how the noumenal is related to the phenomenal view of man in Kant's moral theory. Here it is significant that already the very obligation to form a state presupposes the existence of a "natural law" concerning personal property (1797a, p. 74), which is established on the basis of a legal postulate of practical reason (1797a, p. 56f): For all material things, it must be possible that they be owned. This postulate refers, in turn, to the necessity of making practical use of such things (Kan, 1797a, p. 57). Obviously, this necessity concerns humans' basic needs, for the satisfaction of which the ability to use things is indispensable. Such needs, moreover, also require that unavoidable social interaction, which supplies the starting position for Kant's formulation of the obligation to form a state (1797a, p. 43). If, then, such needs play a decisive role in the moral grounding of the state, why should they not play an equally basic role for extending the authority of such a state to use (unconsented-to) force (and infringe on members' negative right to un-invaded property), in order to satisfy the basic needs of those who are unable to do so for themselves?

Yet in Kant's account of negative rights, humans' noumenal rationality is the only source (1786, p. 64 ff) of moral obligations. This account leaves no room for other such sources.[59] To be sure, humans' rationality is always conceived as being (contingently, but undeniably) embedded in a (phenomenal) embodiment (1786, p. IX), which introduces needs and desires and makes worldly (and social inter-) action indispensable. It is in view of this presupposed embodiment, after all, that bodily integrity and property (Kant, 1797a, p.163) played their role for determining areas for individual self-determination (and thus for the obligation to respect, and for the formation of a state rendering that respect conceivable in the first place). The central point of Kant's morality, however, is to assert persons' noumenal rationality precisely over and against the "pathological" egoism (1786, p.17), which comes with the animal life (1786, 84f) of bodily (and psychological) needs and desires. That asserting, accordingly, imposes an ascetic struggle, through which humans' basic needs are kept from repudiating humans' higher vocation (Kant, 1786, p. 85). The fact that humans (egoistically) tend to care for their survival, thus, is normatively irrelevant, or even a moral impediment: one should rather die than compromise one's moral integrity (Kant, 1788, p. 282f).[60] Accordingly, no moral justification has been provided for Kant's admission of an obligation of the state to (violate autonomy respect in order to) care for those in need.

2. Beneficence

The issue of beneficence raises the question as to how the morality, which the categorical imperative establishes for individuals, is related to the metamoral legitimacy of the state. So far, that legitimacy had concerned the state's function for rendering the categorically required respect for persons, and thus for the worldly autonomy resources they are entitled to, conceivable. Can state funded beneficence be integrated into that account? In what sense could it contribute to such conceivability?

Kant himself includes beneficence (at least in the sense of rescue for those in need of perishing) under what is required by the categorical imperative (1786, p. 56).[61] To take up the categories developed in the first part of this essay: Kant not only supplements humans' moral responsibility (in the sense of accountability) by the normative element of rational impartiality (discussed above). He also endeavored to integrate altruism. Is this move legitimate? Does it imply that, just as the state is indispensable for the possibility of the categorically required respect, so it is indispensable for the categorically required rescue-beneficence?

Of course, unlike private (state of nature) respect, private beneficence is not impossible. So the state cannot be argued to be as indispensable in view of beneficence as it was in view of respect. Could one establish a stronger parallel by arguing that, just as private respect is possible among those who privately agree on property lines, but impossible with everyone, so private beneficence is possible among those closely related, but impossible with regard to all? So that, just as generalized respect requires a state, so does generalized beneficence? Yet in the former case the state is the condition for the possibility for any one to even know how to respect (not only everyone, but already) anyone. By contrast, in the latter case the state's being a "condition" for altruism, as this could concern not any one's ability to rescue anyone, would have to concern exclusively his ability to rescue (pretty much) everyone. It thus would introduce a regard for efficacy, which Kant (rightly, in his purely rationalist framework) excludes from all considerations of morality (1786, p. 15).

Kant himself admits that respect is required by the categorical imperative in a different way than beneficence. Whereas social interaction is strictly speaking impossible (in any time-spanning way) without the first, it is not in the same sense impossible without the second (Kant, 1786, p. 57): Rationally generalizing (as the categorical imperative in its first formulation requires, 1797a, p. 25) one's socially interactive behavior while not keeping one's promises and (in that and other ways) trespassing on others' autonomy is incompatible with the general possibility of socially interacting behavior. By contrast, rationally generalizing one's social behavior (Kant, 1786, p. 19) while failing to help others in need is not inconsistent in that sense (Kant, 1786, p. 56). Social interaction as such, after all, can continue peacefully and fruitfully even while those in need keep perishing at neighbors' doorsteps.[62] Not offering beneficence does not involve a moral agent in any implicit contradiction, which would repudiate his rationality.[63] This is why Kant admits that not including beneficence under the moral duties (in the narrow sense) would merely be "undesirable" (in view of phenomenal needs, and thus of what is irrelevant for morality in the narrow—and at the same time elated—sense).

If beneficence is thus not required by the categorical imperative in the sense in which respect for autonomy is, one is no longer tempted to take the state to be authorized to enforce the "external aspects"[64] of the former in the same way in which the state had to be shown authorized to enforce the external aspects of the latter. It becomes especially significant that, were the state to enforce the former, this would happen at the cost of violating the latter. Only a very strong parallel between the two cases, or only a proof that morality would be inconceivable without public beneficence, could overrule that consistency threatening "inconvenience".

3. The duty to care for one's phenomenal needs

In his theory of the virtues, Kant posits a duty to care for one's self-preservation (1797b, p. 70) and natural development (1797b, p.15). If this nature-related (in the naturalistic sense of the term) duty could somehow be linked with man's rational morality, then the fundamental condition for the possibility of deriving even just natural entitlements to beneficence from others, or to social support, could be fulfilled: there would be a connection between what can rationally be claimed as unconditionally obligatory and what concerns empirical embodied humans' phenomenal needs and potential. The needed "biological and psychological dimension of humans' moral dignity" would have been established. Given that there are degrees in which the obligatory securing of one's self preservation and development of one's potential can be accomplished, it becomes at least conceivable that engaging the state's efficiency resources (in order to secure a higher degree of virtue) can also be covered by what is morally required, and that social rights can be rationally grounded after all.

In order to evaluate that possibility, this third sub-section must explore the relationship between the morality of the categorical imperative and the theory of virtues, and of both in view of the state as the addressee of human rights claims.

Kant's theory of the virtues principally imposes two purposes on moral persons: one's own perfection and others happiness (1797b, p. 13). It requires treating others and self differently. That required difference contrasts with the (in the narrow sense) morally obligatory impartiality (which requires treating oneself no different than others). If Kant's moral theory (now in the virtue-encompassing sense of the term) is not to suffer from inconsistency, positive virtue-duties must be of a different class than those native-egoism-informed strivings, which the categorical imperative is designed to check. And indeed, where as the categorical imperative demands that one altogether sacrifice (1788, p. 278 f) one's native partiality and replace it by rational impartiality, the altruism imposed by the second positive duty, just as the struggle against egoism imposed by the first duty, is not intended to have persons altogether sacrifice their native partiality for themselves (1797b, p. 18). Kant's theory of the virtues (unlike his morality in the narrow sense) does not require (and even forbids) self-sacrifice (1797b, p. 27). These duties are intended to have persons merely curb their partiality: man, considered not as a rational but as an empirical being (with body-linked needs and desires) naturally tends to benefit himself. As far as others are concerned, he prefers to demand their moral improvement (rather than working at his own). It therefore makes rational-higher-nature-promoting sense to curb these egoistic drives through the two counteracting virtue-commands (1797b, pp. 3ff, 46f, 51). The goal is to develop that dispassionate (Kant, 1797b, p. 51) rational impartiality between self and others, which the ability to obey the categorical imperative already presupposes. This is why Kant's theory of morality, understood in its comprehensive sense as including the virtues, not only requires (negatively) that persons stay within what is morally licit. It requires also that they develop, in order to become capable for the sacrifices such "staying within" may involve (1797b, p. 176f). The virtues serve the purpose of morality in the narrow sense; they provide the ascetical or therapeutic means guiding the moral person's life-long striving (Kant, 1797b, p. 53) towards the end of moral perfection (Kant, 1797b, p. 176).

The duty to preserve oneself and even keep oneself out of need forms a component part of the duty to develop one's moral strength (Kant, 1797b, p. 14f): embodied rational beings can hope to morally progress in their ability to obey the categorical imperative only if they keep themselves out of the more violent sorts of temptation (Kant, 1786, pp. 12; 1797b, p. 18).[65] Engaging this duty for the cause of establishing social rights would have to presuppose that the morally (in the wide sense of the term) obligatory concern for one's own moral progress somehow implies a concern for the progress of humanity, and that this latter concern in turn imposes engaging the efficiency resources of the state. The virtues would have to be so closely linked with morality in the narrow sense that the state could not provide the conditions for the possibility of the latter without providing those of the former. One might then take Kant's endorsement of the state's function for furthering moral progress (1796, p. 86 note)[66] as a license to extend that state's meta-moral function to the promotion of such moral progress through support of the virtues. The state's function for making (categorical) morality possible would then be extended from the narrow "rendering its realization theoretically conceivable" to the wider "rendering its realization practically more likely". The state would make morality possible not only in the sense of providing a legal framework for the former, but also in the sense of instituting a social system which, in keeping everyone out of the more violent temptations, promotes the latter.

In order to accomplish all of this in the context of the Kantian theory, two alternatives present themselves: Either (1) one integrates the third formulation of the categorical imperative into the virtuous regard for humanity's moral progress, or (2) one offers a morally self-interested interpretation for claims made by Kant, where he himself goes beyond the merely ascetical interpretation of the virtue of beneficence.

(1) In its third formulation, the categorical imperative imposes on all willing that "humanity" be willed along "as a purpose", or to consider "humanity" never only a means but always also as an end (1786, p. 66f). Since Kant's categorical imperative imposes restraining rather than committing actions, the third formulation must be adjusted to this negative pattern: it then requires checking all intended actions in view of whether the maxims guiding these actions (not only can be generalized so as to ensure

rational impartiality, but also) are compatible with such an end (1786, p. 82f). Humanity here appears as an imposed purpose, which must, so to speak, be willed along with any other purpose one sets for oneself (Kant, 1786, p. 69).[67]

Suppose that positive end can be interpreted in the light of Kant's theory of the virtues. This would require that the virtue duty of each moral agent to pursue his own perfection could somehow imply a concern for the perfection of humanity (loc.cit). Just as each moral agent must care for his basic needs in order to protect himself from temptations, so he would have to care for everybody else's basic needs so as to protect them from temptations. It would follow that each moral agent must engage the state for securing such general moral progress by satisfying basic needs. The connection between rational moral responsibility (in the sense of accountability) and of altruism, which was found to be indispensable for a rational derivation of social rights, would then have been provided through the intermediary of rationality-imposed impartiality and generalization. This intermediary would also permit to limit the required altruism to precisely that equality of achieved living conditions (or chances), which effectively protect against the temptation to envy, and which the modern theory of social rights implies.

But of course the presupposed implication between the virtue duty to preserve oneself and a duty to preserve others does not hold. The possibility and moral necessity of generalizing from self to all is restricted to humans' noumenality. It is not in view of their noumenality that humans can perceive each other as needing to morally progress. Their noumenality is mutually recognized. It constitutes an, as it were, ideal heaven of higher-nature, towards the implementation through real world action of which each embodied empirical person of this phenomenal world is called to strive. As embodied and empirical, each lives a separate life, each thrown into his private ascetic labors. That noumenal heaven itself, on the other hand, derives no further enhancement from the number of phenomenal humans' success in these labors. Noumenal humanity is "as a whole" embodied in each individual, and each of them recognizes it as "the same" in each other individual. Imposing humanity's progress as a purpose (even in the positive sense stipulated here) can only mean not actively interfering with others in such a way that their progress is jeopardized, for such acting would jeopardize one's own moral progress. (A heavenly concern for phenomenal man's moral progress, and for the numbers of those who "make it" is conceivable only, where the "noumenal" is re-instated as a man-loving God.)

(2) In an exclusively ascetic context of benefiting others, one could be content with giving away goods that no one cherishes but oneself, just in order to hurt one's own emotional attachment to these goods. No thought would have to be wasted concerning whether others need, or could morally profit from, those goods. It would be virtuous for a drug addict to widely share his stuff, and thus, in a certain way (which admittedly differs from that prohib-

ited by the categorical imperative) to instrumentalize others for the purpose of improving himself.

Kant disapproves of such an interpretation (1797b, pp. 17, 27). On what grounds can he do so? The categorically imposed (narrowly moral) concern for humanity's perfection has just been shown not to imply a concern for humanity's realized moral progress. So the reason cannot lie in the evil consequences such drug sharing might have for such progress. Perhaps Kant thought that leading others into temptation could lead to rendering them a temptation to oneself. Doing so would repudiate the (subordinate) duty to keep oneself out of temptation. Keeping oneself out of temptation then must impose some concern for keeping others from becoming a temptation for one-self. The second virtue duty must include a concern for at least discouraging the moral regress of those one benefits. Accordingly the state, with its resources for general basic needs satisfying, could more efficiently discourage such regress. Instituting a beneficent state would be required by one's duty to morally improve oneself by keeping oneself out of temptation by keeping others from regressing, and thus from becoming a temptation for oneself. The connection between rational moral responsibility in the sense of accountability and of altruism, which was found to be indispensable for a rational derivation of social rights, would then have been provided through the intermediary of the virtue duty of furthering one's own moral progress. Even the function of the state for securing every one's survival, which had to be discounted in the context of morality in the narrow sense, could be rehabilitated in view of that interpretation of the virtues.[68]

But the ascetical purpose served by the second duty to morally improve oneself would be defeated if what serves the purpose of that duty (namely caring for one's phenomenal well-being and that of others) was implemented by force (Kant, 1797b, p.176). In particular, taking care of one's worldly needs is obligatory not in terms of securing the conditions under which others would be forced to supply those needs. It is obligatory in terms of shouldering responsibility and hard work, and thus of applying counter-forces to embodied humans' natural lethargy. (Even with regard to the obligation of the state to care for those in need, which Kant illegitimately endorsed, he added precautionary remarks that such help should not encourage laziness, 1797a, p.188)

Moreover, a political implementation of such needs satisfaction (in self and others) would go at the expense of that categorically obligatory autonomy respect, for the sake of which the use of political force was justified in the first place. Implementing a virtue duty through means that violated that respect thus also violates the fundamental principle determining the relationship of the virtues to morality in the narrow, categorical sense: that what satisfies the latter limits what can be done in pursuit of the former (Kant, 1797b, p. 15). More particularly: on the level of individual morality (in the narrow sense) and the cultivation of the virtues, both (being related as the end to the means) are (*a fortiori*) reconcilable. The virtues occupy, so to speak, the free space that is left for action after all the (narrowly moral) freedom-compatibility checks have been completed. By contrast, on the level of the state, there exists no such free space. Financing a social system would repudiate the liberty-protecting, autonomy-respect-securing implications of that state's meta-moral function. The means-end relationship between the virtues and morality in the narrow sense would on this level be defeated: rather than engaging the cultivation of the virtues as a training ground for increased ability to respect others' autonomy, that cultivation would violate the required respect.

III. Conclusion

The initial question posed by this essay concerned rational grounds for engaging commitment to human-rights as a criterion determining moral limits to the toleration of cultural diversity in bioethics. Given the patent irrationality of bioethical norms in international human rights documents, as exposed in a particularly prominent example that was analyzed in the first part of this essay, this question had to be re-focused: Is at least the granting of social rights morally obligatory in a rationally compelling sense? Only if it is, so it was argued, can one recognize as morally legitimate not only the (forceful) implementation of these rights (in any democratically settled arbitrary fashion) within a given state, but also the forming of cross-culture compromise agreements for biomedical cooperation between states (which imply additional force used against partner states' individual members). Within the framework of the Kantian moral theory, as discussed in the second part, social rights could not be accommodated. Humans' moral dignity could not be shown to include that psycho-biological dimension, which would have permitted to extend that concept's ability to ground negative freedom rights to the grounding of positive social rights. A fortiori, the very cultivating of health care rights turned out to be a mere "cultural thing" after all.[69]

In particular, the accountability implication of moral responsibility, which underlies Kant's (philosophically legitimate understanding of) human dignity, could not be linked in any rationally intelligible (let alone compelling) way with that altruism implication, which is endorsed by present day human rights advocates. Accordingly, *a fortiori* no society-wide extension of that altruism (to "societal solidarity"), which supplements the (post-traditional) European variety of Western human rights endorsement, can be rationally defended against non-Western (or traditionally minded Western) cultures restricting altruism (or hierarchizing it with regard) to particular communities. Nor can the post-Enlightenment individualism implied in that societal altruism be claimed to be more valid than the traditionalist character of other cultures of altruism. As a result, the invocation, in the literature of human rights advocating, of a world wide, if vague (Andorno, 2002, p. 960), agreement about human dignity, runs aground. The differences in what members from different cultures understand by that term are so fundamental, that engaging that term amounts to engaging an empty formula or, in Capaldi's words, an intellectual platitudinarianism (Capaldi, 2005, p. 4), behind which differences in values and interests can be veiled.

But then one cannot help to conclude with Petroni (2006, p. 257) that granting social rights is incompatible with granting freedom rights. If the general ability of Kant's moral theory for grounding the latter, which the second part of this essay has defended, could withstand closer scrutiny (a task that goes beyond this essay), then granting the former would even have to count as a violation of human rights. States found guilty of such violation should find themselves classified as also falling beyond the limits of what can be morally tolerated. They could hope to be protected against the implied permission of, and even obligation towards, forceful intervention (cf. note 5) only by appeal to Kant's distinctly peace-preserving concern for the autonomy-guided character of moral and legal progress (1797a, pp. 231, 235; 1796, p. 11). At the very least (so we must conclude), no social-rights-granting state could claim any secularly good moral reason, when threatening to interfere (whether through the pressure of public opinion or physical violence) with other states' "failing" (or, as we should better say, innocent) in that regard. Cultivating human rights in the encompassing European sense of the term is indeed a merely "cultural thing". It must be understood as a way of adjusting Europe's culturally particular "Christian roots" to Europe's increasing secularization by reducing their fruits (or should we say "sprouts"?) to solidarity and equality. It represents the attempt to establish a social-justice inspired "peace on earth". Unfortunately, this very culture stands in the way of both, a more effectively "un-peace defying" secular restriction to autonomy rights in a sense which Engelhardt's libertarianism (2006, p. 25 f) or Petroni's reference to Buchanan and Frey has indicated (2006, p. 40 f), and of that more traditionally Western Christian culture, which sustains (at least in those willing to join) a (non-secularly) reasonable hope towards a more content-rich peace.

Notes

1. In the convention against discrimination against women, such unsettling is consciously endorsed. "A change in the traditional role of men as well as the role of women in society and in the family is needed" (Office, 1979, Preamble), see also Article 5, 10 c, h. Given the emphasis this document lays on the integration of women in work and public life, thus separating them from their function as transmitters of cultural traditions, it is surprising to find that document at the same time endorsing the right of "peoples" to self-determination (Preamble). Equally profound invasions into cultural integrity, normative traditions and family life are envisaged by the convention on the rights of the child (Office of the High

Commissioner, 1989, especially Art.13, 14.3,15-17.19. 24.2, f, 24.3, 28.1, a, 29.1 c-2., 30, 31.2), by the draft for the universal instrument in bioethics, which undertakes to identify "practices contrary to human dignity" (UNESCO 2003c # 54), and by the Addendum to the declaration on genetic data, with its emphasis on partner states' efforts towards human rights based bioethics education (UNESCO 2003d, Art.24)

2. To quote just one obvious example: Against the UN financed and coordinated lobbying for a "right to family planning" grew especially in the Third World (Kaupen-Haas, Rothmaler, 1997, p. 14). An extreme position is defended by H. Sakamoto: he disputes even the very notion of individual rights (1999, p. 194). But even independently of such principal objections, international human rights monitoring is perceived by many states as bothersome, and as a threat to their sovereignty (Pocar, 1993, # 17f, see also # 37f for successor states).
3. This universal character of human rights is emphasized by Pocar (1993, # 7f) as well as by the invocation of a "common ground" for all humans in The United Nations Economic and Social Council (2002) #1.
4. One recent affirmation of that claim received particularly "global" media attention: In his visit to Peking University, Jürgen Habermas confessed his faith that reason does not stop at cultural borders. (Blume, 2001)
5. Examples for the wide spread (if tacit) acceptance of such not only supervisory (Pocar, 1993 #9) and public pressure (op.cit. # 23), but even world-police enforcement implications of international human rights agencies' authority can be found in *Global Summit of National Bioethics Commissions: Tokyo Communique* (1999). The Commission (1995) speaks of an "adjusting" of traditional norms of the law of nations, a "reconsidering" of concepts of sovereignty (op.cit. pp. 3, 12 f). It thus – if implicitly - endorses potentially forceful interventions on the international level (*op.cit.* p. 6, see also Knowles, 2001) To be sure, these latter implications are reserved for cases in which states violate the fundamental "negative" human rights (i.e. apply torture, or commit crimes against humanity such as in ethnic "cleansing" endeavors). Yet the majority of authors contributing to these issues does not distinguish in any principal manner such violations of individuals' right to autonomy from violations of—say—women's right to not be discriminated against (not only publicly but also privately) or rights of children. A recent typical example of such indiscriminate human rights-endorsement, which links polities' legitimacy with their compliance with international human rights declarations in this comprehensive sense, and endorses (in addition to threats of withheld international aid) actively (through support of NGOs and opposition parties) de-stabilizing governments that fail to comply, is Buergenthal, 2004, p.196 ff). (But already the French Declaration (1789) stipulates (Art. 16) that only constitutions granting human rights deserve the name. Only states, so we must conclude, which engage such constitutions are partners in the law of nations' mutual acknowledgement game that morally precludes the use of force.)

   Given these implications concerning the limitation of states' sovereign status, I would argue against the claim made by Joseph Boyle (2005, p. 10) that the global affirmation of human rights does have a global impact: not – and here I agree with him, in terms of policy implementation, but in terms of a threat.
6. It will probably not be difficult for readers to agree that only a secular account of human rights is a liable candidate for universal acceptability: it is generally believed (I think) that while all humans have some sort of secular existence (and

commitment), not all humans are religious. Secularity is thus generally seen to present a minimal common denominator of humanity. (The problem is only: how much can one say about this denominator. This essay argues: very little.) Other readers will probably not agree so readily that Kant is the most important representative of such a secular account. In this volume, for example, Joseph Boyle defends a theory of natural law that claims to ground its conclusions on the nature of practical reasoning. The problem, however, with claims about nature, is that they always presuppose decisions concerning relevance and concerning value (what traits should represent true nature, and what degenerate or perverted nature, see for example Boyle, *op.cit.* p. 22f). These presuppositions cannot themselves be rendered universally compelling outside of a very particular religious context. (This is also why John Locke, another frequently favored candidate, ultimately is not helpful: much of his ethical conclusions simply continue natural law thinking.) The beauty of Kant's account lies in its transcendental nature: since he makes very few factual claims (one being that humans understand themselves as morally responsible), there is little to quarrel about with him. Most of his theory involves hypothetical "condition-of-the-possibility-of…." exploring, that is, a free play with ideas which claim to illuminate what all—as a matter of fact—agree to be valid. Nor are these factual claims invoked as a ground: the appeal of his theory can simply be restricted to those who acknowledge the claims. No moral theory needs to worry about critics who consider the whole undertaking of devising a moral theory pointless.

7. See also his *Zum Ewigen Frieden* (1796, pp. 35, 104, 112).
8. To be sure, the concept of morality that informs Kant's vision of a world-wide polity is restricted in view of the requirements of legal justice (1796, p. 107). Since that justice however in turn rests on a specifically moral understanding of human dignity, Kant's ideal of a peace securing global confederation (1796, p. 38) implies the quest for a globalized morality (1796, p. 97). It is exclusively considerations of feasibility that keep Kant from recommending a world state in the proper sense of the term (*op.cit.* 63), which he theoretically would endorse as the rational solution to the problem of peace and moral progress (1797a, p. 228).
9. Even though Kant himself was opposed to democracy, he understood by that term a mere majority rule. His endorsement of republicanism (1796, p. 25, 60; 1797a, p. 212 f) rests on that government's granting human rights. It thus also covers present day constitutional democracies.
10. See—for a particularly recent and official example—the draft to the European Constitution, Preamble, Preamble to Part II, Article II, 1 (Intergovernmental Conference, 2004).
11. That "securing" is to operate not only within any one polity as a realization of what that polity is morally called to. Even beyond thus constituting a moral community of all polities, the moral call is also addressed to what turns tout to be a moral community of all individuals on earth (Commission, 1995 p. 7). Andorno, even though he realizes the culture-sensitivity of bioethics (2002, p. 962), still believes in the possibility of working out culture-diversity-transcending universal principles, which can give rise (so he assumes) to "an international biomedical law" (*op.cit.* p. 959). Similarly, UNESCO 2003c endorses "laws accompanied by effective controls" (#38).
12. Cf. United Nations, 1997, Preamble. When generally acknowledged human rights

were first affirmed as politically binding in the post revolutionary constitutions of the 18th century, their existence was simply drawn from the theological natural law tradition, and posited for politics as what constitutions (according to the ancient republican ideal) are ontologically about (Declaration 1789, Art.16). The acknowledgement of such rights was also recommended as a way to promote harmony between government and the governed, and thus as a means for rendering government more effective (op.cit. Art.2). Human rights thus served a function similar to that which had previously been fulfilled by divine authority and the promotion of the common weal. Similarly, even before dignity was attributed to humans generally (but instead linked with desert, position, or birth), human life and integrity was considered somehow sacred (with exceptions, such as the life of captives, slaves, the new born and the incapacitated old). It is only within the secularized polities of modernity that a reason had to be given for the inviolability imposed by the previous sacredness. Human dignity, along with its roots in the (culturally domesticated) Judeo-Christian tradition, provides that secular reason.

13. The distinction between positive (claim-rights) and negative (defensive) rights is not as straightforward as the distinction between "economic, social and cultural rights" on the one hand and "civil and political rights and freedom" on the other hand suggests (United Nations, 1997, Preamble). The right to freedom from "fear" (*loc.cit.*) is negative, if that fear concerns others' trespasses on one's rights, it is positive if it concerns the disasters of life. "Economic" and "social", just as "cultural rights", can be understood in either a negative or a positive sense. Political participation rights occupy an ambiguous position in-between. Even civil rights and political freedom, as Angelo Petroni pointed out to me, have a "positive" side to them with regard to the extent of state funded efforts that are undertaken to protect these negative rights. Despite these problems of separation in practice, both kinds of rights can be distinguished in theory. (See also his discussion, 2005, p. 25 ff.)
14. A particularly straightforward statement to this effect is provided by The United Nations Economic and Social Council (2002) # 52.
15. The UN General Assembly report (United Nations 2001 § 11) emphasizes the need to pursue bioethical and human rights issues in combination (see also the response of the WHO, op.cit. Addendum II). The UNESCO (2003c, #5, 8) even holds modern bioethics as a whole to be "indisputably founded on the pedestal of the values enshrined in the Universal Declaration of Human Rights".
16. A good summary of Jürgen Habermas' presentation of this disagreement is given by Bayertz (2006, p. 212). Bayertz himself emphasizes that it is in particular the market which is evaluated differently in both Western cultures: We might summarize this opposition thus: in Europe the market is suspected of degrading morality and thus undermining human dignity, in the US it is seen as an expression of a commitment to achievement and as encouragement to freedom and responsibility, thus serving as a support of human dignity. (This difference has been developed in depth in Cherry's essay (2006, pp. 105-108) Disagreements concerning human rights and the market are also mirrored in disagreements about the meaning of "liberalism", as that theory which claims to harness human rights to the promotion of liberty (Capaldi, 2006, pp. 128-129,132-133,137).
17. As Ulrich (quoted by Kurt Schmidt, 2006, p. 182) puts it concisely: a "satisfactorily socially balanced society" is the here perceived to be the goal of a polity.

18. The emphasis on non-discrimination among human rights advocates derives from the French Revolution's commitment to an equality that was placed (unlike in America) in a context of the ideal of "fraternity". Whereas the principle of equality in its basic sense concerns governments' policy of treating all citizens alike (or indiscriminatingly) when applying the laws, or, insofar as governments distribute benefits, of securing "equal access", - the "fraternal" context has been perceived to impose on governments the additional duty to enforce, on the one side, non-discrimination even among citizens, and, on the other side, a solidaric network of economic sharing which aims at equalizing individuals' starting position in their struggle for economic achievement.
19. The WHO speaks of the possibility of reaching a "reasoned consensus" (United Nations 2001, Add. II), thus leaving the interpretive bias undetermined. UNESCO (2003c #7) mostly endorses the first interpretation, when it affirms a "need for universal ethical guidelines covering all issues", which "should guide public policies... on these issues" (*op.cit.* #10). Quite accordingly, this draft of a "universal instrument in bioethics" in its first four parts emphasizes as the most important values not cultural self determination, but rather "benefit-sharing and equal access to the advances of science and technology for all humanity" (*loc.cit.*). The issue of freedom is here raised in the context of the freedom of science (#12). Where that issue is extended to parents' authority over their children (#12) and to end-of-life autonomy (#13), the plurality-tolerant impact of these concessions are immediately relativized by reference to (supposedly universal) "pre-eminent needs and interests of the children" and to the fact that people look for "guidance to ease the burden on their conscience" respectively. In both cases general norms (governing "needs and interests" and providing such guidance) are appealed to. Thus "cultural sensitivities" are to give way to a "broad consensus" (#12, 14), where consensus is understood as a result of a regard for something objectively normative. There is, in the context of stem cell research, an awareness of "cultural pluralism" (*op.cit.* #32). But it is not clear how a "universal instrument of bioethics "of the "harmony" (#33) sort suggested, which is even to "take the lead in identifying an ethical framework", could recognize the human rights implications of such pluralism. The general reflections of the fifth part of the document contain at least a nominal recognition of "many different ethics" (#37) as "an expression of human freedom." But already in the subsequent section it is claimed that moral rules from different backgrounds "can develop by enrichment and consensus thus contributing to common universal values", a phrase which entirely repudiates that recognition.
20. As Joseph Boyle's interpretation of the natural law indicates, there are understandings of reason that allow for both a regard for moral truth and for discussion and a process of consensus-development as the way to determine that truth. I have given a more thorough account of these different understandings, which also accommodates the bad compromises Boyle classifies as "accommodation" (2005, p. 317) in Delkeskamp-Hayes (2004, p. 149-153). For two related but somewhat different approaches to these differences see Solomon (2005, pp. 27ff, 355) and Wildes (2005, pp.11ff, 369).
21. For the consequences of such policies for the principle of liberty see Petroni (2005, pp. 24, 263).
22. Independently of such a reason, which explains how intelligent human rights advocates could have been blind to the tension between both accounts, one can, of

course, contemplate on reasons in the sense of motives, which may have suggested it as advisable for such advocates to hide the incompatibility. In the field of biomedicine, negotiations are often conducted between partners from more and less developed countries. Global bioethics declarations combine the promise of access to urgently needed health resources and benefit from scientific progress for the latter with the call towards universal ethical compliance with standards endorsed by the former. (The most forceful example is UNESCO 2003c; see especially # 14 and 16.) More developed states (or inter-state agencies) offering such cooperation are in a position to more effectively refuse what the other side more urgently needs. It may thus be a matter of strategic interest to the former that this inequality in bargaining power is de-emphasized in the respective documents. Such de-emphasizing is evident from the fact that crucial details, such as the securing of patent rights and the deriving of material benefit from research, come up only in the small print portions of the texts (see for instance UNESCO 2003a, Annex A §§ 20, 31, and UNESCO 2003c #25, and 17, with further comments on "compulsory licensing"). At the same time, such de-emphasizing is also served by appeal to a supposedly universal human dignity, and hence morality. The side-by-side reference to agreement processes and universal values in the human rights documents thus makes—in a somewhat sinister sense of the term—"sense".

Such duplicity, on the other hand, has not gone un-noticed. Newly placed international appeals to human rights and dignity already raise suspicions concerning a hidden purpose of introducing merely new international resources for serving developed countries' interests. A good summary of reasons supporting such suspicions is offered in Qiu (2002, p. 80). A further illustration of such advantage-taking can be found in the convention against discrimination against women: here acknowledgement of "the right of peoples under alien and colonial domination and foreign occupation to self-determination and independence", and thus the offer of an at least potential political support for those who are in a particularly vulnerable position, is combined with the imposition of substantial, culture-threatening changes which those favored "peoples" will have to undergo (cf. note 1). Cultural autonomy rights are to be had only at the price of cultural self destruction. Similar trade-offs are suggested by the commitment to preventing "stigmatization, discrimination and other forms of injustice" (UNESCO 2003c # 21, 23, 24) against which underdeveloped countries must be protected. The promised "recognition of researchers from developing countries as full and equal partners in biomedical studies" and of a raise in standards for "benefits accruing to participant communities and countries" and for equitable access (#22, 26f) come only at the price of partner states' commitment to safety standards for genetically modified organisms (*op.cit.* #36) and their willingness to comply with the *Universal Instrument,* which again contains serious challenges for cultural plurality (#22). (None of this is to deny, of course, that there are ways of asserting cultural relativism which also serve as an ideological veneer for securing the interest of medical researchers from developed countries, who are, as in the example mentioned by Beauchamp (1997, p. 38), engaged in using subjects from underdeveloped countries.) For a criticism of this position however, see Nuffield Council 2002, pp. 94f, 139f)

This strategy of diverting attention from one's superior bargaining position by appealing to an existing normative consensus binding all people could, of course, be accepted as morally innocuous, and could defeat the charge of engaging a merely ideological cover for normative colonizing, if the rock bottom human rights core of those contingently negotiated bioethics standards in fact did command that claimed rational compelling-ness, which is the subject of this essay.

23. Commission (1995, p. 5) Office of the High Commissioner 1980, Preamble. An expression of this celebrating is also the extension of individual rights to cultures' rights (United Nations, 1997, Art. 1.1)
24. See the UN Resolution 1514, as quoted by Nowak (1989, p. 5ff).
25. See also (1997b), # 159. A complementary endorsement of countries' authority to lower protection levels appears in the declaration on human genetic data, where the privacy of genetic information can be overruled by law (UNESCO 2003a, Art 14.b), and where nationally different ways of regulating pre-implantation genetic diagnosis are acknowledged (UNESCO 2003b #60-61).
26. The problem addressed here is thus situated at an even deeper level (concerning the relationship between the individual and the state) than that addressed by Petroni's criticism of European Union legal harmonization, where the issue is Europe-wide centralization rather than inter-state cooperation (2005, p.3ff)
27. The Universal Declaration on the Human Genome similarly invokes public debate as a way of sorting out the "distinctive nature" in which each people develops (UNESCO 2000 Preface). It seems to thereby also endorse the idea of state implemented cultural identities.
28. A high priority for equality characterizes Denmark, where state funded insurance is part of the social insurance system (van Kemenade, 1993, p. 31). Societal diversification and freedom are emphasized in Luxemburg (with insurance determined by government, employers, and trade unions, *op.cit.* p.62), Germany (which also involves the medical profession's association, *op.cit.*, p. 43), and Belgium (where national insurance is managed by non-governmental private sickness funds, half of them catholic, the other socialist or liberal, as well as by local—Dutch versus French—communities, *op.cit.*, p. 27 f). Other differences in the extent to which market forces are permitted to influence health insurance reflect the weight given to individual responsibility and to a high technical standard (from none in Luxemburg, *op.cit.* p. 62, all the way up to France with 60% for supplementary funding, *op.cit.* p. 38). Patients' involvement in payment (from "all pay and get reimbursed" in France, (*op.cit.* p.39) to "no pay" in Germany, (*op.cit.* p. 46), Luxemburg (*op.cit.* p. 62) and Denmark (*op.cit.* p. 31)), also show different priorities with regard to individuals' responsibility. The relevance respectively given to freedom of access becomes obvious from the extent to which specialists and hospitals can be visited independently or only upon referral by the general practitioner: mostly those patients (in France, *op.cit.* p. 29, and Belgium, p. 29) who get to pay (at first), also get to choose freely, whereas those who do not pay (in Denmark, p. 32, and Germany, p. 44) also need referrals.
29. To be sure, in Germany a new law was passed on 28 May 1993, which declared the financing of abortions through public insurance unconstitutional. Yet the 1995 "Schwangerenhilfegesetz" determines that these insurances are to pay if the aborting woman's income is below a certain limit. This limit is higher than the one qualifying individuals for social security. Moreover, income from husbands or partners is not taken into account, nor does the income of parents matter, if the woman is underage. In addition, §3 #5 stipulates that the "Persönlichkeitsrecht" of the preg-

nant woman must be respected in the course of her applying for public support. As a consequence, her claims to such support are not examined (Hefty, 2004). Among the German states, Nordrhein-Westfalen ranges highest with 96% of all abortions fact financed by public insurance (average percentage 80-90%). So far, protests by the pro-life lobby "Bundesverband Lebensrecht" against the public (i.e. enforced) financing of actions that are officially classified as not legal has remained fruitless (Hefty, 2003).

30. While no physician can be forced to personally practice killing on demand or medically supporting suicide (at least the Belgian law provides physicians with a conscience clause, cf. Albert, 2002, sect. 14, just as in Germany no physician can be forced to perform abortions), all physicians are forced to refer patients desiring such services to other, more accommodating colleagues. All are thus forced to accept the burden of complicity with what their consciences condemn.
31. Christian hospitals cannot forbid their physicians to accede to euthanasia requests by their patients. In Belgium, this restriction of religious hospitals' spiritual self-determination operates on several levels. First, there was a parliamentary discussion concerning the advisability of withdraw public funding from hospitals that refused to offer voluntary euthanasia services. Second, one Roman Catholic hospital in Flanders is reported to have denied a request for such euthanasia. After the responsible minister threatened to withdraw hospital's public license, no more resistance was offered (Fittkau, 2004, p. 42). Third, the Belgian legislature has stipulated that only newly drawn up work contracts, if they contain a provision against such acceding, are legally binding. It has, however, denied Christian hospitals the right to require such renewal from their presently employed physicians. But even in regard of newly hired physicians, it is unclear whether such stipulations are binding. The European Union's moral commitment to human rights imposes safeguards against discrimination, which includes discrimination on the grounds of religion in hiring contracts. As Schuck (2002, p. 277 f) has shown, the European Anti-discrimination article (integrated as article 13 into the EU-contract in 1996), while being supplemented by a rule that secures the Union's religious communities' liberty to restrict hiring policies to members (in 2000), has restricted this rule to clerical positions. Social institutions, even if operated by churches or religious communities, are considered by European law as economic entities, and thus are subject to the anti-discrimination ruling (Schuck, 2002, p. 278; see also Vachek, 2000, p. 110). The principle of religious freedom could be invoked for defending special hiring policies of Christian health care institutions only if Union law could be brought to subsume "medical care in such institutions" under "exercise of religion in the narrow sense of the term". It is unlikely that this will happen.
32. Depending on economic ups and downs and election results, people will have a right to eye lenses, gold fillings, rehabilitative gymnastics or cosmetic operations, or else they will not have that right. Such changes are illustrated by growth rates in the total health expenditures: For the years 1991 to 1992, the difference between Denmark (-1.5%) and Germany (+ 3.6%) indicates that in the first case, rights were being a little deflated, in the second case (discounting inflation) still increased. (Health Affairs, Fall 1994, p. 101).

    In what concerns general budget decisions, we find differences in percentage of the gross domestic product spent on health in 1992 ranging from 9.4 in France to 6.5 in Denmark (with an OECD average of 8.1), which is corroborated by the per capita amounts spent (in $) of 1.745 in France and 1.163 in Denmark (with 1.374 as average). (Health Affairs, 1994, p. 101) Whether this difference is due to the fact that the French are sicker or that they use their resources less efficiently, still a *prima facie* difference in comparative priority given to health care can be noted. Similarly, in 1997, the national per capita health spending in Denmark was $1,848, whereas in Germany it was $2,339 (average 1.728), which reflects a difference in GDP percentage of 7.4 versus 10.4% (average 7.5), (Health Affairs, 1999, p. 179).

Cultural differences in favouring either the state or the individual become visible in view of hospital ownership: differences range from "all publicly owned" in Denmark (*op.cit.* p. 32) to the Netherlands with 88% private ownership (p. 66).

33. It is only in the *Explanatory Report* (Council, 1997b, # 26) that health care rights are explicitly distinguished: unlike negative rights, they do not create individual entitlements, which can be invoked in legal proceedings against the state.
34. At one place, positive rights (such as that to benefit from progress) are also declared to be merely "important" aims (Council, 1997b, # 23). But this is not helpful either. It suggests, that humans' negative rights to life and bodily integrity can be limited (or solidarity earmarked) in view of merely "important aims".
35. The convention against the discrimination of women (Office, 1979) acknowledges women's function as mothers and safeguards of family welfare (Preamble), but does not seem to notice that granting them equal rights to work (Art. 11.2) and "maximum participation" in the development of their countries (Preamble) may jeopardize their ability of serving that function.
36. States are not the exclusive addressees (United Nations, 1997, Preamble). A similar extension to individuals seems endorsed by the invocation of the "intellectual and moral solidarity of mankind" (UNESCO, 2002, Preamble).
37. Individualism is, of course, only one of the contested issues. As Engelhardt shows, Christian and non-Christian cultures also differ with respect to their implicit assumptions concerning the normative implications of nature, thus giving rise to conflicting moral guidance in the field of gene technology (2006, p. 22ff).
38. Concerning Islam, a recent portrayal can be found in Nagel (2004, p. 133), where the opposition to Western individualism is highlighted, concerning Confucianism see Tao (2006), Fan (2006, p. 4ff, 12ff) and Engelhardt (2006, p. 25).
39. This is, of course, an overly simplified picture. Non-Western cultures are no monolithic blocs, but have their own moral diversity problems, which are even enhanced by Western modernization influences. There is a huge literature on the problem of traditional values being politically abused by non-Western governments. Still, the misuse of a principle does not repudiate the principle.
40. "Solidarity" as in UNESCO 2003c # 54.
41. Obviously in the West the insufficiency of mere individualism has long been recognized, and has elicited "communitarian" reactions. But while in the West the evils attending absolute individualism are supposed to get "remedied" through politically enforced, society-spanning communality, non-Western (or traditionally minded Western) opposition to that individualism favors traditional communities, the political protection of which is sought only at a secondary level. To be sure, Western social democracies also cultivate a rhetoric that praises familial integrity and neighborhood cohesion. But the internal dynamic of granting autonomy rights even to those unable to consent, along with the provision of nation-wide social services, in effect authorize governments' intrusion in family life and erodes com-

munal responsibility structures. In this connection it is ominous to see how the endorsement of non-discrimination of women, offered in exchange for acknowledged cultural self-determination even of non-autonomously constituted cultures, recommends those very work-integration favoring child-care facilities (Art. 11.2,c) and social security programs (Art. 14.2 c), which expose children to educational conditioning along the lines of the politically privileged "mainstream" culture and which have already exerted their family-eroding influence in the West respectively. (For an analysis of this influence in the case of German social legislation, see Schwab 1993, Schwab 1994, or Borchert 2002.)

42. Analogously, no-longer-persons could enjoy the ex-post effects of their previous prospective rights for determining how they will wish to be treated when no longer competent.
43. Non-Western cultures consider such specimens of human life merely as a part of nature (Sakamoto, 1999, p. 195).
44. Once human dignity has been linked (in a way that is in turn hard to understand) with the uniqueness and diversity of the human genome (UNESCO 2000, Article 2b), of course, not granting person status and rights bearer-ship to those who are genetically unable to attain moral personhood counts as human rights violating discrimination (op.cit. Art. 6). (Given that document's emphasis on non-discrimination on genetic grounds, it is surprising to find it remaining silent on the practice of selecting only genetically promising fertilized ova for implantation.)
45. For the issue of profiting from genetic research, a parallel problem with respect to those unable to consent (in the proper written form) is addressed by UNESCO 2003a, Annex A, §§ 27-9, and UNESCO 2000, Art. 5e.
46. See also UNESCO 2003c #28f. A kindred problem arises with the prohibition to derive financial gain from one's genome (UNESCO 2000, Art 4).
47. Most hard or hazardous bodily labor that threatens one's bodily integrity (and shortens life expectancy), after all, is altruistically motivated.
48. Even though one would be unhappy (for more than one reason) to have an alcoholic sell his kidney in order to subsidize his addiction, the existence of such risks does not justify as a matter of principle (and in a secular context) keeping a father from selling his kidney (a mother from renting out her uterus) in order to finance the children's education.
49. A similar case of moral paternalism is the ban on parents' (non-medicine-related) choice of sex when it comes to implanting in-vitro fertilized ova (Art. 14). This ban seems to rest on the conviction that wanting a baby is dignified, whereas wanting a girl is not.

    Alternatively, the fertilized eggs' right to protection against sexual discrimination is invoked. But this invocation disregards the fact that fertilized eggs which will not be implanted on the basis of their sex still owe their very existence to parents' decision to undergo (the ordeal of) technology-assisted reproduction in the first place. That is, without that sexually biased decision, those discarded eggs would not even have made it into the fertilization stage. Unless one entertains some hypothesis concerning rational souls on a waiting list for embodiment, and being disadvantaged if they happen to catch the wrong (egg-) body, there seems for such in-ovated potential persons no ground (and certainly no secularly assessable one) on which to complain. As discrimination is proscribed only with regard to rights, one would have to posit a right to existence among those rational souls, in order that sexual discrimination could even be affirmed. Moreover, since that type of reproduction (IVF) is implicitly permitted by the *Convention,* and since not implanting fertilized ova that are genetically deficient is also permitted, there is—from a human rights standpoint with extended bearer-ship—no reason why sexual discrimination should be treated differently than genetic discrimination.

A similar disregard for the existential selection context can be found when genetically damaged parents opt for selecting a child with the same genetic damages: such choice is considered un-ethical because it leaves the "lifelong and irreversible disadvantages" of such a child un-considered (UNESCO 2003b). The authors seem to imply that for such a child, it is altogether better never to make it into (post fertilization) existence.

50. The societal concern, that permitting organ sale will expose those already disadvantaged to pressure by their families, can be obviated by instituting legally required counseling services, such as have been developed—for instance—in Germany with regard to abortion. It is interesting that concern about social pressure has not moved the European Council to prohibit voluntary euthanasia and physician-assisted suicide in the Netherlands and Belgium.
51. Another motive for proscribing organ sale should be noted in passing. Physicians' involvement in organ sale may be perceived as threatening that corporate normative identity, to the preservation of which the medical profession might wish to claim a right of its own. But from a human rights standpoint, professional self-determination does not cover a monopoly on bio-technological services: Just as abortion clinics and beauty enhancement surgery have already set up biotechnological parallel structures to the traditionally understood practice of medicine as a healing mission, so commercial organ transplantation clinics could cater to the traditional-medicine-transcending needs of organ donors (and perhaps even recipients).
52. Of course, such an "encompassed dimension" could again suggest that all species-human life formed a continuum of biological development, which would link humans' moral personhood with the very beginning of their physical existence. As a consequence, rights-bearership could again be extended to all species-human life. Moreover, biological and psychological integrity, which also preserves autonomy resources, might even be philosophically ratified as an obligation-imposing value. The two problematic assumptions, which had involved the Bioethics Convention in its more bio-medicine specific inconsistencies (which even went beyond the difficulty of coordinating positive and negative rights as such) and thus defeated that document's ability to provide criteria for limits to culture-tolerance), might well be found compatible with an account of the human condition which claimed a Kantian universal rationality. The project of endorsing such a rationality will therefore from the very start have to be protected against such rationality-defeating implications.
53. Similarly, Kant himself extended human-rights-bearer-ship to (only potential person) infants (1797a, 112). He also considered autonomy resources and bodily integrity as a value that must be protected even against their owners (1797a, p. 116 f, 193f; 1797b, p. 73). Kant thus personally endorsed commitments, which, as our analysis of the Convention has shown, render bioethics inconsistent.
54. This twofold approach is already present in Rousseau's appeal to "humanity" as implying liberty and morality, and constituting inalienable rights (1764, chap.4).

Kant merely systematized its transcendental implications: one must regard humans on the one hand as they appear empirically to themselves and others, and on the other hand insofar as they accept the implications of what they cannot but suppose (freedom, 1786, 98), when they enter the moral discourse. Concerning the possibility of such a noumenal self-understanding, Kant's analysis of human experience and scientific understanding in the First Critique has opened a space: the category of causality extends only to phenomena, not to the things in themselves (or noumena, 1787, p. 235).

55. In the context of a rationalist moral theory that has cut the link between what is rationally normative and what is biologically desirable, the only normative significance physical survival could theoretically carry would have to be derived from the fact that it sustains persons' rational existence. This argument appears, in fact, in Kant's refutation of the legitimacy of suicide (1797b, p. 73). But in another part of his theory, he himself repudiates this possibility: In order to secure some motivational power for his moral law, he must solve the problem that the world does not tend to reward those who have led a life of moral renunciation (1788, p. 204 f). Kant therefore renders the hypothesis of an (how so ever unknowable) immortal soul (1788, p. 220) and of an (equally unknowable yet surely) desert-rewarding God (1788, p. 224) morally obligatory (1788, p. 226). But if people, or rather their normatively relevant "rational humanity", must be assumed to (somehow) survive in the shape of such souls, their (normatively relevant) rational existence cannot be made to depend on their embodiment.

To be sure, persons' physical existence is indispensable for their advancing in moral perfection, and thus for realizing that "vocation", which the hypothesis of an (otherwise unknowable) God renders at least conceivable. As far as the argument against suicide goes, even this is not sufficient for opposing altruistic sacrifice of one's life: for on the grounds of Kant's moral theory there is no higher level of moral perfection than the ultimate victory of respect for the moral law and faithfulness to the purpose of humanity's moral progress this law imposes than such total sacrifice of phenomenal egoism. Accordingly, Kant always emphasizes that it is better to accept death than to violate the categorical imperative.

Looking now at humans below that level of moral perfection, and thus at their vast majority, could the dependence of persons' moral progress on their physical existence be invoked for justifying the institution of force against the non-consenting, - given that such force is indispensable for gaining security (at least) against trespasses on persons' lives? To grant such a possibility would be to allow violating the moral imperative (never to use—or institutionalize—force against a person without his consent) for the sake of making moral progress possible. It would involve Kant's rationalist morality in a contradiction.

56. Usually the necessity and moral legitimacy of the Kantian state is derived from the state's function of rendering everyone's autonomy compatible with that of everyone else (1797a, p. 33; 1797b, p. 7): since every one ought to respect every one's autonomy (or freedom), and since the state makes it possible for every one to do what he ought to, therefore every one ought to form a state.

On a second look the matter is less clear. Whose moral concern, more particularly, is it supposed to be that he (or it) secures autonomy compatibility, in order for a state to be necessary? Individuals as rational beings have no need for such securing: Their ability to be moral (to respect the moral law in not invading others' privacy or disrespecting their autonomy) does not seem jeopardized by the fact that everybody else keeps beating up on everybody else, including himself (at least in a *prima facie* sense, which will be corrected further down). Of course, as phenomenal beings with an interest in healthy bones and un-invaded vegetable gardens, they must welcome an institution that renders autonomies compatible, thus protecting bones and gardens. But such a regard for consequences is (rightly) excluded from Kant's moral and aprioricallly rational account of the state.

If autonomy compatibility is the state's concern, then any inability to secure that compatibility effectively is an argument against the state's moral legitimacy. But deficiencies in this regard are inescapable: legal sanctions deter some, but by no means all. Could one say that the state is the more morally legitimate the more efficiently it deters trespassers? But then locking all its members away would secure the most moral legitimacy.

The term "render compatible" should therefore better be understood in the sense of determining entitlements which is suggested by the interpretation offered in this essay: as a condition for the possibility of individuals being able to extend the required respect.

57. Whereas acting a-morally merely indicates that the agent has—as it were—put his moral autonomy aside (just as in sleep, or when running a race, tasting a mushroom sauce or engaging in any other intensely phenomenal activity), but does not imply a denial (in the serious sense of betraying his autonomy), acting immorally amounts to just such a betrayal.

58. This retaliative understanding is profoundly at odds with present day, human rights theory based understandings of punishment. Yet the latter rest on an empirical anthropology that regards persons as phenomena, not as noumena. Since a rational foundation for individual freedom rights could be had only in view of noumena, ("correctively") violating respect for them by reference to certain (educative, re-socializing) goals (that concern them as phenomena) would at least not be sufficient. (The retaliative understanding can, of course, be supplemented by such a view, as the theory of virtue suggests.) As commitment to human rights was found to require a transcendental foundation, it must accommodate that foundation's retaliative view of punishment.

59. The tendency of human rights theorists to claim support from Kant for their endorsement of social rights can be understood as arising from several seductive misperceptions:

The first of these was addressed already in note 49: surely, if it could be a moral concern of the state to secure its members' survival, social rights could be derived for those members. But the state is no moral agent of its own. Independently of historical contingencies, its moral justification rests on its serving a function for rendering morality possible. Morality presupposes, but does not in turn require, social interaction. Hence morality cannot be invoked for keeping humans alive in sufficient numbers so as to render their social interaction indispensable and advantageous, thus giving occasion for the necessity of a state. It is not a Kantian move to have a state implement its own moral indispensability.

Second: clearly, what makes social interaction possible is respect for every partner's autonomy. As the meta-moral function of the Kantian state consists in making the latter possible, such a state will also make the former possible. Social interaction in turn is indispensable for embodied persons' ability to satisfy their physical needs. These premises are easily taken to prove that a public rescue (or welfare) system, which may also satisfy embodied persons' needs, is indispensable in a Kantian state. The fallacy becomes obvious if one remembers that respect for moral autonomy was morally obligatory not because it makes survival-useful interaction possible. The one merely coincides with the other. The argument, which establishes that the state is there for the sake of the one, is therefore not sufficient to establish that the state is also there for the sake of the other.

Third: respect for persons' autonomy also embraces leaving their bodily integrity and property un-invaded. To respect an embodied person's autonomy amounts to respecting what he is entitled to as resources of real-world-transforming (as distinguished from mental) action. This embracing (or amounting-to) is conditioned by the fact that, on this earth, persons come as embodied (and with needs). But the rationale behind the obligation to respect was to concern persons' noumenal rationality exclusively, not their physical subsistence. Hence nothing follows for the state's obligation to use force for securing that subsistence. (Nor could, of course, the invocation of human dignity support a Kantian case for social rights.) Kant's "human dignity" concerns persons' moral accountability, or their ability to restrain their actions by a regard for the moral law, exclusively. Respecting that dignity cannot be made to extend to providing all with "dignified living conditions", which again envisage man on the phenomenal level.)

60. Kant explicitly opposes suicide. But his discussion is restricted to suicide for non-noble motives: humans do not own their bodies (1797a, p. 96). So they cannot simply dispose of them at will. In a sense, embodied humans thus live as hostages to the noumenal rationality they embody. Humans are also bound by duties towards others, from which they cannot simply escape (1797b, p. 71f). Kant also forbids even altruistic self-sacrifice (1788, p. 282). Still, on the basis of his theoretical commitments and against what Kant wishes to affirm, suicide and sacrifice for moral motives ought to be counted as a person's ultimate victory over any natural tendency to preserve his life (at any cost). It ought to be considered morally praiseworthy. (Kant's casuist questions (1797b, p.74f) and his, implicit, endorsement of soldiers' sacrificing themselves for their country (1788, p. 282) betray his uncertainty in the matter.)

61. Kant's morality (in the narrow, categorical-imperative sense of the term) is, more precisely, second-order. Kant affirms this with respect to the law (1797b, p.7). But as the law constitutes the enforceable aspect of what the categorical imperative imposes (as a "natural law", 1797a, p. 24, which I call morality in the narrow sense), it also holds for that imperative's morality (as can also be gleaned from *op.cit.* 25). What is morally imposed (and legally "enforced") are not certain ways of acting, but certain ways of restraining one's actions. In what concerns morality exclusively, these restraints must result from a regard for the moral law, as that law imposes precisely that noumenal impartiality (of not making exceptions for oneself, 1786, p. 57f), which befits a rational being that understands itself in terms of its rationality. For beneficence to fit under the categorical imperative, one therefore would have to reconstrue the imperative to help those in need as the imperative to restrain one's native pursuits (or the disposal of one's resources) in such a way as to support rescue endeavors, thus adjusting the positive duty to help to the negative framework of Kant's morality (in the narrow sense), - and such a reconstruction would be really hard to render persuasive.

62. A problem would arise only in case one would be the only survivor. But this again would only be a practical problem for the survivor (he would have trouble fending all for himself), not a moral one. There exists no moral imperative that one must keep that (naturally indispensable) social interaction going, which the moral imperative is designed to restrain. Once there is no more occasion for such restraining, even the ascetical support of the virtues is no longer necessary. Hence even the goal of moral progress cannot be invoked for any imperative that could impose efforts to keep people alive for the sake of keeping social interaction going.
63. In trying to prove beneficence to be required by the categorical imperative, Kant appeals to the fact that, were oneself in need, one would wish to be rescued (1786, p. 56): He concludes from this fact that one should therefore "impartially" offer that same rescue to others in need. But such hypothetical wishes (with regard to receiving help if one is in need) are (at least *prima facie,* as in note 43) morally irrelevant in the rationalist context of his theory.
64. As Kant rightly insists, the state can concern itself only with external actions, not with attitudes of the mind (Kant, 1797a, p. 47).
65. Accordingly, Kant's argument for including beneficence under what is required by the categorical imperative, which had to be discarded in the narrowly moral context (cf. note 48), can (so it may seem at present) be rehabilitated in the virtue-context, where phenomenal man's strivings against his phenomenal nature are to be supported: Insofar as it is a virtue duty to care for one's self preservation, it is also a virtue duty to request others' rescue-beneficence, and therefore (for impartiality-reasons) a categorical duty to acknowledge others' right to request that same rescue-beneficence from oneself. But even if this would work (irrespective of the problem that Kant's morality is negative), it would still not permit rendering the state an agent in forcefully implementing that rescue-beneficence, towards which each individual moral agent is obligated.
66. Taking such a function seriously would not already involve one in violating Kant's verdict against teleological foundations for the legal system (1793, p. 234). It may be that this verdict concerns only the institution of such a system, but does not preclude accepting utility as a consequence of having instituted it.
67. To be sure, "as an end" can also mean considering all humans as rational beings in the sense of their ability to set ends for themselves. In this case, the third formulation of the categorical imperative amounts to the second, which requires that one refrain from instrumentalising others (whose autonomy one must respect by granting them, according to the first—generalization imposing—formulation, equal rights with those one claims for oneself). But in the present context we must explore if that phrase could also take up the positive (altruistic- responsibility) meaning in which beneficence is treated in the theory of virtues.
68. Even Kant's remark that one must work at one's (not only moral, but also "technical") improvement in order to be better able to serve others (1797b, p. 112), would make sense in view of the general development of the arts and sciences, which is indispensable for satisfying every one's basic needs. Moreover, it would even make sense to engage the state for contributing to that aspect of its population's moral progress as well. Apart from propriety, safety and general decency which Kant foresaw (1797a, p. 185f), public education, a high standard of health care and scholarly institutions, a liberal endowment of arts and culture seem the obvious candidates. Here again, we are presented with a moral context in which services, which

today are construed as a matter of (positive) right, could be accommodated under the heading of a moral-progress-oriented utility notion of individual rights.

69. It is revealing that some human rights endorsing documents speak of "faith" in such rights (Office 1979, Preamble), thus invoking a religious dimension that fits both with that endorsement's lacking rationality credentials and with human rights' advocates temptation towards crusading zeal. Thus, even though Capaldi's concept of Enlightenment philosophizing implicitly excludes Kant's theory (which pointedly opposes materialist reductionism), he may in the end be right in claiming that the Enlightenment project, here understood as the attempt to sell as universal what is really particular, is "totalitarian" (2005, p. 9).

References

Albert, King of Belgium. (2002). 'Act on euthanasia,' *Ethical Perspectives,* 9(2).

Andorno, R. (2002). 'Biomedicine and international human rights law: In search of a global consensus,' *Bulletin of the world health organization,* 80 (12).

Bayertz, K. (2006). 'Struggling for consensus and living without it: the construction of a common European bioethics,' in H.T. Engelhardt, Jr. (ed.) *Global Bioethics: The Collapse of Consensus.*

Beauchamp, T.L. (1997). 'Comparative Studies in Japan and America,' in K. Hoshino (ed.) *Japanese and Western Bioethics.* The Netherlands: Kluwer Academic Publishers.

Blume, G. (2001). 'Gefährliche Fragen,' *Frankfurter Allgemeine Zeitung,* 26 April, p. 47.

Buergenthal, T. (2004). Legitimität von Regierungen und die Menschenrechtsrevolution, in Nolte, G., & Schreiber, H.-L. (eds.). *Der Mensch und seine Rechte,* Wallstein Verlag, Göttingen.

Borchert, J. (2002). Wozu noch Familie?' *Die Zeit* 03

Boyle, J. (2005). 'The bioethics of global biomedicine: A natural law reflection,' in
Bulletin of the World Health Organisation, 80(12), 959 ff.

Capaldi, N. (2006). 'Manifesto: Moral diversity in health care ethics,' in H..T. Engelhardt, Jr., *Global Bioethics: The Collapse of Consensus, pp. 131-135.*

Cherry, M. (2006) 'Preserving the possibility for liberty in health care,' in H..T. Engelhardt, Jr., *Global Bioethics: The Collapse of Consensus, pp. 95-130.*

Commission on Global Governance, The. (1995), *Our Global Neigbourhood,* [On-line]. Available: www.asiawide.or.ip.

Council of Europe. (1997a). *Convention for the Protection of Human Rights and Dignity of the Human Being with regard to the Application of Biology and Medicine: Convention on Human Rights and Biomedicine,* Adopted by the Committee of Ministers on 19 November 1996. Directorate of Legal Affairs, Strasbourg, [Online]. Available: http://conventions.coe.int/treaty/en/treaties/htm/164.htm.

Council of Europe. (1997b). *Explanatory Report to the Convention for the Protection of Human Rights and Dignity of the Human Being with Regard to the Application of Biology and Medicine:*
Convention on Human Rights and Biomedicine, Directorate of Legal Affairs, Strasbourg, [On-line]. Available: http://conventions.coe.int/treaty/en/Reports/Html/164.htm

Declaration of the Rights of Man and of the Citizen (1789), [On-line]. Available: http://www.hightowertrail.com/Declaration.htm.

Delkeskamp-Hayes, C. (2004). 'Societal consensus and the problem of consent: Refocussing the problem of ethics expertise in liberal democracies,' in L,

Rasmussen, (ed.). *Ethics Expertise*, pp. 139-164. Dordecht, The Netherlands: Springer

Delkeskamp-Hayes, C., *Justification of Political Power,* forthcoming

Engelhardt, H.T. (2006). 'The search for a global morality: Bioethics, the culture wars, and moral diversity,' in H.T. Engelhardt, Jr. (ed.) *Global Bioethics: The Collapse of Consensus.*

Fan, R. (2006). 'Globalization: Communitization or localization,' in H..T. Engelhardt, Jr., *Global Bioethics: The Collapse of Consensus, pp. 271-299.*

Fittkau, L. (2004). 'Die Betroffenen können nicht klagen,' *Frankfurter Allgemeine Zeitung,* 31. March, p.42.

Global Summit of National Bioethics Commissions: Tokyo Communique (1999), Eubios Journal of Asean and International Bioethics 9, [Online]. Available: http://www.biol.tsukuba.ac.jp/~macer/communique.html

Hawkins, D. & Humes, M. (2002). 'Human rights and domestic violence,' *Political Science Quarterly,* 117 (2).

Health Affairs, (1994) Fall, Vol. 13, No 4

Health Affairs, (1999) May–June, Vol. 3

Hefty, G.P. (2003). 'Rechtswidrig, aber öffentlich finanziert,' *Frankfurter Allgemeine Zeitung,* 12. Sept.

Hefty, G.P. (2004). 'Die Subventionierung der Abtreibungen,' Mehr als vierzig Millionen Seuer-Euro im Jahre 2003, *Frankfurter Allgemeine Zeitung,* 1st Jan..

Inter Action Council (1996) *Report on the Conclusions and Recommendations by a High-level Expert Group on "In Search of Global Ethical Standards"*, Vienna, Austria, [Online]. Available: http://www.cgg.ch/

Intergovernmental Conference (ed.). (2004). *Draft Treaty establishing a constitution for Europe* (86/4), [Online]. Available: http://gandalf.aksis.uib.no/%7Ebrit/EXPORT-EU-Constitution/Draft-EU-Constitution-June-2004/index.html

Kant, I. (1786). *Grundlegung zur Metaphysik der Sitten,* (2nd edition). Riga: Johann Friedrich Hartknoch.

Kant, I. (1787). *Critik der reinen Vernunft,* (2nd edition). Riga: Johann Friedrich Hartknoch.

Kant, I. (1788). *Critik der praktischen Vernunft.* Riga: Johann Friedrich Hartknoch.

Kant, I. (1793). 'Über den Gemeinspruch: Das mag in der Theorie richtig sein, taugt aber nicht für die Praxis,' *Berlinische Monatsschrift,* September, pp. 201-284

Kant, I. (1796). *Zum Ewigen Frieden,* (2nd edition). Königsberg: Friedrich Nicolovius.

Kant, I. (1797a). *Die Metaphysik der Sitten,* Erster Theil, Rechtslehre. Königsberg: Friedrich Nicolovius.

Kant, I. (1798). *Die Metaphysik der Sitten, Erster Theil, Rechtslehre,* (2nd edition). Königsber: Friedrich Nicolovius.

Kant, I. (1797b). *Die Metaphysik der Sitten, Zweiter Theil, Tugendlehre.* Königsberg: Friedrich Nicolovius.

Kaupen-Haas, H., & Rothmaler, C. (Eds.).(1997). *Moral, Biomedizin und Bevölkerungskontrolle.* Frankfurt: Mabuse Verlag.

Knowles, L. P. (2001). 'The lingua franca of human rights and the rise of a global bioethic,' *Cambridge Quarterly of Healthcare Ethics,* 10.

Küng, H. (1996). *Yes to a Global Ethic.* New York: Continuum Publishing Company, [Online]. Available: www.uni-tuebingen.de/stiftung-weltethos/dat_eng/st_3_e.htm.

Macer, D. (1994). *Bioethics for the People by the People,* Eubios Ethics Institute 1994 Christchurch, Tsukuba, USA

Nagel, T. (2004). 'Erst der Muslim ist ein freier Mensch! Die Menschenrechte aus islamischer Sicht,' in Nolte, G., Schreiber, H.-L., (Eds.). *Der Mensch und seine Rechte,* Göttingen: Wallstein Verlag.

Nowak, M. (1989). *Uno-Pakt über bürgerliche und politische Rechte,* CCPR Kommentar

Nuffield Council on Bioethics (ed.) *The ethics of research related to health care in developing countries,* [On-line]. Available: http://www.nuffieldbioethics.org/filelibrary/pdf/errhdc_fullreport.pdf

Office of the High Commissioner for Human Rights. (1979). *Convention on the elimination of all forms of discrimination against women,* [Online]. Available: http://www.un.org/womenwatch/daw/cedaw/

Office of the High Commissioner for Human Rights. (1989). *Convention on the rights of the child.*

Petroni, A. (2006). 'Perspectives for freedom of choice' H..T. Engelhardt, Jr., *Global Bioethics: The Collapse of Consensus.*

Pocar, F. (1993). 'Enhancing the universal application of human rights standards and instruments,' in United Nations, General Assembly (ed.). *Status of publication of preparations, studies and documents for the world conference,* [Online]. Available: www.unhchr.ch/Huridocda/Huridoca.nsf/TestFrame/da9fdf34ef1a9a8c802568c7005a19dd?Opendocument

Qiu, R-Z. (2002). 'The tension between biomedical technology and Confucian values,' in J. Tao (ed.) *Cross-Cultural Perspectives on the (Im)Possibility of Global Bioethics,* pp. 71 ff., Dordrecht, The Netherlands.

Rousseau, J-J. (1762). *The social contract or principles of political right,* [Online]. Available: http://www.classicreader.com/booktoc.php/sid.2/bookid.615/

Sakamoto, H. (1999). 'Towards a new "Global Bioethics,' *Bioethics,* Vol. 13 no. 13(5).

Schmidt, K. (2006). 'Lost in translation – bridging gaps through procedural norms,' in H..T. Engelhardt, Jr., *Global Bioethics: The Collapse of Consensus.*

Schuck, M. (2002). 'Verwirklichungssformen der Religionsfreiheit in Europa,' *Zeitschrift für evangelische Ethik* 46(4).

Schwab, D. (2003). 'Wertewandel und Familienrecht,' *Schriftenreihe der Juristischen Studiengesellschaft Hannover* 22.

Schwab, D. (2004). *'Konkurs der Familie? Familienrecht im Umbruch'* C.H. Beck'sche Verlagsbuchhandlung München.

Solomon, D. (2006). 'Domestic disarray and imperial ambition: Contemporary applied ethics and the prospects for global bioethics,' in H..T. Engelhardt, Jr., *Global Bioethics: The Collapse of Consensus, pp. 335-361.*

Tao, J. (2006). 'A Confucian approach to a "shared family decision model" in health care: reflections on moral pluralism,' in H..T. Engelhardt, Jr., *Global Bioethics: The Collapse of Consensus, pp.154-179.*

UNESCO. (2000). *The universal declaration on the human genome and human rights: From theory to practice,* [Online]. Available: http://www1.umn.edu/humanrts/instree/Udhrhg.htm

UNESCO, General Conference. (2003a). *Draft international declaration on human genetic data,* 28 August, [Online]. Available: http://unesdoc.unesco.org/images/0013/001302/130223e.pdf

UNESCO, International Bioethics Committee. (2003b). *Report of the IBC on pre-implantation genetic diagnosis and germ-line intervention,* [Online]. Available: http://unesdoc.unesco.org/images/0013/001302/130223e.pdf

UNESCO, International Bioethics Committee. (2003c). *Draft report on the possibility of elaborating a universal instrument on bioethics,* [Online]. Available: http://unesdoc.unesco.org/images/0013/001302/130223e.pdf

UNESCO, General Conference. (2003d). *Draft international declaration on human genetic data, addendum,* [Online]. Available: http://unesdoc.unesco.org/images/0013/001312/131204e.pdf

United Nations, The, General Assembly. (1948). *Universal Declaration of Human Rights,* [Online]. Available: http://www.un.org/Overview/rights.html

United Nations, The. (1997). International covenant on economic social and cultural rights, [Online]. Available: http://www.unhchr.ch/html/menu3/b/a_cescr.htm-42k.

United Nations, The, General Assembly. (2001). *Human rights questions: human rights questions, including alternative approaches for improving the effective enjoyment of human rights and fundamental freedoms,* [Online]. Available: http://www.icrc.org/Web/Eng/siteeng0.nsf/iwpList112/305786EE947B69EB41256C780028EDa9

United Nations, The, Economic and Social Council. (2002). *Report of the United Nations High Commissioner for human rights and follow-up to the world conference on human rights,* [Online]. Available: http://www.hrw.org/un/unchr-statement.htm

Vachek M. (2000). *Das Religionsrecht der Europäischen Union im Spannungsfeld zwischen mitgliedstaatlichen Kompetenzreservaten und Art 9 EMRK,* Studien und Materialien zum öffentlichen Recht 11, Frankfurt.

Van Kemenade , Y.W. (1993). *Health care in Europe,* National Council for Public Health, Zoetermeer, The Netherlands.

Wildes, K. (2006). 'Global bioethics and the limits of practical reason,' in H..T. Engelhardt, Jr., *Global Bioethics: The Collapse of Consensus, pp.362-379.*

Preserving the Possibility for Liberty in Health Care

Mark J. Cherry

> There is, perhaps, no stronger contrast between the revolutionary times in which we live and the Catholic ages, or even the period of the Reformation, than in this: that the influence which religious motives formerly possessed is now in a great measure exercised by political opinions. … so now political zeal occupies the place made vacant by the decline of religious fevour, and commands to an almost equal extent the enthusiasm of men. It has risen to power at the expense of religion, and by reason of its decline, and naturally regards the dethroned authority with the jealously of a usurper.
>
> *Lord Acton 1859*

I. Incommensurable Conceptions of Liberty

H. Tristram Engelhardt, Jr. and Corinna Delkeskamp-Hayes's rich and insightful essays illustrate the ways in which the recent history of medical morality and bioethics discloses a profound shift in moral commitments within the dominant intellectual culture. These changes have been especially prominent in medicine. Where once abortion had been forbidden, it is now widely practiced. Where once physician-assisted suicide and euthanasia were rare, they are now emerging as accepted practices in Belgium, the Netherlands, Oregon, and Switzerland. As Engelhardt and Delkeskamp-Hayes each note, the prevailing intellectual culture reflects the vision of a liberal, social-democratic, cosmopolitan polity, which in turn shapes aspirations

H.T. Engelhardt, Jr. (ed), *Global Bioethics* (pp. 95–130).

for a truly global bioethics. This vision encompasses, as Engelhardt documents, harmonization of health care, thereby requiring considerable taxation to accommodate the redistribution of wealth, goods, and services necessary to guarantee a universal standard of care, including the availability of abortion and euthanasia services, perhaps through licensure or legal operational requirements, regardless of physician choice or institutional religious integrity (e.g., as Roman Catholic or Orthodox Jewish). The hope has been to establish a single, content-full, canonical bioethics, thereby justifying a global approach to health care policy and law.

This comprehensive vision also embodies deep skepticism regarding market-based financing and distribution of health care. The market is frequently caricatured as decreasing altruistic sentiments, eroding a sense of community, lowering scientific standards, limiting personal and professional freedoms, as well as legalizing hostility between patients and physicians. Profiting from the provision of health care is viewed as morally suspect. The forces of the market, it is believed, bring on more harm than benefit.[1] The profit motive is not regarded as leading to the wise use of resources, nor is the market considered a place that rewards responsible free decision-making, while providing tutelage concerning the limitations of the human condition. The market is seen as starkly limiting, rather than enhancing, human liberty and responsible behavior; that is, as restricting, rather than preserving, the possibility for liberty and moral choice in health care. Thus the prevailing accounts of western bioethics inevitably seek command and control, top down national and international regulation of the standard of care as well as of new areas of research and technological development. Western bioethics has come to possess a national socialist, liberal, statist character (Engelhardt, 2006, pp. 19-20).

This central and forceful criticism of the market as failing to preserve human liberty and the conditions which sustain moral choice, such that significant national and international regulation is necessary to protect the most fundamental rights and interests of persons, is pervasive and requires careful assessment. It will serve as the focus of this paper.

To begin, at least four distinct conceptions of liberty compete to frame the foundations of a global bioethics. (1) Liberty$_1$ as the entitlement to *realize* one's abilities and choices; i.e., to achieve one's own understanding of the good life. (2) Liberty$_2$ as acting according to an ideal, rather than an actual, account of free choice, informed by rationally discoverable universal moral norms. (3) Liberty$_3$ as lived human flourishing; i.e., a content-full way of life, fully embedded within a particular cultural or religious context. (4) Liberty$_4$ as freedom from interference, as expressed in the existence of significant forbearance rights—i.e., rights to be left alone and protected from nonconsensual use of oneself and one's private property. Developing a morally authoritative "global bioethics", which sustains liberty and the possibility for diverse moral choice, will only be possible when the arguments for and implications of the various conceptions of liberty have been sorted through, and the unsustainable set aside.[2]

Liberty$_1$ and liberty$_2$ each frame core moral assumptions of the liberal, social-democratic, global aspirations of western bioethics. Each supports the imposition of uniform systems of health care and guarantees of equality in the provision of medical services. Whereas the first underscores universal access to comprehensive health care as central to the preservation of the conditions for achieving one's own understanding of the good life (section II), the second judges global establishment of particular biomedical standards, moral principles and precepts, as grounded in human moral rationality (section III). Moreover, each manifests an immanent displacement of what were once theological matters: concerns, such as the sanctity of human life, human flourishing, and human dignity, have been relocated within a fully secular context and have thereby been set adrift from traditional metaphysical anchors of meaning. Thus, as I will argue, while *prima facie* endorsing liberty and diversity, each privileges a particular, fully secular, concept of moral choice and human flourishing, prioritizing individual autonomy understood in terms of fair equality of opportunity, self-determinism, and freedom from constraints on the pursuit of self-fulfillment.

Such a worldview is at core incompatible with traditional religions and cultures (e.g., Orthodox Judaism, Orthodox Christianity, and traditional Confucianism). Traditional religions and cultures experience morality as part of a living phenomenological world. Here, liberty$_3$ can be encapsulated, *grosso modo,* as a way of life embodying virtue. Rather than developing action guiding principles or ranking central values, the focus of the moral life is to develop and sustain the cardinal elements of human flourishing, which itself varies from tradition to tradition and culture to culture. Whereas certain moral positions will be more-or-less compatible with a virtuous way of life, medical morality and bioethics will not be reducible to moral principles which generate such choices. Nor, will their moralities be reducible, without significant loss of content and moral distortion, to secular accounts of the right and the good. Rather, the moral life is the living experience of true human flourishing (section IV). Here the search for moral truth and human good is grounded with a metaphysical anchor; e.g., God or metaphysical conception of human nature. The challenge, however, for establishing a global bioethics is that religious and cultural moral diversity runs deep. The national and international political landscape compasses persons from diverse and often fragmented moral communities, with widely varying moral intuitions, evaluations, and commitments. All do not hear the same God, possess the same appreciation of Divine revelation, or metaphysical understanding of human nature. One comes to appreciate the significant plurality of fundamentally different, incompatible, and often mutually antagonistic moral visions and moral rationalities, within which complex bioethical issues are addressed. Which mode of life or experience of human flourishing should guide bioethical decision-making and define the standard of care? Whose bioethics should guide the creation of national law and international treaty?

Whereas the vision of western liberal, social-democratic, bioethics offers the hope of a communality binding all persons and the resolutions of biomedical moral controversies through universal moral norms, as this paper argues, this hope is chimerical. This cosmopolitan vision offers only the false promise of a global moral consensus, while failing to acknowledge the deep cleft between traditional religious and cultural moral communities and its own robust post-traditional aspirations. Judging among the rival versions of moral inquiry to guide the establishment of universal bioethical content, therefore, either straightforwardly begs the question of such moral content or arbitrarily embraces a particular moral vision—whether traditionally religious or post-traditionally liberal social-democratic. As a result, the foundations for a morally authoritative global bioethics must be found elsewhere. This brings the discussion, finally, to a consideration of the implications for morally authoritative bioethics grounded in an understanding of liberty[4], freedom from interference, as expressed in the existence of significant forbearance rights (section V).

II. Liberty as the Entitlement to Realize One's Abilities and Choices (Liberty$_1$)

Whereas all individuals are exposed to the vicissitudes of nature, some will through unforeseen fortune fair better than others, remaining relatively free from disease and major suffering. Others will be born with congenital defects or genetic disorders, confront crippling illness, or through accident or chosen risk become injured or maimed. The healthy, talented and intelligent have natural advantages over those who are sickly, less talented, and less intelligent. As a working group of the International Bioethics Committee (IBC) of UNESCO notes:

> Health has a dual moral value: it is essential for the quality of life and life itself and is instrumental as a precondition for freedom. When disease prevails, the destiny of a person (and even of a nation) is left to external factors and powers and may enter into an irreversible vicious circle of regression. The inequality between the rich and the poor—at the level of individuals, communities and nations—is becoming increasingly deeply felt in the area of health and health care, thereby contributing to the desperation and injustice that continues to increase and prevail in other health-related fields such as food, income and education (Working Group of the IBC, 2003, p. 4, para. 15).

Healthy individuals generally spend a less significant portion of their physical resources and personal time on health care, allowing for the pursuit of other opportunities. Moreover, talent and intelligence is positively correlated with higher income, higher status jobs. Such advantages, in turn, are statistically correlated with an increase in the quality and quantity of life (Iglehart, 1990; Wilkins, Adams, & Brancker, 1989a).

$Liberty_1$ frames such inequalities as social injustices, because some are less able to realize their positive entitlements to secure their own understanding of the good; and, in turn, assumes that these injustices ought to be redressed through redistributive state action. As Rawls urges, our natural talents, abilities, and health, are to be appreciated as arbitrary from a moral point of view (1999, pp. 63-64) and, indeed, as common assets for the creation of social benefit (1999, p. 87). Thus, insofar as each do not have an equal chance at realizing their own individual understanding of the good, justice requires state action to mitigate the influence of social contingencies and natural fortune (1999, p. 63):

> As health care services and medicines become increasingly more expensive, access to them by poor populations becomes more severely compromised. While poor people have as much need for these medicines as everybody else, many do not have the resources to guarantee access. In the context of the dreaded diseases currently confronting the world, the obligation to find new and effective ways of dealing with the situation has truly acquired immense ethical significance (Working Group of the IBC, 2003, p. 4, para. 16).

The international community, it is argued, possesses both moral responsibility and legitimate moral authority to equalize access to health care products and services (Working Group of the IBC, 2003, p. 4, para. 16). Markets for the production and allocation of health care, must be thoroughly constrained within political institutions, which themselves guarantee fair equality of opportunity, access, and outcome. Market systems are decried as advantaging the wealthier and healthier members of society.[3]

Norman Daniels encapsulates this concern as the need to sustain more than the conditions of formal liberty, as freedom from constraint, but to guarantee material liberty, as expressed in fair equality of outcomes. For example, while universal suffrage grants the wealthy and the poor identical voting rights, the wealthy have greater ability to select candidates, as well as to influence public opinion and elected officials. In terms of actual impact on outcomes, political liberty has greater worth for the wealthy (Daniels, 1976, p. 256; 1996). The underlying concern is for equal worth of personal and political liberty, especially concerning the material and social conditions necessary to eliminate natural and social disadvantages, so that each may enjoy fair equality of outcomes in terms of the freedom to fulfill their potential, however individualistically defined. In moral theoretical terms, this consideration can be construed as a teleological, consequentialist, or goal-oriented moral concern. It is an affirmation of the value of individual liberty or autonomy, not merely as a forbearance right, but as a claim right.

Often encapsulated as equal rights to self-determination (International Covenant on Economic, Social, and Cultural Rights, 1997, p. 1, art. 1, para. 1), such liberty rights are held to include, without being limited to: rights to work as one chooses (p. 3, art. 6, para.1)—with taxpayer financed primary, secondary, and higher education, as well as vocational and technical training (pp. 3, 5-6; art. 6, 13 and 14); to promotion within the work environment as well as paid time off for rest, leisure, holidays, and maternity leave (pp. 3-4, art. 7 and 10); as well as to the "highest attainable standard of physical and mental health" (p. 5, art.12). As this short list of examples illustrates, equal worth of liberty is, in turn, argued to depend on sufficient levels of economic equality as well as personal health and welfare (Callahan, 1987, pp. 136-137; Sulmasy, 1996, p. 317). Wide-ranging welfare entitlements to adequate employment opportunities, education, and health care are underscored as necessary to successfully secure individual abilities and choices. Preserving personal capacities for forming, revising, and achieving one's own goals and objectives requires removing, as much as possible, the physical, mental, and social, handicaps of illness, disease, and disability. In particular, because health care helps guarantee the chance to enjoy the normal range of human opportunities, access to adequate health care as a basic human entitlement, without income-based barriers, is given special status as foundational to preserving liberty and fair equality of opportunity.[4] Each is understood as possessing an equal basic entitlement to realize one's own understanding of the good life, fully unhampered by the fortunes of nature and social choice.

Prima facie, such an ethos embraces religious and cultural diversity. Difference in moral, cultural, and religious expression is, after all, the likely outcome of the search for individual meaning and understanding of the good. International statements continue to affirm basic rights to freedom of thought, conscience, religion, and expression. However, moral and religious viewpoints must not take on an exclusionary character. Toleration, understood in the thick political sense as a willingness to affirm other religions and lifestyles as potentially equally as good as one's own, is central to sustaining this moral vision of a social-democratic, liberal, cosmopolitan polity (see Rawls, 1993, pp. 58-62, 194ff; Engelhardt, MS 28). Viable political negotiation towards substantial moral concessions requires such toleration as a civic virtue, since the values realized in practice will not be those that particular persons would choose, but rather the values chosen and ranked in the course of legislative discussion and compromise. Real disparity of belief threatens the possibility of reaching broad and meaningful political agreement. To engage in such comprehensive compromise, participants must free themselves from too deep of an involvement with any particular values and principles; they must not be burdened with the constraints of traditional religions and cultures.

Contemporary liberalism thus excludes from public political debate on controversial moral issues the voices of those informed by a thick moral or religious view. As Rawls notes, to secure political agreement public debate must "...avoid disputed philosophical, as well as disputed moral and religious questions" (1999, p. 394). As a result, in its very advocacy of tolerance, liberalism is strikingly intolerant of a wide range of traditional moral positions (see Khushf, 1994; Engelhardt, 2000; Cherry, 2002a; 2002b). In *Political Liberalism*'s brief discussion of abortion, for example, Rawls argues that agents who accept the humanity of the fetus can do so only on the basis of a "comprehensive doctrine", which, precisely because it rules out abortion, is "unreasonable" from the standpoint of public reason and thus unacceptable in the public square (Rawls, 1993, p. 243). While officially endorsing the goods of moral pluralism, such a perspective embraces a superficial secular understanding of religion and culture in which the search for meaning is individualized[6] and diversity may only be affirmed as akin to variation in aesthetic taste: at best, the expression of personal or group idiosyncrasy; cultural stops for the secular cosmopolitan tourist.

Consider its implications for private associations, such as traditional religions, dedicated to developing and sustaining particular understandings of the good in the public space. Sustaining wide-ranging welfare entitlements requires significant taxation and redistribution of the time, talent, goods, and resources of all members of society, defeating individual or group claims to have exclusive use of private property. "Property" is recast as a social benefit to be redistributed as needed to preserve fair equality of opportunity and outcome, thereby ensuring equal worth of liberty. Ownership rights are conveyed insofar as they promote these special goods. The burden of proof is removed from governmental and other authorities, who would continually interfere in private use of one's property, and placed on those who would freely utilize personal property with consenting others. There exists, e.g., international encouragement for the systematic violation of property rights and patent protections in favor of potentially increasing access to pharmaceuticals:

> As important as the concern about access to health care might be, some of the most promising efforts to provide solutions have been controversial. Some countries have claimed that they should be allowed to infringe drug patents in emergencies. For instance, economically struggling governments have resorted to "parallel importation" to allow the purchase of cheap supplies from countries with weak patent laws, thereby undermining the commercial interests of transnational companies that rely on the observance of patents to protect their investments. Other governments have tried a system of "compulsory licensing", enabling them to license a local generic manufacturer to make drugs more cheaply or to buy a generic version from another country (Working Group of the IBC, 2003, pp. 4-5, para. 17).

The products of private enterprise, indeed, the goods and services of all, are the means through which to create and finance a universal system of welfare entitlements. Guaranteeing equal access to health care regardless of personal income, social status, or geographical location, requires significant redistributive taxpayer financing. Guaranteeing fair equality of outcomes requires state-based health care distribution, uniform standards of care, and universal rather than regional or local regulation.

Such systems, however, carry significant financial as well as medical costs. Governmentally financed health care predictably lowers the standard of care. Canada, for example, ranks last among developed countries for access to MRI technology, resulting in diagnostic degradation (e.g., restricted access to MRI increases the risk of death and disability due to stroke) (Rankin, 1999, pp. 89-92). Those over 65 years-of-age consume 42.7% of Canada's total health care expenditures while only accounting for 12.5% of the population. Adjusting for the age of its population, relative to other countries, Canada spends a greater percentage of its GDP on health care than any other industrialized, universal access, OECD country. Yet, Canada ranks 10th among such countries in the percentage of expected disability free years, 7th in the prevention of death by preventable causes, and 6th in the incidence of breast cancer mortality. Queuing times for specialty consultations and procedures continues to increase. Waiting time between general practitioner referral and specialist consultation swelled from 7.3 weeks in 2001-02 to 8.3 weeks in 2003. Waiting time between specialist consultation and treatment rose for Canada as a whole between 2001-02 and 2003, from 9.2 to 9.5 weeks, with the shortest waits experienced in Ontario (7.1 weeks) and the longest in Saskatchewan (23.0 weeks) (Esmail & Walker, 2004, p. 3). Similarly, Canada forbids the use of one's private resources to purchase better basic care. Unlike Canada, all six of the OECD countries that experience fewer years of life lost from preventable causes, have private alternatives to the public health care system (Esmail & Walker, 2002, pp. 5-6).[7] Since all health care must be purchased within the Canadian governmental system, it is not possible for entrepreneurial physicians or even benevolent charity organizations privately to provide regional centers of medical excellence.[8] Governmentally sustained mediocrity thereby also gives rise to significant losses in private incentive.

This vision of equal worth of liberty, fair equality of opportunity and outcome, embodies an egalitarianism of envy—a jealous hubris that some might fair better than others—and appears more apt at reducing misery than at creating excellence; more apt to ensure all some access to health care, even at a lower standard of care, than to generate tremendous insight and medical genius. It is a prioritization of equal worth of liberty over market efficiency, regional centers of excellence, or higher total standards of care. Whereas free market economies have historically produced greater prosperity, even with inequalities, here, political creation and enforcement of the privileged conceptions of liberty and equality trump greater availability of high technology medicine, reduction of suffering, and years of life saved.

State-based health care distribution also gives rise to important moral costs. Significant redistributive taxation to support universal access to health care is hardly compatible with respecting real moral difference. As an example, traditional Roman Catholics consider financing abortion as being complicit with evil. Since the right to abortion is widely endorsed in western bioethics as central to gender equality and the equal liberty of women—Rawls, e.g., refers to restrictive abortion laws as "cruel and oppressive" (1993, p. 243f.)—respect for such expression of individual liberty is given priority over deeply held religious objections. Authoritative Catholic teaching forbids obtaining or performing abortions, as well as cooperating with or enabling others to obtain abortions (McHugh, 1994, p. 496). Yet, such religious objections are set aside in pursuit of the greater liberty for those whose life plans and personal values affirm abortion as liberating women from patriarchy and enforced pregnancy.[10] (Abortion is covered by public expenditure as part of the Canadian health care system.)[11] Those who object to the provision of particular services, such as abortion, find themselves coercively compelled into participating in their purchase.[12]

Rights not to participate in the propagation of services which one conscientiously opposes, to utilize private property only in ways which one believes to be morally acceptable, are, at best, insecure and limited. As Delkeskamp-Hayes notes,

> To be sure, public health care can be provided only if all (can be forced to) contribute. As its provision will always be particular, some losses in moral diversity are unavoidable. Acknowledging a right to health care, merely as such, implies accepting such losses. ... In Germany, the reform of home care for the elderly or helpless forced religious orders (which had long been integrated into a system of subsidiary cooperation) to discontinue their no-pay charity services. ... In Belgium and the Netherlands, even religious hospitals are unable to hinder their staff from responding to patient demands for euthanasia (pp. 56-57).

Such losses, she rightly notes, are not negligible; traditional moral and religious communities are coerced into supporting that which they know to be gravely evil: offering, providing, and financing abortion, physician-assisted suicide, *in vitro* fertilization, sex reassignment surgery (Schmidt, 2002) and so forth. Even those who on moral or religious grounds oppose or do not wish to provide any such services, are implicated in their financing.

As Lord Acton recognized, safeguarding private property is central to preserving true liberty. Private property protects one's liberty of conscience and choice regarding the use of oneself, one's talents and abilities. Yet, even when defense of conscience does not directly arise, property is always exposed to interference; it is the constant object of public policy (Acton, 1988, p. 572). To paraphrase John C. Calhoun, such taxation enriches and strengthens those hostile to traditional cultures, practices, and religions, while impoverishing and weakening those who would wish to pursue traditional ways of life. Coercive taxation to support what one understands to be deviant moral visions impoverishes one's own ability to sustain a traditional religious understanding; it suppresses moral disagreement and privileges a particular moral viewpoint (1992).[13]

In summary, liberty1 as the equal entitlement to realize one's abilities and choices creates *pro-forma* space for certain types of idiosyncratic moral difference, akin to aesthetic variation in life-style and cultural expression. Substantive moral diversity, however, is ruled out in pursuit of political compromise regarding the material, psychological, and social conditions necessary to preserve equal worth of liberty. As Engelhardt and Delkeskamp-Hayes illustrate, true believers, i.e., those who denounce others as wrong, attempt to convert, or refuse to see central religious or moral beliefs as the appropriate subject of political compromise, are perceived as dangerous and threatening. To forge consensus, different religious perspectives may not appear to have an exclusionary character. Any serious validity claim, that is not at the same time presented as a matter of personal idiosyncrasy, is seen as endangering social cohesion. When traditional constraints collide with the post-traditional individualistic search for self-determination one encounters controversy rather than compromise. Consider Engelhardt's examples:

> … the role of third parties in reproduction (the traditional Christian judgment that the use of donor gametes involves a form of adultery), the propriety of abortion (traditionally forbidden by Christianity), the propriety of cloning (Christianity traditionally requires all sexual activity and reproduction to occur within the marriage of one man and one woman) … and the appropriateness of using animals in research (post-traditional rejection of humans as the masters of creation), as well as the licitness of physician-assisted suicide and euthanasia (traditionally, Christianity rejects such interventions) (Engelhardt, 2006, p.33).

Acknowledging substantive moral diversity requires recognizing the existence of moral opposition, thereby exposing the aspirations of the liberal, social-democratic vision, including state-based health care, to the significant likelihood of failure.

III. Liberty as Ideal, Rather Than Actual, Free Choice (Liberty$_2$)

If liberty is understood as acting in accord with an ideal, rather than actual, account of free choice, informed by universal moral norms, then insofar as particular bioethical standards can be canonically established, they may be legitimately imposed through national law and international treaty. Here, autonomy is not understood as acting on one's own wishes and desires, but rather as acting in accord with right reason. As Engelhardt notes, much of bioethics has sought top-down guidance framed in terms of a "... rationally discoverable vision of morality, justice, and proper conduct, which authorizes state or international governmental authority to constrain and direct citizens, groups, and communities", rather than social space for expression of diverse religious and moral beliefs (p. 22). In moral theoretical terms, as Engelhardt and Delkeskamp-Hayes each argue, this consideration can be appreciated as the vision of the universal legislator of Kant's categorical imperative, who derives an understanding of appropriate human choice from a particular account of moral rationality and rational volition.

Through appeal to core values, e.g., human dignity, and to central principles, e.g., beneficence, justice, and autonomy, bioethics is believed to transcend regional, cultural, and religious differences, binding all nations and peoples. Consider:

> Perhaps the two most distinctive features of international instruments relating to biomedicine are the very central role given to the notion of "human dignity" and the integration of the common standards that are adopted into a human rights framework. This is not surprising if we consider that human dignity is one of the few common values in our world of philosophical pluralism. Moreover, in our time, a widespread assumption is that the "inherent dignity ... of all members of the human family" is the ground of human rights and democracy [United Nations, Universal Declaration on Human Rights, Preamble]. It is indeed difficult, if not impossible, to provide a justification of human rights without making some reference, at least implicitly, to the idea of human dignity (Andorno, 2002, p. 960).

Human dignity is cited as a universal value, which while vague, none-the-less provides justification for substantive and far reaching human rights and welfare entitlements. The expectation is that through such universal values, secular moral reason discloses a communality of all persons, justified not in faith but in reason. The hope is to reveal a universally accessible secular basis for human moral community, justifiable without appeal to particular religions or cultures, traditional moral commitments or insights. Citing objective, rational analysis, freed of the particularities of religious belief and cultural practice, as Engelhardt and Delkeskamp-Hayes note, such appeal is held to ground particular, content-full moral conclusions. Thus, bioethics seeks universal declarations on prenatal diagnosis and selective abortion and physician-assisted suicide, the ethical status of the human genome, the use of animals in research, embryo experimentation, third-party assisted reproduction, the sale of human organs for transplantation, and so forth. Moreover, appeal is made to the existence of a so-called "global moral consensus", which denies the existence of real moral difference, while announcing the secular equivalent of orthodox religious belief.[14]

This compelling moral language—"human dignity", "objective reason," "global consensus" and so forth—rhetorically shifts the burden of proof to those who disagree. Dissenters are thereby made to appear as mean-spirited, idiosyncratic or superstitious, as acting in "bad faith" or as fundamentalist adherents of irrational dogma. As Engelhardt argues, western bioethics continues to give political and institutional expression to the Enlightenment hope that ethics and thus bioethics "...should liberate from unjustified customs and constraints, those contrary to the demands of universal moral reason" (Engelhardt p. 20). Choosing other than in accord with "right reason" and the purported "moral consensus", whether in adherence to traditional religious commitments or to advance diverse secular accounts of the good, is characterized as acting under a false consciousness or as the victim of exploitation, social, cultural or patriarchal despotism. Such harmonization across diverse segments of national and international populations is not characterized as limiting legitimate diversity or restricting individual liberty but rather as returning individuals, families, and communities to the appropriately objective standards of rationally disclosed morality. In this fashion, bioethicists have been elaborating an international bioethics to guide court decisions, public deliberation, clinical decision-making, and legislative action, as well as international convention and treaty. Moral disagreement is to be shunned, if not actively persecuted.

Yet, substantial moral diversity remains. As Engelhardt and Delkeskamp-Hayes each make clear, the acrimonious bioethical controversies—abortion, physician-assisted suicide, cloning, embryo experimentation, health care resource allocation, and so forth—illustrate that within medicine there exists, as always, foundationally different accounts of the moral life. Indeed, rather than justifying a morality to which no rational being could deny assent, liberal social-democratic bioethics straightforwardly adopts a particular moral content so as to secure specific moral judgments: a content to which reasonable rational dissent is surely possible. To ignore such fundamental differences, while claiming a "global moral consensus" sufficient to establish this particular moral vision, engages in what might be termed coercive moral colonialism.

Consider the sale of human organs for transplantation as a heuristic example. Regardless of the underlying reasons or likely personal or social advantages, selling human organs for a profit is held to be exploitative and degrading, morally analogous to slavery, as well as incompatible with basic human values, such as human dignity, and important social goods, such as equality and a spirit of altruism. The human body, it is argued, should not be treated as property (Scott, 1990). Financial incentives are believed to coerce the poor into selling parts of their bodies. In 1970, the Committee on Morals and Ethics of the Transplantation Society held that "the sale of organs by donors living or dead is indefensible under any circumstance" (1970) and the World Health Organization's "Guiding principles on Human Organ Transplantation" prohibits giving and receiving money for organs. The WHO urges member states to legislate forbidding the commercial trafficking of human organs (WHO, 1991). Similarly, the International Bioethics Committee of UNESCO urged: "...there is an equally important need for the preservation of choice, personal liberty and human dignity, which would be offended if the disposable parts of the human body were considered commodities or bargaining tools" (Working Group of the IBC, 2003, p. 7, art. 28). In the United States, Title III (Section 301) of the federal "National Organ Transplant Act" makes it unlawful for any persons knowingly to acquire, receive, or otherwise transfer human organs for valuable consideration. Morally acceptable uses of the body are those which are viewed as protecting "… a central element of the undefined, yet widely endorsed demand for respect for the human body and for human dignity" (Nuffield Council on Bioethics, 1995, para 6.4). Selling human organs for transplantation has been rhetorically characterized as the extreme of human greed.

However, many parts of the body, including redundant internal organs, blood, and regenerative tissue can be removed without destroying oneself or reducing adequate human functioning. While donating such parts as blood, sperm, and bone marrow, has become more-or-less routine, assuming a suitably sterile environment and an appropriately talented surgical staff, even removing redundant internal organs (e.g., a kidney), whether for donation or sale, is less risky than many other occupations. Such medical activities are consistent with personal health, and the practice of saving lives supports the respect of other persons. Those who participate engage in a life-saving activity, perhaps even heroically, at some risk to themselves, which is intended to alleviate suffering. Opponents of an organ market typically reflect a vision of social justice which brings into question the good fortunes of those who have more opportunities, wealth, and resources to purchase more extensive health care.[16] It is a vision marked by envy towards those who fair better, whether through accidental chance or personal choice. Moreover, it is unclear why greed ought to be condemned or altruism praised from a secular perspective. Dissent to the so-called "global moral consensus" opposed to the sale of human organs for transplantation, appears not merely reasonable, but fully rational. Given the significant potential of the market to increase access to life sustaining organs, to reduce human suffering and death—after all, roughly 5,000 people die every year in the United States alone, while queuing for needed organs (see www.UNOS.org)—such dissent may even be seen as morally compelling.

How then should public policy be crafted? Should one simply acquiesce to the personal preferences or deep moral intuitions of academic bioethicists, current biomedical convention, or claims to global moral consensus? Or should one seek moral content to guide public policy through appeal to intuitions, consequences, casuistry, the notion of unbiased choice, game theory, or middle-level principles? All such attempts, Engelhardt argues, confront insurmountable obstacles: one must already presuppose a particular morality so as to choose among intuitions, rank consequences, evaluate exemplary cases, or mediate among various principles, otherwise one will be unable to make any rational choice at all. As he points out, even if one merely ranks cardinal moral concerns, such as liberty, equality, justice, and security differently, one affirms different moral visions, divergent understandings of the good life, varying senses of what it is to act appropriately (Engelhardt, p. 40ff.). Appeals to "human dignity" will similarly fail to provide the necessary justification. Some will seek to preserve human dignity through universal access, single-tier health care, others will understand the dignity of access to the market and economic freedoms. From a general secular perspective, the guarantee of property rights and free collaboration would appear to be core to human respect and dignity, despite inequalities. Once secularized and thereby cut off from any particular metaphysical anchor (e.g., God), the dignity of humans is no more and no less than what humans make of it (see Engelhardt, 2003). In general secular terms, it is impossible to break through the seemingly interminable bioethical debates to truth.

Given such circumstances, the claims of ideal rational choice theory, e.g., Rawlsian hypothetical contractors, to "global moral consensus", or to rationally discoverable moral truths are implausible. As already noted, many retain hesitations regarding embryo experimentation and abortion, even though these are practices which society permits and bioethics as a field generally endorses. Even the assumption that "human dignity" possesses moral import, presupposes a particular moral understanding regarding licit uses of oneself and the limits on permissible consensual interaction with others.[17] Because of divergent understandings of the good life and of what should actually count as doing good, one cannot appeal to canonical accounts of "beneficence" and "human dignity". Such sentiments appear to be remnants of Christian sentiments that cling to the fabric and language of western society (Engelhardt, 2000; Torcello & Wear, 2000), often misconstruing and distorting their origins. Christianity, albeit shorn of its metaphysical foundations and transcendent concerns, provided the moral content and culture for much of traditional secular moral judgment. Stripped of their traditional religious foundations, however, such judgments embody emotionally volatile, but rationally indefensible, moral intuitions. The political strategy is evidently to deny or discount the significance of such disagreement, discounting or marginalizing those who disagree as non-mainstream or radical, or even dismissing alternate views as simply wrong or hopelessly irrational. The aspirations of contemporary liberal bioethics to impose a particular "rational" moral content as the foundation of public policy, therefore, straightforwardly begs the question.

IV. Liberty as Lived Human Flourishing (Liberty$_3$)

As already noted, the universalistic claims of western bioethics embody thick understandings of the values of liberty, autonomy, and equality which are incompatible with the often taken-for-granted assumptions of traditional religions and cultures. Drawing on quite different metaphysical and ethical assumptions, traditional religions and cultures, e.g., Orthodox Christian or traditional Confucian, shape moral conclusions that are at odds with those that western bioethicists endorse. Moral understandings, particular accounts of human flourishing, accepted social roles, including appreciations of gender and sexuality, expressed in often taken-for-granted norms of human form, behavior and grace, mark the conceptual frameworks which underlie public policy. As the widening gulf between traditional moral understandings and contemporary bioethical judgments illustrates, there does not even exist a unique canonical account of human nature from which to draw content-full understandings of licit and illicit biomedical conduct. Whereas western bioethics focuses on the individual and is almost always expressed in discursive terms, within traditional cultures and religions bioethics is part of a living phenomenological world: it is part of a way of life. In moral theoretical terms, $Liberty_3$ can be appreciated as an experiential, embodied, living account of full human flourishing.

Consider a central tenet of liberal western bioethics: the principle of equality. Julia Tao notes that this obsession of the liberal cosmopolitan west is set aside within traditional Confucian ethics:

> Confucian care ethics rejects universal love. Instead, Confucius himself also urges that a person ... should start from one's parents and siblings and then extend to other people. ...There is no requirement to treat everyone equally with the same impartial treatment. ... Our obligations are defined by our relationships (2002, pp. 54-55).

As Qiu Ren-Zong elaborates, for Confucianism "Keeping familial integrity and orderly familial relations may be even more important than keeping bodily integrity..." (2002, p. 77).

Similarly, autonomy understood as free individualistic choice, is fundamentally incompatible with traditional Confucian understandings of essential moral relationships.

> Values seem to be shared by different moral communities or cultures, but their meanings differ among them. Autonomy in Western culture means decisions made by an independent person, but in Confucian culture it means decisions made by a family incorporating the person (Qiu, 2002, p. 84).

Here, Father Thomas Joseph's reflections on the hostility of western liberal bioethics to the traditional family are also helpful:

> One of the difficulties in attempting to reinvigorate the family is one of its very strengths: families bring within them concrete substantive moral commitments. Substantive commitments divide a society. They ingrain a moral pluralism. In addition, some critics are especially concerned about the family's connection with religious faith because of their commitments to rendering society ever more secular (Joseph, 2002, p. 61).

The robust, content-full visions of human flourishing available within traditional religions and ways of life cannot be captured or recreated within the secular vision of cosmopolitan liberal moral theory. Traditional

Confucians and Christians, for example, understand the pursuit of a fully flourishing human life as situated within the thick expectations of family structures rather than in disinterested commitments to the pursuit of social justice, equality, fairness, civic duty or generalized solidarity. From such living moral perspectives, however otherwise different from one another, western liberal cosmopolitan bioethics is appreciated as stark and impoverished.[18]

As noted, in western bioethics, the burden of proof is weighed against traditional families and ways of life. Whereas the family plays a central role in traditional cultures and religions, its place in western bioethical decision-making is evermore marginalized. Western health care policy and law is framed in terms of individualistic consent, reflecting the centrality of the individual, and ensuring adequate opportunity for persons to free themselves from familial constraints. As Engelhardt argues:

> ... [C]onsider the contrast between those who favor autonomous individualism and those who would give moral priority to family life. Those who regard autonomous individualism as the presumptively appropriate relation among persons would require any deviations to be established by explicit statement and agreement. For example, patients would be presumptively treated as autonomous individuals willing and committed to choosing on their own, unless they explicitly demanded to be regarded and treated within a traditional family structure. ... On the other hand, if one considers life within a traditional family structure as the presumptively appropriate relation among persons, the burden of proof shifts. Persons are approached as nested within the thick expectations of traditional family structures, unless they explicitly state that they wish to be regarded and treated as isolated individuals (2002, pp. 24-25).

Consent in traditional cultures and religions is typically paternalistic and family-oriented, where patients may not even know their diagnosis, much less personally consent to treatment (Alora & Lumitao, 2000). Western bioethics, on the other hand, seeks legal requirements for patient-oriented confidentiality and informed consent to protect individual autonomous decision-making, shielding personal information from spouses, children, parents, and other relatives. Securing equal worth of liberty requires liberating morality and personal choice from traditional viewpoints, cultural practices, and religious beliefs. The goal is a secular ethic that begins with the privileged presumption of the sovereignty of the individual—individualistic autonomy and equal worth of liberty.

Those committed to such a goal often perceive ideologically directed state-based civic education of children as crucial for redressing practices incompatible with the privileged conceptions of equal worth of liberty and fair equality of opportunity. Again consider Rawls:

> ... a long and historic injustice to women is that they have borne, and continue to bear, a disproportionate share of the task of raising, nurturing, and car-

> ing for their children. … These injustices bear harshly not only on women, but also on their children and they tend to undermine children's capacity to acquire the political virtues required of future citizens in a viable democratic regime. Mill held that the family in his day was a school for male despotism: it inculcated habits of thought and ways of feeling and conduct incompatible with democracy. If so, the principles of justice enjoining democracy can plainly be invoked to reform it (2001, p. 166).

This goal is echoed in the United Nations' "Convention on the Elimination of all Forms of Discrimination Against Women." The Convention held that states ought legally to require education to combat what it perceived as inappropriate and unequal treatment of women:

> States shall take all appropriate measures:
>
> (a) To modify the social and cultural patterns of conduct of men and women, with a view to achieving the elimination of prejudices and customary and all other practices which are based on the idea of the inferiority or the superiority of either of the sexes or on stereotyped roles for men and women;
>
> (b) To ensure that family education includes a proper understanding of maternity as a social function and the recognition of the common responsibility of men and women in the upbringing and development of their children, it being understood that the interest of the children is the primordial consideration in all cases (1979, p. 4, art. 5).

In Rawlsian terms, state education of children is required to prepare the young "... to be fully cooperating members of society and enable them to be self-supporting; it should also encourage the political virtues so that they want to honor the fair terms of social cooperation in their relations with the rest of society" (Rawls, 1993, p. 199). The political virtues include toleration and mutual respect, together with a sense of fairness and civility (1993, p. 122). Such education teaches children "...such things as knowledge of their constitutional and civic rights ... to insure that their continued membership [in their parent's religion] is not based simply on ignorance of their basic rights or fear of punishment for offenses that do not exist" (1993, p. 199). Accordingly, the family must be subject to significant governmental regulation to ensure proper attitudes and beliefs.

Decisions regarding core curriculum in education are made with the express intention of diffusing this particular societal and civic, fully secular, culture. As Amy Gutmann comments:

> Some kinds of social diversity ... are anathema to political liberalism. Civic education should educate all children to appreciate the public value of toleration. The basic political principles of liberalism, those necessary to protect every person's basic liberties and opportunities, place substantial limits on social diversity. ... The limits on racial and gender discrimination, for example, enable many people to pursue ways of life that would otherwise be closed to them by discriminatory practices at the same time as they undermine or at least impede some traditional ways of life (1995, p. 559).[19]

Since the focal point of the moral life is autonomous self-determination, the celebration of free individualistic choice is appreciated as integral to the good life for persons.[20] The hope is that through such education the choice to remain in a traditional community or family can be shown to be morally deficient and thus progressively discouraged (Engelhardt, 2002, p. 25).[21] The liberal cosmopolitan ethos simply presumes the sovereignty of the individual, rather than the family, which in traditional forms is pejoratively caricatured as an institution of repression, injustice, and despotism.[22]

There is growing evidence that the civic education endorsed by the liberal cosmopolitan vision has had a significant impact on traditional religion. In a 1999 survey by the National Catholic Reporter, approximately 72% of Catholics responded that one could be a good Catholic without following the Vatican's teaching on birth control; 65% believed that one could be a good Catholic without following the Vatican's teaching on divorce and remarriage; and 53% responded that one could be a good Catholic without following the Vatican's teaching on abortion. Nearly 50% responded that individual choice should be the final arbiter of the morality of abortion, homosexual activity, and sexual relations outside of marriage more generally. Indeed, 23% reported that one could be a good Catholic without even believing that Christ rose from the dead, and 38% without believing in the Transubstantiation of the Eucharist (D'Antonio, 1999). Similarly, in one survey of Protestant pastors, 17% supported laws in favor of assisted-suicide, with over 33% of those surveyed who were also associated with the National Council of Churches in favor (Christian Century, 2000, pp. 948-949). Such data represent a striking departure from traditional belief and practice.

Here Hegel's account of why determinative moral content requires the specification of a particular context is illustrative: "Because every action explicitly calls for a particular content and a specific end, while duty as an abstraction entails nothing of the kind, the question arises: what is my duty? As an answer nothing is so far available except: (a) to do the right, and (b) to strive after welfare, one's own welfare, and welfare in universal terms, the welfare of others" (1967 [1821], p. 89, §134). Nothing particular follows from the general notions of duty, the right, and so forth. Thus, political struggles inevitably concern not merely which policies will best achieve desired objectives, but which objectives are themselves desirable, for whom, given what set of criteria; that is, which moral understanding should be established (e.g., pro-life or pro-choice, individualistic or family-oriented approaches to health care decision-making), utilizing which school of practice (e.g., allopathic, homeopathic, naturopathic, chiropractic, and so forth), at what standard of care (e.g., guaranteed equal access for all, or regional deviations and varying levels of insurance coverage). Even to sort useful information from noise, one must already possess a moral sense, standards of evidence and inference. That is, as Hegel noted, one must first specify a particular moral context within which to make moral distinctions and judgments. Removing or ignoring the theological and cultural particularities which mark religious and moral differences thereby eliminates any context for assessing the content and veracity of moral claims.

The aspirations of liberal cosmopolitan bioethics are thus revealed as especially insidious because they are subtly invasive, suggesting that one ought to side with the claims of "rationality", "expertise", and "consensus", i.e., with general secular bioethical "orthodoxy", over against what one may know in the fullness of a particular moral community to be true. To premise governmental and institutional policy on individualistic understandings of autonomy, or concerns for social justice and equality, simply begs the question, substituting post-traditional liberal individual-oriented ethical constructs for traditional family-oriented moral commitments. Those who choose to live within thick moral communities confront a governmental and institutional environment that is hostile to traditional understandings of moral goods and important family relationships.[23]

Outside of an appeal to an all encompassing moral and metaphysical viewpoint, outside of a particular moral context, moral truth appears deeply ambiguous. Without the presupposition of particular content, one cannot morality distinguish among different accounts of the nature of the good life, much less provide definitive guidance on how to proceed when the right and the good conflict. The inevitably post-modern character of contemporary bioethics, to which Engelhardt refers, is simply the recognition of the foundationally irresolvable character of such moral pluralism in general secular terms.

V. Forbearance Rights and the Freedom to Venture and Fail (Liberty$_4$)

The more general secular reason is unable to disclose a universal, content-full moral understanding of health care, or to secure justification for political authority to impose such a vision without begging the question, the more one must seek alternative foundations. Liberty$_4$ understood as freedom from interference, as expressed in the existence of significant forbearance rights, where persons are free to venture with others, open to the possibility that one's choices may lead to success or failure, will support the existence of a free-market in health care. In moral theoretical terms this consideration can be construed as a deontological moral concern, one focused on a right making condition that governs independently of a concern to realize a particular good, or a positive balance of benefits over harms.

Here, moral authority will not be drawn from assertions of so-called "moral consensus," ideal theories of rational action, or even deep moral intuitions regarding consequences, human rights, or cardinal moral concerns, but rather from the agreement of the parties to collaborate. Collaborators need not agree regarding the background ranking of values or moral principles, cultural or religious assumptions; they need only affirm the content of their agreement. No value standard or order must be presumed, just the recognition that collaboration is possible through agreement. Agreement or permission is the ground of the moral justification of such collaboration.

Forbearance rights create strong protections against battery, i.e., nonconsensual touching or use of one's person or property, defining a sphere in which one is morally immune from interference, protecting self-interest and self-preservation in the private use of person and property. Such rights describe side-constraints prohibiting nonconsensual interference, which hold against other persons, as well as society and state. Here the market is central for understanding authoritative human interaction. Market transactions and contractual relationships draw moral authority from the consent of the participants to be bound by their agreement. The parties to the transactions, themselves, freely convey authority to the enforcement of the specified conditions. Moral authority to interfere in the free interaction of consenting persons is created by, and thus limited to, the actual agreements of actual persons. The market is not affirmed as in itself good; rather, the idea of the market is the creation of social space for unencumbered personal interaction. The market is simply the result of respecting the moral authority of persons over themselves and their private property. Consequently, health care will not be appreciated as possessing any special priority or value: it will simply be among the many ways in which one may express oneself in peaceable consensual collaboration with others.

Liberty$_4$ grounds significant private property rights, where persons have exclusive control of their property, subject only to the constraints of prior agreements and the avoidance of using persons, and their property, who do not choose to participate.[24] Alienation, whether through abandonment, donation, exchange, or sale, is morally licit, if freely chosen. Provided that both vendor and purchaser freely agree to the transaction, property may be utilized for fun, beneficence, or profit, including the financing and purchase of health care. Absent actual agreement, forbearance rights act as side-constraints, defeating the claims of others, persons and governments, to have any entitlement to the time, talent, or property of individuals. Particular values or special considerations, such as equal positive worth of liberty or equal ability to impact political outcomes, fair equality of opportunity, benefits to others, or judgments of irrational choice, fail to establish moral authority either to create universal health care systems or to forbid consensual transactions for various types and standards of health care, shaped by varying moral commitments and taken-for-granted background assumptions.

Individuals, families, or communities, including traditional religious communities, would be free to contract for (1) various types of health care (e.g., allopathic, homeopathic, naturopathic, chiropractic, and so forth), with (2) particular standards of care (e.g., regional variations and varying levels of insurance coverage), (3) shaped through divergent moral commitments [e.g., Engelhardt's vision of Vaticare, Atheistcare, Islamicare, Jewishcare, and Texicare (p. 46)] and (4) framing presuppositions regarding health care practices (e.g., individual vs. family or community oriented consent, or varying concepts of health and disease (Cherry, 2000; Sadegh-Zadeh, 2000)). Imposition of all-encompassing uniform systems of health care, guarantees of equality in the provision of health care services, and the search for global standards regarding the foundations of health care policy violate basic human liberty: forbearance rights expressed as peaceable consensual interaction in the market.

The rights of persons will foreclose what many envision to be worthwhile goals. In contrast to $liberty_1$ as the entitlement to realize one's abilities or $liberty_2$ as ideal rational choice, forbearance rights recognize persons as only entitled to their own private resources and those additional resources which they are able peaceably to convince others to donate or sell to them. Basic human rights to health care, much less to the general amelioration of losses due to bad luck, individual choice, disease, ill health, or other misfortunes, do not exist.[25] Seen in this light, financing personal health care choices through coercive taxation, clearly forces those with substantive ethical commitments or content-full understandings of the good life, to be complicit in the purchase of health care services which they hold to be at best deviant (e.g., chiropractic or naturopathic), if not evil (e.g., abortion or embryo-research). Insofar as freedom is not merely one value among others, or a good which may be valued more or less along with other goods, but rather functions as a side-constraint, one may not injure, steal from, tax, defraud or otherwise coerce non-consenting others, even to produce good consequences. This would violate their status as free and responsible agents. One may not utilize persons, absent actual permission, merely as the means to benefit others.

Morally authorized statutes are confined to the protection of persons' rights to forbearance, protection of individuals from battery, and to those additional policies to which actual persons give actual consent. Persons, and organizations of persons, may be held responsible for nonconsensual acts of violence, fraud, and breach of contract, since such actions violate the rights of persons not to be touched or used without permission.[26] As a consequence, governments, even democratically elected majorities, do not possess moral authority to enforce uniform standards, to finance universal access or to regulate equal distribution of health care. Governmental authority created by the express agreement of those governed is also limited to the extent of such agreement. So grounded, the state would have the general character of a limited democracy. It would have no general moral authority to interfere in the medical marketplace. Forbearance rights make implausible interventions to forbid persons from freely using personal resources with consenting others, including the purchase of various types and levels of health care. Note, though, that the market is not being endorsed as a good in itself, nor are free choice and moral diversity celebrated in themselves as special goods. Rather, the market defines social space for peaceable consensual human interaction. As Engelhardt encapsulates the view, here morality exists as the "... marketplace of moral ideas and moral understandings within which each peaceably pursues his own ends without sharing a common, content-full moral vision or concrete view of justice" (p. 23). Respecting the freedom of persons defaults to protecting liberties of association, contract, conscience, and religion, and thereby to protecting the possibility of substantial moral diversity, including divergent incommensurable instantiations of liberty$_3$ (e.g., Orthodox Christian and Confucian).

Market incentives encourage persons to raise resources to further personal as well as social interests and goals, including the development of efficient and effective production and dissemination of health care. While often perceived solely in terms of pursuit of profit, the market does not preclude altruistic action. Churches and other charitable organizations could play a significant role in creating health care resources for the poor. Again, consider the sale of human organs for transplantation as a heuristic. One might envision individuals donating rights in organs directly to local churches, which would guarantee high quality health care for surgery and minimize other risks associated with donation. The organs could then be sold to the rich to raise funds to purchase health care, food, and medicine, or be made available for transplantation to the poor. One could imagine a group such as "Mother Theresa's Organs for the Poor" generating resources to provide health care for the impecunious. Such organizations could raise money to provide health care to those who could not otherwise purchase resources. One might think of creating "Catholic Kidneys International" to raise funds. Or, "Mother Theresa's Non-Profit Organs Inc.", brokering organs from the poor in developing countries to advantage those poor. The market creates social and political space to explore additional opportunities and incentives for organ procurement and allocation, without thereby forbidding other types of incentives and opportunities.

Freely chosen, market-based, health care financing, procurement, and distribution, respects the liberty of persons to pursue their own deep moral commitments. The market creates social and political space for the free interaction of individuals. It secures the possibility of diversity within particular states as well as for the emergence of a worldwide network of non-geographically based communities with their own particular understandings of moral probity, including bioethics, health care policy and institutional restrictions (Engelhardt, p. 23). Substantial moral diversity will likely exist: not due to any endorsement of diversity's value—indeed, it may be bitterly regretted—but because moral authority does not exist to foreclose peaceable consensual interaction. Coercively taxing others to create a comprehensive state-based health care system is prohibited, not because of the simple ascription of positive individual rights, but because of the lack of moral authority to so tax (see Bole, 2004). The permission of the parties to collaborate creates, rather than discovers, moral authority. Unlike $liberty_1$ as the right to realize one's abilities and choices or $liberty_2$ as ideal rational choice, $liberty_4$ understood as freedom from interference actually carves out and protects social and political space for the possibility of moral diversity in health care.

VI. Concluding Reflections on the Market and the Preservation of Liberty

An additional concern regarding the ability of the market to preserve liberty is that since obligations are imposed because of the parties manifesting consent to the agreement, such consent must be autonomous (see generally Prosser, 1971, p. 613). Here one must assess the possibility for autonomous consent to health care choices in the medical marketplace. One might argue that actual autonomous choice either does not exist, or may in some fashion be invalidated. For example, many argue that health care should not be considered a commodity to be distributed through market mechanisms because patients do not fully comprehend the implication of various health care options and are thereby precluded from making autonomous choices. "[M]arkets assume relationships of equality and independence. However, the relationship between a doctor and a patient is characterized by profound *inequality* and vulnerable *dependence* on the part of the patient" (Sulmasy, 1996, p. 313). While ignorance is not generally held to invalidate all choices and contracts, the claim is that the failure to understand significant life threatening risks associated with the provision of health care may be sufficient to raise the standard of proof for consent.

It is unclear, though, that markets fare worse regarding autonomy and free informed consent than other strategies for providing health care. Ignorance as a barrier to consent does not respect the distinction between universal, governmentally created, health care systems and market-oriented multi-tier health care systems. State-based systems simply replace marketplace choices and consumer preferences with bureaucratic policy crafted through political compromise and the universalistic claims of bioethicists to "moral expertise", enforced through coercive taxation and governmental regulation. Those living within governmental systems are usually ignorant of the full financial and empirical costs of the plan, such as the likely negative impact of extensive taxation on the economy, and lower standards of care due to implicit rationing and patient queuing. Voters are rarely, if ever, adequately informed of the likely impact of their choices.[27] Insofar as ignorance rules out autonomous choice in the health care marketplace, it similarly rules out "democratically" chosen social medical insurance plans.

Yet, not all private purchasers of health care will be ignorant of the various risks, nor will all be irremediably so. Insofar as persons are free to venture and fail, the market encourages the development of individual responsibility. It provides tutelage regarding the limits of the human condition and individual ability, as well as the ways in which past agreements can constrain future choices. Opportunities to receive consultation, to read through various plan documents, to learn from past mistakes, as well as to choose among moral and medical experts for consultation, prior to purchasing a particular plan, should ameliorate such concerns.

Coercion by need or other external circumstances similarly fails to meet the burden of proof to nullify the agreed to transaction. While it is true that the poor, in virtue of their poverty, have a narrower range of choices, in itself this situation does not invalidate free choice. As external conditions are admitted to defeat the claim that a sale or purchase was freely agreed to, they will also destroy the possibility of a market in any product, much less in health care. Every transaction would be subject to mutual reciprocal claims of external coercion (e.g., regarding food: coercion by hunger vs. coercion by the need to make a living selling groceries). Defeating the permissibility of the transaction requires demonstrating that one of the parties coerced the other or that circumstances rendered valid consent impossible. In the latter case, the parties are not directly in the relationship of coercer and coerced. Nor are there obvious grounds for holding that the circumstances of the external constraints of nature would render either party incompetent to choose. Other values may be offered peaceably to persuade persons not to enter into certain types of transactions or to motivate different choices, but free choice would in general trump. Much more would have to be made out to show that valid agreement would not be possible.

Finally, if the threat of significant harm increases the standard of proof for consent too greatly, this raises the additional concern that other important freedoms will be ruled out as well. Consider, for example, the circumstance where without a job one would starve or need to take a job which carries substantial risks (e.g., home roofing or oil-platform construction). Would autonomy be impossible in such circumstances? Or consider the possibility of harms due to poor choice in marriage. Yet, here significant peaceable manipulation abounds (e.g., seduction, offers of various financial or personal incentives). Even if some ought to be excluded from choosing among the various types of health care insurance programs, providers, standards of care, and services, for reasons of irremediable ignorance (e.g., the mentally disabled), Engelhardt and Delkeskamp-Hayes each makes clear that blanket prohibitions, universal bioethical declarations, violations of traditional religious and cultural beliefs, and paternalistic governmental decisions, in short, the imposition of a particular secular bioethical orthodoxy, do not serve the interests of liberty; such restrictions foreclose rather than enhance the possibility of moral diversity in health care.

Notes

1. Richard Titmuss provides one of the classic denouncements of the medical marketplace, regarding the sale of blood and blood products for transfusion: "... the commercialization of blood and donor relationships represses the expression of altruism, erodes the sense of community, lowers scientific standards, limits both personal and professional freedoms, sanctions the making of profits in hospitals and clinical laboratories, legalizes hostility between doctor and patient, subjects critical areas of medicine to the laws of the marketplace, places immense social costs on those least able to bear them—the poor, the sick and the inept—increases the dangers of unethical behaviour in various sectors of medical science and practice, and results in situations in which proportionately more and more blood is supplied by the poor, the unskilled, the unemployed, Negroes, and other low income groups and categories of exploited human populations of high blood yielders. Redistribution in terms of blood and blood products from the poor to the rich appears to be one of the dominant effects of the American blood banking system" (1971, pp. 245-246).

   Consider also Edmund Pellegrino on markets and managed care: "I refer here to how the books are 'balanced', and profits reaped—by the denial of claims, cutting of payments to physicians and hospitals, erecting new barriers to care, disenrolling patients and physicians who cost too much, and refusing grievances and appeals by defining medical necessity and experimental therapy ... I refer, too, to the legitimation of self-interest and profit-making on the part of physicians, investors, and managed care organizations" (1998, p. 106).
2. The power vested in the medical and bioethical community has become increasingly significant. Its authoritative judgment is sought on nearly all aspects of life: from copulation and birth, appropriate diet, sexual behaviors, and methods of child-rearing, to abortion, infanticide, suffering, and death. This is the medicalization of life. Judged solely in terms of expenditures, health care commands nearly one out of every seven dollars in the United States. In 2003 this amounted to 1.7 trillion dollars, some 15.3% of the Gross Domestic Product (GDP) (Rovner, 2004). Increasingly significant investment of personal and social resources is driven by a perceived technological and moral imperative to ameliorate the consequences of age, injury and disease, and thereby extend life and alleviate suffering. Moreover, bioethical expertise serves as the basis of expert testimony in courts of law (see, e.g., Morreim, 1997; Wildes, 1997) and is widely sought in the framing of public and institutional policy. Witness the broad advisory role of the President's Council on Bioethics in the United States, as well as the European Bioethics Convention, which sought not merely to explain or analyze moral issues but to justify political resolutions.
3. The United States Catholic Bishops have urged: "Our nation's health care system serves too few and costs too much. ... Every person has a right to adequate health care. This right flows from the sanctity of human life and the dignity that

belongs to all human persons, who are made in the image of God. Health care is more than a commodity; it is a basic human right, an essential safeguard of human life and dignity (Conference of Catholic Bishops, 1993, p. 1).

4. Consider: "Because health care is a fundamental good, the moral ideals of justice, equality, and community require that the health care system be universal, comprehensive, and equitable in the sharing of benefits and costs" (Brock & Daniels, 1994, p. 1189). "Health care needs are basic insofar as they promote fair equality of opportunity. Health care for children is especially important in relation to other social goods, because diseases and disabilities inhibit children's capacities to use and develop their talents, thereby curtailing their opportunities" (Kopelman, 2001, p. 202).

   Similarly, Article 3, of the Council of Europe's "Convention for the protection of human rights and dignity of the human being with regard to the application of biology and medicine: Convention on human rights and biomedicine" states: "Parties, taking into account health needs and available resources, shall take appropriate measures with a view to providing, within their jurisdiction, equitable access to health care of appropriate quality" (1997, p. 2, art. 3).
5. The United Nations' "Convention of the Rights of the Child" (adopted 1989, with entry into force September 2, 1990), for example, held "The child shall have the right to freedom of expression; this right shall include freedom to seek, receive and impart information and ideas of all kinds, regardless of frontiers, either orally, in writing or in print, in the form of art, or through any other media of the child's choice" (p. 6; art. 13). Moreover, that "States Parties shall respect the right of the child to freedom of thought, conscience and religion" (p. 6; art. 14).
6. This ethos is similar to Habermas's concept of a *herrschaftsfreier Diskurs,* where all whose interests are touched by a course of action have a voice in stating their particular needs: "Citizens are politically autonomous only if they can view themselves jointly as authors of the laws to which they are subject as individual addressees" (1995, p. 130). Habermas admits that his model of political discourse requires that all participants free themselves from too deep of an involvement with any particular values and principles: "... the truth claims of all reasonable worldviews have equal weight, where those worldviews count as reasonable which compete with one another in a reflexive attitude, that is, on the assumption that one's own truth claim could prevail in public discourse in the long run only though the force of better reasons" (Habermas, 1995, p. 125). They must not be burdened with the absolutist constraints of traditional religions and cultures.
7. Australia, Iceland, Japan, Norway, Sweden, and Switzerland.
8. Consider critical care: Because of the significant expense of such intense and technologically sophisticated care, it may not be economically feasible to provide universal, unlimited access to all those who might receive some marginal benefit. Choices regarding the use of ICU resources will have to be honestly faced. If the choice is to forgo access since it cannot be provided equally to everyone, this will lower the standard of care, permitting the death and suffering of many salvagable patients. Even different macro-allocations to health care, and within health care to critical care units, will result in significant variation in outcome. When comparing critical care in the United States and Great Britain utilizing the APACHE III scoring system, for example, outcomes of intensive

care are qualitatively and quantitatively lower in Britain than in the United States (Pappachan, Miller, Bennett *et al.*, 1999; Wood, Coursin, & Grounds, 1999).

9. As Alexis de Tocqueville frames this concern: "After having thus successively taken each member of the community in its powerful grasp and fashioned him at will, the supreme power then extends its arm over the whole community. It covers the surface of society with a network of small complicated rules, minute and uniform, through which the most original minds and the most energetic characters cannot penetrate, to rise above the crowd. The will of man is not shattered, but softened, bent, and guided ... Such a power does not destroy, but it prevents existence; it ... compresses, enervates, extinguishes, and stupefies a people, till each nation is reduced to nothing better than a flock of timid and industrious animals, of which the government is the shepherd" (1994, vol. II, p. 319).

   Here also, John Stuart Mill's illuminates the ways in which governmental and social paternalism inhibit the creation of genius: "Persons of genius, it is true, are, and are always likely to be, a small minority; but in order to have them, it is necessary to preserve the soil in which they grow. Genius can only breathe freely in an *atmosphere* of freedom. Persons of genius are, *ex vi termini,* more individual than any other people—less capable, consequently, of fitting themselves, without hurtful compression, into any of the small number of moulds which society provides in order to save its members the trouble of forming their own character" (*On Liberty,* Chapter 3, p. 11).

10. As Suzanne Poppema encapsulates: "I'm an abortion doctor ... What I do is right and good and important. Perhaps my story will appall some, but it also may inspire others, particularly the young women who need to know that the struggle between feminism and the patriarchy has not been in vain" (1996, p. 11).

11. According to "Health Canada", in British Columbia, Alberta, Ontario, Newfoundland and most facilities in Quebec, hospital and clinic fees for abortion are paid by the province. In the other provinces and territories, only abortions performed in hospitals are funded. [On-line.] Available: http://www.hc-sc.gc.ca.

12. In *Planned Parenthood v. Casey* (505 U.S. 833, 857-859 [1992]), for example, the court argued that in *Roe v. Wade* the significance of individual control over the self and to personal bodily integrity has been correctly applied to a woman's right to choose abortion: "... if *Roe* is seen as stating a rule of personal autonomy and bodily integrity, akin to cases recognizing limits on government power to mandate medical treatment or to bar its rejection, this court's post *Roe* decisions accord with *Roe*'s view that a state's interest in the protection of life falls *short of justifying* any plenary override of individual liberty claims." Concerns to preserve the unborn living fetus, even in cases of late term, partial birth abortion, which require that enough of the fetus' head be delivered to allow its brain to be vacuumed out, prior to removing the now dead fetus, failed to satisfy the burden of proof necessary to override the significance of individual authority over one's body. Respect for individual control over one's body, they argued, is of greater significance than preserving life.

13. John C. Calhoun noted that "The effect, then, of every increase is to enrich and strengthen the one and impoverish and weaken the other. This, indeed, may be carried to such an extent, that one class or portion of the community may be ele-

vated to wealth and power, and the other depressed to abject poverty and dependence, simply by the fiscal action of the government; and this too, through disbursements only – even under a system of equal taxes imposed for revenue only. If such may be the effect of taxes and disbursements, when confined to their legitimate objects – that of raising revenue for the public service – some conception may be formed, how one portion of the community may be crushed, and another elevated on its ruins, by systematically perverting the power of taxation and disbursement, for the purpose of aggrandizing and building up one portion of the community at the expense of the other" (1992, p. 19). Taxing traditional Christians for support of abortion rights, enhances the liberty of those who wish access to abortion, at the expense of the former.

14. There has even been the attempt to assert authority over bioethical professional training and competency assessment. See, for example, the American Society for Bioethics and the Humanities publication: *Core Competencies for Health Care Ethics Consultation* (1996), which itemized areas of competence, skills, and desirable personal traits for bioethics consultation.
15. The following are representative examples:

    1) The pronouncements of the Barcelona Declaration, which enumerated basic human rights to autonomy, dignity, integrity, and vulnerability (1995). Here, respecting personal autonomy is spelled out in terms of protecting and enhancing individual capacities for the "creation of ideas and goals of life", "moral insight, 'self-legislation', and privacy", "reflexion and action without coercion", "personal responsibility and political involvement", and informed consent (Sass, 2001, p. 219). Similarly, dignity, integrity, and vulnerability are explicated in terms of preserving the material, psychological, and social conditions for individuals to achieve their own abilities and goals. Respecting dignity requires ensuring that individuals are able to express "autonomous action", individual integrity compasses the "basic condition of the dignified life, both physical and mental … respect for privacy and in particular for the patient's understanding of his or her own life and illness…" (Sass, p. 220). Respecting persons, here, consists in appreciating the finitude and fragility of human life, which in turn is seen as grounding a general obligation to care for those who are perceived as vulnerable (Sass, p. 220). Thus, all must be guaranteed the material conditions as well as psychological and social support necessary to ameliorate physical, social, and health disadvantages. Each possess basic human rights to state assistance sufficient "to enable them to release their potential" (Sass, p. 220).

    2) The United Nations published guidelines on "HIV/AIDS and Human Rights" (1996), which specifically calls for unfettered access to abortion: "Laws should also be enacted to ensure women's reproductive and sexual rights, including the right of ... means of contraception, including safe and legal abortion and the freedom to choose among these, the right to determine number and spacing of children..." Failing to provide safe and legal abortion as a matter of positive right is understood as a violation of basic human rights.

    3) The Council of Europe's "Convention for the Protection of Human Rights and Dignity of the Human Being with regard to the Application of Biology and Medicine: Convention on Human Rights and Biomedicine" (1997), which held signing parties to protect the dignity and identity of all human beings, guaranteeing everyone, without discrimination, respect for integrity and other rights

and freedoms regarding the applications of biology and medicine. Such rights and freedoms included: individual-oriented free and informed consent, restrictions on the use of genetic testing, protections for human research subjects, and prohibitions on the sale of human organs for transplantation.

4) UNESCO's Universal Declaration on the Human Genome and Human Rights (1997).

16. As Engelhardt notes: Such opponents raise "...the specter that commercialization will threaten important ideals of equality. The premise is that purchasing organs will allow the rich to have access to treatment not available to the poor" (Engelhardt, 1999, p. 293).
17. Suggestions that moral guidance is to be found in respect for human vulnerability or social solidarity presumes background moral assumptions regarding appropriate expressions of beneficence. For example, some argue that protection of the vulnerable commands all to participate in the establishment of a totally encompassing welfare state, including universal single-tier governmentally regulated health care. Those who disagree are to be coerced into participation. Others argue that such concerns require understanding persons as free to refuse to be complicit in what one sees as evil, with beneficence, including basic welfare needs, limited to acts of private charity. Whose account should guide policy? Does "solidarity" command that all accept and participate in embryo experimentation and human cloning, or that all contribute through general taxation to its continued development? How with "respect for human vulnerability" should one respond to those who suffer with long term illness and disability: with encouragement towards an end in assisted suicide or towards baptism, rebirth, and redemption? Since secular reason cannot comprehend pain, disease, disability, and death as meaningful apart from the loss of the pleasures, beauty, and engagement of this world, suffering can only be experienced as surd. Thus, while some see assisted suicide as a justified act of kindness, love, and mercy, which preserves human dignity, others understand it to be murder and the complete denigration of personal dignity. It is unclear why "solidarity", "human dignity" and "human vulnerability" requires those who abhor such practices either to participate in or to finance assisted suicide.
18. Similarly, traditional Filipino culture does not share Western obsessions for individuality, equality, and personal autonomy. Instead, the family is the basic social unit: it is the primary means of financial and emotional support, education, career, and health care. As Kuan and Lumitao note: "Family interests take precedence over those of the individual members" (2001, p. 23). Families as a whole participate in successes, honors, and shames. As a result, Filipino health care does not support patient-based confidentiality or individual-oriented informed consent. Consent is fully family-oriented: "When a family member falls ill, he or she is considered to be in need of protection from the harmful effects of knowing the diagnosis, as well as the stress of decision-making. Family members automatically take the role of patient advocate, even requesting that the patient not be told the diagnosis. The dominant authority figure (the mother or father) together with older extended relatives take it upon themselves to talk with the physician and decide among treatment options" (2001, p. 24). Benevolent paternalism is thoroughly characteristic of the Filipino medical context.
19. As Will Kymlicka notes, this is precisely why traditional religious communities

seek to find exemption from such requirements: The aim is "...to integrate citizens into a modern societal culture, with its common academic, economic, and political institutions, and this is precisely what ethnoreligious sects wish to avoid. Moreover, the sorts of laws from which these groups seek exemption are precisely the sorts of laws which lie at the heart of modern nation-building—for example, mass education" (2001, p. 37).

20. John Harris encapsulates the position: "... we need to remind ourselves of the point of valuing liberty—freedom of choice. The point of autonomy, the point of choosing and having the freedom to choose between competing conceptions of how, and indeed why, to live, is simply that it is only thus that our lives become in any real sense our own. The value of our lives is the value we give to our lives. And we do this, so far as this is possible at all, by shaping our lives for ourselves" (1995, p. 11).
21. As Rawls acknowledges, the concern to support equal worth of liberty through fair equality of opportunity even tends towards the dissolution of the family: "The consistent application of the principle of fair opportunity requires us to view persons independently from the influences of their social position. But how far should this tendency be carried? It seems that even when fair equality of opportunity (as it has been defined) is satisfied, the family will lead to unequal chance between individuals. ... Is the family to be abolished then? Taken by itself and given a certain primacy, the idea of equal opportunity inclines in this direction" (1999, p. 448).

    Similarly, the United Nations' "Convention on the Elimination of all Forms of Discrimination against Women" specifically sets as a goal the systematic changing of the traditional roles of men and women, and of the family (1979, p. 2, Preamble).
22. Such an ethos is not morally neutral. Consider, for example, the claim that appropriate procreative autonomy requires sweeping access to prenatal screening technology to detect genetic abnormalities, such as trisomy 21, which causes Down's Syndrome, coupled with unfettered access to non-therapeutic abortion. Genetics counseling, it is argued, should cover all of the various options, including the appropriateness of abortion (Becker, 2002, pp. 118-124). The goal of such counseling is "... to empower her (the pregnant woman) to informed and independent decision-making as to which course of action to take at each step in the screening and testing process .... It is assumed that the woman's autonomy is best respected if the service empowers her to independent decision-making..." (Becker, 2002, pp. 119-120). The benefits of screening are seen primarily in terms of informed choices regarding selective abortion. Indeed, in the United States failure to inform pregnant women of the possibility of non-therapeutic abortion has exposed genetic counselors to civil liability under the law of torts (Milunsky & Annas 1976). Such suits typically allege malpractice on grounds of either "wrongful life" or "wrongful birth". Civil claims for "wrongful life" involve parental suit on behalf of the child alleging that his nonexistence would have been preferable to his current existence with defects, such that his existence is a wrong done to him as a result of the negligence of the genetic counselor. Under a wrongful birth civil suit, the parents allege emotional and financial harms associated with caring for a defective newborn, whom they would have chosen to abort if they had been informed of the appropriateness of the option. Such

legally supported torts, require counselors to encourage patients to seek abortions based on quality-of-life judgments, even if in violation of deeply held religious convictions (Atkinson & Moraczewski, 1980, pp. 27-29). As Becker notes in passing, however, most surveys find that over 90% of trisomy 21 diagnosis cases end in abortion (2002, p. 115). Significantly increased incidence of abortion is the undeniable result of prenatal testing and genetics counseling. Here, authoritative state endorsement gave a powerful voice to secular individualistic autonomy.

23. Qui Ren-Zong argues that as western bioethics has become the basis of "global bioethics", and it has thereby become the basis for imperialistic war: "A so-called global bioethics may borrow some canons of morality from existing bioethics or invent something new. The fact is that Western bioethics is dominant in the world. So, the newly articulated global bioethics may be tainted with a strong color of Western culture, or may be just ... another version of Western bioethics within the clothes of global bioethics. When it is imposed on the non-Western communities or heretic communities within Western culture, this constitutes ethical imperialism. Now the warning has become reality. When some country or a number of countries makes a military action somewhere using the excuse of protecting the universal value of human rights, it is claimed that it is an ethical war, but it is a war of ethical imperialism" (2002, p. 85).

    Here, one might also consider the established European norms on minority rights, as adopted by the Organization for Security and Co-operation in Europe (OSCE, 1990) or the Framework Convention for the Protection of National Minorities adopted by the Council of Europe (1995). According to an OSCE report: minority rights "are matters of legitimate international concern and consequently do not constitute exclusively an internal affair of the respective State" (quoted in Kymlicka & Opalski, 2001, p. 4). Failure to accommodate to the western liberal cosmopolitan understandings of liberty is seen as a violation of basic human rights and, thereby, justification for international response.

24. Blackstone, reflecting on the common law of England, argued: "There is nothing which so generally strikes the imagination and engages the affections of mankind, as the right of property; or that sole and despotic dominion which one man claims and exercises over the external things of the world, in total exclusion of the right of any other individual in the universe (1803, book 2, p. 1). The nature of property rights, their character, scope, and form, was drawn from the nature of persons. Under the traditional law of torts, the person includes any part of the body as well as anything attached to it and practically identified with it. Violation of a person included nonconsensual contact with the individual's "...clothing, or with a cane, a paper, or any other object held in his hand..." (Prosser, 1971, p. 34). Interest in the integrity of the person included his body and all the things intimately associated with it. As such, property is an extension of the person and is protected as part of the individual's forbearance rights against battery, unauthorized touching or use.

25. Note, such an account is consistent with understanding persons as free to choose to participate in insurance schemes which created welfare rights for the poor, ill, or disadvantaged, however "disadvantaged" is defined. One could imagine Atheistcare as including rights to third-party assisted reproduction, human cloning, abortion, organ vending for transplantation, and assisted sui-

cide, to protect those "disadvantaged" is such areas of life, while members of Vaticare might accept lower standards of care in deference to providing more care or equal care for the poor. State authority would not exist to force insurance plans to offer compatible comprehensive levels of coverage. In general, it would be an illicit use of force to compel either participation or taxpayer financing of any such scheme, even through majority democratic rule. The moral authority to interfere with such rights is limited to peaceable consent among persons and communities.

26. As Locke notes, governments which use the property of their citizens without permission are not conceptually different than thieves: "Wherever law ends, tyranny begins, if the law be transgressed to another's harm; and whosoever in authority exceeds the power given him by the law, and makes use of the force he has under his command to compass that upon the subject which the law allows not, ceases in that to be a magistrate, and acting without authority may be opposed, as any other man who by force invades the right of another" (1690, p. §202).
27. Here independent clinical outcome studies, such as those based on the APACHE III scoring system, will be important for exposing the hidden costs. Such data allows one to compare outcomes across large populations of ICUs and patients, tracking quantitative and qualitative outcome. In short, it tracks the vectors of the cost-benefit curve, allowing honest assessment of the benefits and harms of allocating medical and financial resources to critical care.

References

___. (2000). 'Protestant pastors support death penalty,' *Christian Century*, September 27-October 4, 948-949.

Acton, L. (1988). *Essays in Religion, Politics, and Morality*, (Ed., J. R. Fears). Indianapolis: Liberty Classics.

Alora, A., & Lumitao, J., (eds.) (2001). *Beyond a Western Bioethics: Voices from the Developing World.* Washington, D.C.: Georgetown University Press.

American Society for Bioethics and Humanities (1996). *Core Competencies for Health Care Ethics Consultation.* Glenview: American Society for Bioethics and Humanities.

Andorno, R. (2002). 'Biomedicine and international human rights law: In search of a global consensus,' *Bulletin of the World Health Organization*, 80(12), 959-963.

Atkinson, G., & Moraczewski, A. (Eds.) (1980). *Genetic Counseling, the Church & the Law; A Task Force Report of the Pope John Center.* St. Louis: Pope John XXIII Medical-Moral Research and Education Center.

Becker, G. (2002). 'The ethics of prenatal screening and the search for global bioethics,' in J. Tao (Ed.), *Cross-Cultural Perspectives on the (Im)Possibility of Global Bioethics*, (pp. 105-130). Dordrecht: Kluwer Academic Publishers.

Blackstone, W. (1803). *Commentaries on the Laws of England*, (Ed., G. Tucker). New York: Augustus M. Kelley Publishers; South Hackensack, N.J.: Rothman Reprints, Inc.

Bole, T. (2004). 'The perversity of Thomistic natural law theory,' in M.J. Cherry (Ed.), *Natural Law and the Possibility of a Global Ethics*, (pp. 141-147).

Dordrecht: Kluwer Academic Publishers.
Brock, D., & N. Daniels (1994). 'Ethical foundations of the Clinton administration's proposed health care system,' *Journal of the American Medical Association*, 271(15), 1189-1196.
Calhoun, J. C. (1992). *Union and Liberty: The Political Philosophy of John C. Calhoun*, (Ed., R. Lence). Indianapolis: Liberty Classics.
Callahan, D. (1987). *Setting Limits: Medical Goals in an Aging Society*. New York: Simon and Schuster.
Conference of Catholic Bishops. (1993). *Comprehensive Health Care Reform, Protecting Human Life, Protecting Human Dignity, Pursuing the Common Good.*
Council of Europe. (1997). *Convention for the protection of human rights and dignity of the human being with regard to the application of biology and medicine: convention on human rights and biomedicine.* Oviedo: Council of Europe.
Cherry, M. (2000). 'Polymorphic medical ontologies: Fashioning concepts of disease,' *The Journal of Medicine and Philosophy*, 25(5), 519-538.
Cherry, M. (2002a). 'Coveting an international bioethics: universal aspirations and false promises,' in H.T. Engelhardt, Jr. & Rasmussen, L.M. (Eds.), *Bioethics and Moral Content: National Traditions of Health Care Morality*, (pp. 251-279). Dordrecht: Kluwer Academic Publishers.
Cherry, M. (2002b). 'The search for a global bioethics. Fraudulent claims and false promises,' *The Journal of Medicine and Philosophy*, 27(6), 683-698.
Council of Europe. (1995). *Framework convention for the protection of national minorities.* Oviedo: Council of Europe.
Daniels, N. (1976). 'Equal liberty and unequal worth of liberty,' in N. Daniels (Ed.), *Reading Rawls*. New York: Basic Books.
Daniels, N. (1996). *Justice and Justification*. Cambridge: Cambridge University Press.
D'Antonio, W.V. (1999, October 29). 'Trends in U.S. Roman Catholic attitudes, beliefs, behavior,' *National Catholic Reporter*.
Engelhardt, H.T., Jr. (1999). 'The body for fun, beneficence, and profit: A variation on a post-modern theme,' in M.J. Cherry (Ed.), *Persons and Their Bodies: Rights, Responsibilities, Relationships*, (pp. 277-302). Dordrecht: Kluwer Academic Publishers.
Engelhardt, H.T., Jr. (2000). *The Foundations of Christian Bioethics*. Lisse: Swets and Zeitlinger.
Engelhardt, H.T., Jr. (2002). 'Morality, universality, and particularity: Rethinking the role of community in the foundations of bioethics,' in J. Tao (Ed.), *Cross-Cultural Perspectives on the (Im)Possibility of Global Bioethics*, (pp. 19-40). Dordrecht: Kluwer Academic Publishers.
Engelhardt, H.T., Jr. (2003). 'Introduction: bioethics as a global phenomenon,' in J. Peppin & Cherry, M.J. (Eds.), *Regional Perspectives in Bioethics*, (pp. xiii-xxii). Lisse: Swets and Zeitlinger Publishers.
Esmail, N., & Walker, M. (2002). *How Good is Canadian Health Care*. Vancouver: The Fraser Institute.
Esmail, N., & Walker, M. (2004). *Waiting Your Turn: Hospital Waiting Lists in Canada*. Vancouver: The Fraser Institute.
Gutmann, A. (1995). 'Civic education and social diversity,' *Ethics*, 105(3), 557-579.
Habermas, J. (1995). 'Reconciliation through the public use of reason: Remarks on

John Rawls's *Political Liberalism,' The Journal of Philosophy,* XCII (3), 109-131.
Harris, J. (1995). 'Euthanasia and the value of life,' in J. Keown (Ed.), *Euthanasia Examined.* Cambridge: Cambridge University Press.
Hegel, G.W.F. (1967) [1821]. *Philosophy of Right* (Trans. T.M. Knox). New York: Oxford University Press.
Iglehart, J. (1990). 'Canada's health care system faces its problems,' *New England Journal of Medicine,* 322(8), 562-568.
Joseph, T. (2002). 'Living and dying in a post-traditional world,' in J. Tao (Ed.), *Cross-Cultural Perspectives on the (Im)Possibility of Global Bioethics.* Dordrecht: Kluwer Academic Publishers.
Kopelman, L. (2001). 'On duties to provide basic health and dental care to children,' *The Journal of Medicine and Philosophy,* 26(2), 193-209.
Khushf, G. (1994). 'Intolerant tolerance,' *The Journal of Medicine and Philosophy,* 19(2), 161-181.
Kuan, L.G. & Lumitao, J.M. (2001). 'The family and health care practices," in A. Alora & J. Lunita (eds.), *Beyond Western Bioethics: Voices from the Developing World.* Washington, D.C.: Georgetown University Press, pp. 23-30.
Kymlicka, W. (2001). 'Western political theory and ethnic relations in Eastern Europe,' in W. Kymlicka & Opalski, M. (Eds.), *Can Liberal Pluralism be Exported? Western Political Theory and Ethnic Relations in Eastern Europe.* New York: Oxford University Press.
Kymlicka, W., & Opalski, M. (2001). 'Introduction,' in W. Kymlicka & Opalski, M. (Eds.), *Can Liberal Pluralism be Exported? Western Political Theory and Ethnic Relations in Eastern Europe.* New York: Oxford University Press.
Locke, J. (1980) [1690]. *Second Treatise of Government,* (Ed., C.B. Macpherson). Indianapolis: Hackett Publishing Co.
McHugh, J. (1994). 'Health care reform and abortion: A Catholic moral perspective,' *The Journal of Medicine and Philosophy,* 19(5), 491-500.
Mill, J.S. (1999) [1869]. *On Liberty,* (4th ed). London: Longman, Roberts & Green. [Online]. Available: http://www.bartleby.com/130/.
Milunsky, A., & G. Annas. (1976). 'Prenatal diagnosis of genetic disorders: An analysis of experience with 600 cases,' *Journal of the American Medical Association,* 230(2),232.
Morreim, E.H. (1997). 'Bioethics, expertise, and the courts: An overview and an argument for inevitability,' *The Journal of Medicine and Philosophy,* 22(4), 291-295.
Nuffield Council on Bioethics. (1995). *Human Tissue: Ethical and Legal Issues.* London.
Office of the United Nations High Commissioner for Human Rights and the Joint United National Programme on HIV/AIDS. (1996, September 23-25). HIV/AIDS and Human Rights: International Guidelines. Geneva: United Nations.
Organization for Security and Co-operation in Europe. (1990). *OSCE Handbook.*
Pappachan, J.V., B.B. Millar, & E.D. Bennett. (1999). 'Comparison of APACHE III outcome from intensive care admission after adjustment for case mix by the APACHE III prognostic system,' *Chest,* 115 (3), 802-810.
Pellegrino, E. (1998). 'The good samaritan in the marketplace: Managed care's challenge to Christian charity,' in J. Kilner (Ed.), *The Changing Face of Health*

Care (pp. 103-118). Grand Rapids: Eerdsmans Publishing Company.
Poppema, S. T. (1996). *Why I am an Abortion Doctor.* Amherst: Prometheus Books.
Prosser, W. (1971). *Law of Torts.* St. Paul: West Publishing Co.
Qiu, R.-Z. (2002). 'The tension between biomedical technology and Confucian values,' in J. Tao (Ed.), *Cross-Cultural Perspectives on the (Im)Possibility of Global Bioethics,* (pp. 71-88). Dordrecht: Kluwer Academic Publishers.
Rankin, R.N. (1999). 'Magnetic resonance imaging in Canada: dissemination and funding.' *Canadian Association of Radiology Journal,* 50 (2), 89-92.
Rawls, J. (1993). *Political Liberalism.* New York: Columbia University Press.
Rawls, J. (1999). *A Theory of Justice,* (2nd ed). Cambridge: Harvard University Press.
Rawls, J. (2001). *Justice as Fairness: A Restatement,* (Ed., E. Kelly). Cambridge: Harvard University Press.
Rovner, J. (2004, February 11). 'U.S. health spending increase expected to slow,' Reuters.
Sadegh-Zadeh, K. (2000). 'Fuzzy health, illness, and disease,' *The Journal of Medicine and Philosophy,* 25(5), 605-638.
Sass, H.-M. (2001). 'Introduction: European bioethics on a rocky road,' *The Journal of Medicine and Philosophy,* 26(3), 215-224.
Schmidt, K. (2002). 'Stabilizing or changing identity? The ethical problem of sex reassignment surgery as a conflict among the individual, community, and society,' in J. Tao (Ed.), *Cross-Cultural Perspectives on the (Im)Possibility of Global Bioethics,* (pp. 237-264). Dordrecht: Kluwer Academic Publishers.
Scott, R. (1990). 'The human body: Belonging and control,' *Transplantation Proceedings,* 22(3), 1002-1004.
Sulmasy, D. P. (1996). 'Do the bishops have it right on health care reform?,' *Christian Bioethics,* 2(3), 309-325.
Tao, J. (2002). 'Is just caring possible? Challenge to bioethics in the new century,' in J. Tao (Ed.), *Cross-Cultural Perspectives on the (Im)Possibility of Global Bioethics,* (pp. 41-58). Dordrecht: Kluwer Academic Publishers.
Titmuss, R. (1971). *The Gift Relationship.* New York: Vintage Books.
Tocqueville, A. de (1994) [1835]. *Democracy in America.* London: David Campbell Publishers, Ltd.
Torcello, L., & Wear, S. (2000). 'The commercialization of human body parts: A reappraisal from a Protestant perspective,' *Christian Bioethics,* 6(2), 153-170.
Transplantation Society. (1970). 'Statement of the committee on morals and ethics of the Transplantation Society,' *Annals of Internal Medicine,* 75, 631-633.
United Nations. (1979). Convention of the Elimination of All Forms of Discrimination Against Women. Geneva: United Nations.
United Nations. (1989). Convention on the Rights of the Child. Geneva: United Nations.
United Nations. (1997). International Covenant on Economic, Social, and Cultural Rights. Geneva: United Nations.
Wildes, K. (1997). 'Healthy skepticism: The emperor has very few clothes,' *The Journal of Medicine and Philosophy,* 22(4), 365-371.
Wilkins, R., Adams, O., & Brancker, A. (1989a). 'Changes in mortality by income in urban Canada from 1971 to 1986: Findings of a joint study undertaken by the policy, communications, and information branch, health and welfare

Canada, and the Canadian centre for health information statistics, Canada.'
Wood, K.E., Coursin, D.B., & Grounds, R.M. (1999). 'Critical care outcomes in the United Kingdom: Sobering wake-up call or stability of the lamppost?,' *Chest*, 115(3), 614-616.
Working Group of the International Bioethics Association on the Possibility of Elaborating a Universal Instrument on Bioethics. (2003). Draft Report. Paris: United Nations, Educational, Scientific, and Cultural Organization.
World Health Organization. (1991). 'Human organ transplantation: A report on the developments under the auspices of the WHO,' *International Digest of Health Legislation*, 42(3), 389-396.

Manifesto: Moral Diversity in Health Care Ethics

Nicholas Capaldi

> We oppose the adoption or imposition of uniform codes for moral decision making in healthcare. This opposition extends to regional, national, and global contexts
>
> .

I. Theoretical Arguments Against Uniformity

A. Moral Diversity as Reality

De Facto we live in a morally pluralistic world. The essays by Fan and Tao make this case with regard to non-western cultures, and Bayertz exemplifies diversity even with seemingly homogeneous societies in the EU. There may even be potential conflicts among cultures. In a seminal article and controversy in *Foreign Affairs,* Samuel Huntington (1993) extended into the foreign policy arena some of the domestic debates in the U.S. that have gone on under the name of multi-culturalism. He points out that what we are witnessing is not simply a contrast between a romantic belief in national roots and a more encompassing cosmopolitanism which espouses universal themes. Given the levels of prosperity in new parts of the world, accompanied by the perception, real or imagined, of Western decadence, and the interest in recovering an historical past, there are now *new transnational sentiments* which are neither nationalistic nor cosmopolitan, but informed by "Civilizational" differences. The idea is that Serbia, Russia and Greece are in

H.T. Engelhardt, Jr. (ed), *Global Bioethics* (pp. 131–153).

sympathy, not for reasons of power politics, but because of a shared Eastern Orthodox Christianity. Similarly, Hindu South Asia, Muslim Middle East and Asia, Catholic and Indian Latin America, Confucian China, and Japan are the bases for a "Clash of Civilizations." It would be difficult to understand the anguish within Islamic cultures, for example, without recognizing such conflicts (Scruton, 2002).

Is there a way of overcoming such conflicts and constructing a Global Ethics? At first sight, the answer to this question is 'yes' because prominent international institutions and individuals keep assuring us that this is the case and producing lists of example of global ethics. On second thought, these lists can be summarily dismissed as no more than ritualistic. At best, these lists consist of procedural norms rather than substantive norms. It is not enough for ethicists to agree on a procedural norm, like respect the patient's autonomy, when there are underlying disagreements about the substantive meaning of a norm. Would 'autonomy' mean the same thing in different cultures? It clearly does not mean the same thing to everyone who invokes it even in our own culture! This is why it is so easy to agree on a list and then apply it in conflicting ways. These lists also reflect the full-flowering of intellectual platitudinarianism whose best counterpart is the language of professional diplomacy. These lists are sometimes examples of intellectual imperialism,[1] that is, self-proclaimed universalists too often turn out to be de-racinated intellectuals from the West or those who have been educated in the West or who teach in the West and reflect a kind of rent-seeking by a particular class interest.[2]

The universalist proposals reflect an important dimension of western liberalism. This raises four important questions we need to ask about liberalism. Is there a consensus among western intellectuals about the meaning of liberal universalism? What is the source of its authority (legitimacy)? Can it sustain itself without appeal to some form of transcendence? Is it universalizable or is it a culturally limited and historically transient phenomenon?[3]

Unfortunately, there is no consensus on the meaning of liberalism even among western intellectuals.[4] With regard to its legitimacy, there have been three historically distinct forms of legitimation: pre-Enlightenment, Enlightenment, and post-Enlightenment. During its pre-Enlightenment period, liberalism was justified by appeal either to transcendence, nature, or reason. The pre-Enlightenment version is the one that animates the American Founding (Thomas West). During the Enlightenment, liberalism was justified by an appeal to science. The most significant intellectual development from the point of view of justifying liberalism has been the collapse of the faith in scientism. It is now generally recognized (Rorty, MacIntyre, Gray, Capaldi) that science is not self-legitimating. This has led to what Arendt has called the legitimation crisis at least among secular liberals. The secular response has been to try to justify liberalism simply in terms of conventional assent (Rorty, Habermas, Gray). The other contemporary response is to retrieve the sense of the transcendent for liberalism (Maritain, Novak, and Neuhaus). Moral pluralism seems to be a feature not only of the world in general but even within our own culture. Can liberal culture survive as just one among many if it loses the belief in its own universalizability? Can transcendence be retrieved? Would the belief in transcendence allow for both universalizability and convergence among diverse cultures?

Can the issue of universalizability, that is, whether liberal culture is a potentially useful model for the rest of the world, even be posed except within Western culture? That is, are there even resources in non-Western cultures for dealing with this issue?

B. Moral Diversity Is Inherent in the Human Condition

So far, we have been content to document the de facto existence of moral pluralism. We turn now to considerations of why there is inevitable pluralism. Our account is based on the insights of Michael Oakeshott. According to Oakeshott, there is no such thing as human nature, only the human predicament. By 'nature' he means an objective built-in teleology universally present in all human beings. This he denies. There may be truths about the human predicament but these do not amount to a 'nature' in the classical sense of the term. One fundamental feature of that predicament is human freedom. That is why no individual is a cultural automaton, why any child makes up new sentences, that is, sentences not previously heard. Freedom is part of the ordeal of consciousness within which we create ourselves continually and our understanding of the world based on our experience of it. The way in which this task is accomplished is through learning. However, what distinguishes us from animals is that *we are free to choose how we interpret experience. Experience does not come to us in pre-packaged units.* This is why any reductive scientistic account of the mind or learning (e.g., A.I.) is bound to fail. Our freedom is employed in our imagination and intelligence; these faculties are used in defining ourselves as individuals and in giving meaning to our experience of the world we inhabit; this engagement is called learning and is the source of our humanity. An individual freely chooses meaningful ways of understanding himself and the world around him. We must use our imagination in order to learn. It is the unique ordering of our experience in imagination that makes us unique individuals.

One of the most important ways in which we utilize our imagination is in reconstructing the thought of other persons. What role does our cultural inheritance play in all of this? It is only through interaction with our inheritance that we become who we are. A cultural inheritance is a set of cultural achievements and practices, not a doctrine to be learned. The content of an inheritance can only be conveyed in the form of meanings. The inheritance is re-created through its appropriation; is not homogeneous; there is no final or definitive formulation of it; and within it there are many voices. Postmodernism can add nothing substantive to this Oakshottean account.

One other implication is worth stressing. It follows from what has been said about diversity being inherent that a cultural inheritance can never be definitively formulated. Moreover, every inheritance has to be periodically reformulated to address novel conditions. The problem of diversity is not simply between and among different moral communities but within each moral community.

C. The Inevitability of Moral Epistemological Relativism

Tris Engelhardt has made the following powerful case against the possibility of a philosophical resolution of moral diversity. It is not simply the case that there are significant moral disagreements about substantive issues. Many if not most of these controversies do not appear to be resolvable through sound rational argument. On the one hand, many of the controversies depend upon different foundational metaphysical commitments. As with most metaphysical controversies resolution is possible only through the granting of particular initial premises and rules of evidence. On the other hand, even when foundational metaphysical issues do not appear to be at stake, the debates turn on different rankings of the good. Again, resolution does not appear to be feasible without begging the question, arguing in a circle, or engaging in infinite regress. One cannot appeal to consequences without knowing how to rank the impact of different approaches with regard to different moral interests (liberty, equality, prosperity, security, etc.). Nor can one uncontroversially appeal to preference satisfaction unless one already grants how one will correct preferences and compare rational versus impassioned preferences, as well as calculate the discount rate for preferences over time. Appeals to disinterested observers, hypothetical choosers, or hypothetical contractors will not avail either. If such decision makers are truly disinterested, they will choose nothing. To choose in a particular way, they must be fitted out with a particular moral sense or thin theory of the good. Intuitions can be met with contrary intuitions. Any particular balancing of claims can be countered with a different approach to achieving a balance. In order to appeal for guidance to any account of moral rationality one must already have secured content for that moral rationality.

Not only is there a strident moral diversity defining debates regarding all substantive issues, but there is in principle good reason to hold that these debates cannot be brought to closure in a principled fashion through sound rational argument. As Alasdair MacIntyre put it, "There seems to be no rational way of securing moral agreement in our culture."[5] The partisans of each and every position find themselves embedded within their own discourse so that they are unable to step outside of their own respective hermeneutic circles without embracing new and divergent premises and rules of inferences. Many traditional thinkers find themselves in precisely this position. They are so enmeshed in their own metaphysics and epistemology, so convinced that they are committed to 'reason' when what they are committed to is a particular set of premises and rules, so able to see the 'flaws' in the positions of others who do not accept the same rules, that they quite literally do not understand the alternative positions or even how there can be other positions. More important, they fail to understand the character of contemporary moral debate. What is peculiar about contemporary moral debate is not just the incessant controversy but the absence of any basis for bringing the controversies to a conclusion in a principled fashion. "...philosophy has gone into a deep coma, or, if you prefer, a state of clinical death."[6]

At this point, I am likely to be accused of flirting with or promoting moral relativism or the denying that there is an objective canonical moral truth or a canonical normative account of a subjective truth, or reducing morality to aesthetics or historicism. Nothing could be further from the truth, but the mere fact that such a suspicion is entertained evidences my claim that there is a more fundamental misunderstanding. I am not denying the possibility of moral truth. What I am claiming is that the contemporary world is marked by a moral pluralism that reflects two things: (a) the impossibility of resolving moral controversies by sound rational argument based on generally available *secular* moral premises, and (b) that true moral knowledge presupposes a *personal transformation of the knower.*[7] The special relevance of this is that a large part of traditional or classically-inspired thinking reflects a confidence in 'reason' that can only be understood as misplaced in discursive rationality's capacity to provide a canonical content-full moral understanding of right conduct. What I am suggesting is that we must take seriously *the limits of discursive moral epistemology.*

Moral epistemic skepticism is not the same as metaphysical moral skepticism. Moral epistemic skepticism acknowledges the limits of resolving moral controversies through sound rational argument; metaphysical moral skepticism doubts whether there is moral truth; one can be skeptical about discursive moral rationality's ability to establish a canonical moral understanding without being a metaphysical moral skeptic.

Many within the profession of philosophy think that moral epistemic skepticism can be overcome. Philosophy, in general, has a narrative that is monistic and naturalistic (the world is fully intelligible in its own terms); rationalistic (everything is in principle conceptualizable); impersonal (the ultimate principles of intelligibility have no direct reference or concern for human welfare); and secularly Pelagian (despite the impersonality, humanity can solve its problems on its own). The latest and most powerful and ambitious expression of the philosophic impulse is to be found in the Enlightenment Project.[8] *The Enlightenment Project was the attempt to define and explain the human predicament through science as well as to achieve mastery over it through the use of a social technology.*[9] This project originated in France in the eighteenth century with the *philosophes,* was promoted by positivists in the 19th century, and has come to dominate the intellectual world in the 20th century. The notion that one can formulate an ethical 'theory' and then apply that theory as a form of 'applied' ethics is a notion derived from and promoted by contemporary analytic philosophy. Its analogue is the commonly accepted view that engineering is applied physical science or that medicine is applied biology. Many, but not all, bioethicists, are analytic philosophers manqué (see Solomon).

The Enlightenment Project's attempt to overcome epistemological moral skepticism is as follows. The axiology of the Enlightenment Project (and therefore of the analytic philosophy of bioethical expertise) asserts the primacy of theoretical knowledge. As a consequence of scientism, theoretical knowledge is primary and practical knowledge has a secondary status. The philosophical challenge is not merely to identify the realm of the practical but to explain it theoretically. This leads to a dichotomy of fact and value: (a) Only factual judgments can be true. Value judgments are not truths because they do not refer to structures independent of the observer or agents. This does not, however, in the eyes of supporters of the Enlightenment Project preclude a science of ethics. *Values are a kind of epiphenomenon* (emergent properties to use the current jargon). Given the primacy of theoretical knowledge and the derivative nature of the social sciences, there can be a physical-scientific and/or social-scientific factual account of the *sub-structure* of the context within which *values* function. This is how the realm of the practical will be explained, ultimately, in theoretical terms.

There is a two-tier view of human psychology in which values are epiphenomena with a materialist sub-structure. The relevant explanatory constituents of the sub-structure are physiological drives; that is, there is no real freedom of the will.[10] Liberty is compatible with sub-structure determinism only if liberty is construed as the *absence of arbitrary external constraints,* and where restraints are determined to be arbitrary relative to the fundamental drives. The fundamental drives alleged to exist in the sub-structure are neither culture specific nor conscious level specific but physiological (e.g., seeking pleasure), and therefore more universal. The fundamental drives also seek, it is presumed, some kind of *homeostasis* or maximization that permits negotiation or overruling specific rules (*utilitarianism*). The foregoing conception of liberty leads to a *political conception of ethics*[11] *based on external social sanctions instead of morality (which involves the inner sanction of autonomous agents).*

This substructure allows for a social technology in which *cognition can control volition* because this sub-structure is not dependent upon a perspective; it is a structure that reveals our allegedly basic and universal drives so that we respond automatically (causally) to any information about this structure. This is the science of ethics for which analytic philosophers seek, i.e., this is the level at which we shall find explanations that exhibit realism, causality, and empirical verifiability. Knowledge of this sub-structure is what permits social and political planning.

Many forms of *liberalism, socialism,* and *Marxism* subscribe to this two-tier view of human psychology in which values are epiphenomena with a materialist substructure that is trans-cultural, timeless, and allows for a social engineering that renders human beings compatible and cooperative (homeostasis). This substructure can be appealed to in order to correct surface disagreements and overcome relativism.

The ultimate implications of the Enlightenment Project are totalitarian. What *the political agenda of the Enlightenment Project* amounts to is the following: 1) human beings are, basically, good, not sinful, and the ultimate goal of human existence is happiness in this life (secularization); 2) human beings are to be understood mechanistically, hence evil behavior is exclusively the result of external forces (scientization); 3) social technology can create a utopia by the control of external forces (scientization); 4) society is a hierarchical structure best served by a powerful and authoritarian state supervised by the new clerisy, namely the *philosophes*, or applied ethics experts in our case.

Because this view of philosophy dominates the profession of philosophy it is uncritically accepted by many outside the profession. Unfortunately for those who take this position, the Enlightenment Project has been intellectually discredited.[12] The Enlightenment Project presupposes that physical science is the whole truth about everything and the ground of its own intelligibility. However, science does not have the intellectual virtues claimed for it, for science is not self-certifying. Science cannot provide a naturalistic account. All those who recognize that the Project has failed may be called post-modern, although how they respond to the recognition of the failure varies widely.

More important are the implications of the collapse. Science presupposes the human frame of reference. Any attempt to render the human framework itself intelligible requires a hermeneutical account. Ethics in general and bioethics in particular are part of the human framework and therefore can only be explicated hermeneutically. Any hermeneutical account is ultimately circular. Circularity is both its virtue and its vice. One can explicate one's ethical presuppositions, and while the presuppositions may evolve and change and one can explicate those changes, there is no external position from which one can do this. Simple observation of the current world reveals a plurality of ethical positions, something we have already noted in conjunction with global ethics. Each of those positions can explicate itself, but there is no independent intellectual location from which to evaluate or meta-critique those positions.[13] In short, there is no consensus narrative, neither religious, or metaphysical, or epistemological, from which to resolve ethical and bioethical issues.

One of the consequences of the delegitimation of scientism is *the delegitimation of social technology.* In order to use our ability to control the environment one must have standards. Those standards, unfortunately, have no independent existence. The standards are either themselves the result of external forces or arbitrary. We would have no basis for deciding that we should move the world in one or direction of another. One way that supporters of the Enlightenment Project attempt to evade this conclusion is to assume that the super-structure (epiphenomena) exhibits a normative teleology that is miraculously coordinated with an underlying deterministic structure. I say 'assume' and 'miraculously' because there is no objective evidence of such teleology or a consensus and because there is no reason to believe that any such coordination is entailed by a belief in sub-structure determinism. Even if there were such a miraculous coordination, that coordination could be changed to reflect a different combination of upper level teleology and lower level determinism; and we would still have no independent basis for deciding which coordination to produce.

One other point is worth noting, namely, *the scandalous use of philosophical frameworks to rationalize private agendas.* As Delkeskamp makes clear in her analysis of Kant, many contemporary moral philosophers adopt the language and framework of famous ethical philosophers such as Kant. However, in order to arrive at the public policy implications they favor, it is necessary either to reject premises that Kant embraced or to embrace premises that Kant rejected.[14] Either way, Kant is invoked to defend something that is not Kantian. One may camouflage a normative agenda in philosophical dress but that hardly amounts to the philosophical overcoming of moral epistemological relativism.

D. The Limits of Applied Theory

Joseph Boyle has made the case that even the existence of universalist moral conviction does not entail a "detailed code of bioethics having global reach." There are no rules for the application of rules, no moral epistemological algorithm.[15]

E. Settling for Procedural Normative Agreement

Is there an alternative to relativism and to malignant globalism? We think there is.[16] To the extent that a global consensus is possible, it will be on procedural norms and not substantive norms. In order to make this case I shall provide a narrative; the narrative also serves as an account for the existence of substantive moral pluralism.

Since the Renaissance, the modern western world has endorsed the technological project. By the technological project I mean the view expressed by Rene Descartes in the *Discourse on Method* when he proclaimed that what we seek is to make ourselves the "masters and possessors of nature." Instead of seeing nature as an organic process to which we as individuals conform,

Descartes proclaimed the modern vision of controlling nature for human benefit. It is the same project that Bacon had in mind when he observed that knowledge is power.[17]

The success of the technological project is for the foreseeable future irresistible. It has been a success in two senses: first remarkable technological advantages have been achieved; second, those advantages have enabled subscribers to the project (mostly Western European, American, and East Asian) to "impose" this project on the entire globe. The imposition has not been a simple matter of the powerful imposing on the weak; the weak have come to embrace the project on their own. We understand ourselves to be living in a world which has accepted or is in the process of accepting and coming to terms with the technological project. The issue of global bioethics itself would not have arisen outside of the context of the technological project.

As a second matter of fact, it has been discovered that a free market economy is the most effective means of carrying out the technological project. Markets have been around for a long time, but the concept of the free market did not become an important theoretical construct until the modern period and the rise of the technological project. The crucial theoretical argument for the centrality of a free market was made by Adam Smith in the *Wealth of Nations.* His example of the manufacturing of pins explains how an assembly line of narrowly focused specialists is far more productive. Specifically, forced to focus on one part of a process, creative individuals are led to invent labor saving devices. Another way of putting this point is that the market economy provides the context and the incentives for maximizing creative activity in the technological project. Private property and competition maximize innovation. The practical or empirical argument for the advantages of a free market economy is 1989, the collapse of the Soviet Empire. Everywhere it is now conceded that a free market economy is the most efficient method for conducting the technological project. Economists might give more complex arguments of a purely technical kind, but the fact remains that the market is what works vis-à-vis the technological project.

Again, the idea of a free market economy is a complex one that needs qualification. However, for our purposes a free market means that there is no central allocation of resources and tasks, that resources remain largely in private hands (i.e., private property), and that the government's role with regard to the economy is carefully circumscribed. Rather than employ ideological slogans like the night watchman state or the minimal state, it is more advantageous to recognize that state action (e.g., legal system to enforce contracts and resolve disputes, as well as a legislative system) is always to be justified in terms of whether it serves the interests of a market economy within the technological project. So, for example, the imposed break-up of monopolies is allegedly advantageous to both business and technology.

This leads us to our third important discovery. A free market economy flourishes best under limited government,[18] where limited means restricted to actions that enhance a market economy within the technological project. The most successful instantiations of limited government have come about because of the rule of law, the promotion of individual "rights",[19] where rights are understood to be restrictions upon government action, and religious toleration.

The rule of law, which is not to be confused with the rule of laws, means that the government is itself restricted in what it can do. Usually it is reflected in a constitution which embodies the fundamental values of a polity, that the role of the higher courts or some other body is to review the actions of the executive or new legislation and lower court decisions to ascertain their consistency with those fundamental values, that the norms of due process are not violated; checks and balances are an internal form of limited government. Specifically, in the most successful examples of limited government (Great Britain and the United States, etc.), the constitution embodies the notion of individual rights. In Oakeshott's terminology, in a modern state that is a civil association in which there is no collective good, only the goods of individual members, the laws are not instruments for some collective good or purpose but rather prescribe conditions to be observed by individuals who pursue their own purposes, alone or with others. The laws are neutral or indifferent with regard to whether the purposes are achieved.

In its original Lockean[20] context, rights (e.g., life, liberty, property, etc) are qualified as 'natural' or 'human'. Rights, so understood, are absolute, do not conflict, and are possessed only by individual human beings. Rights are morally absolute or fundamental because they are derived from human nature and God (or later the categorical imperative), and as such cannot be overridden; the role of these rights is to protect the human capacity to choose. Finally, such rights impose only duties of non-interference. So understood, these individual rights limit the government, especially with regard to a market economy.

Pure democracy is looked upon as a potential threat, for it harbors within it the formal notion that what is right is what the majority decides or that the common good is what the majority decides it is on a given occasion. The majority can clearly redefine the fundamental values. It is more accurate to maintain that the purpose of democracy is not to arrive at a substantive value but to make sure that the views of one faction or interest do not prevail above all others. In short, James Madison in *Federalist Paper #10* thinks of democracy as itself part of the checking mechanism. Amartya Sen has subsequently formulated the Sen Paradox to reinforce the idea that democracy leads to incoherence or inefficiency.[21]

In any case, there are two ways available for preventing the misuse of democratic procedure: one is the political machinery of checks and balances and the other is a larger cultural context in which the fundamental values are somehow safeguarded or maintained even in the process of change and reform. Political machinery ultimately depends for its proper use on the larger cultural context. We are, therefore, brought back to the need for a public ethic that preserves something like the doctrine of individual rights.

The notion of individual rights has historically and logically depended upon a larger cultural context in which a substantive ethical consensus has operated. The substantive ethical consensus contains a commitment to **personal autonomy.** By autonomy is meant self-rule.[22] An individual is free to the extent that he/she imposes order upon himself/herself. Personal autonomy is lacking in cases of heteronomy, including the exploitation of others. Although the concept of autonomy is classical in origin, its religious roots are most relevant for the modern period. It is the culmination of the Christian doctrine of free will and responsibility transposed to the civil sphere and as guaranteeing the coincidence of individual good and the common good. Precisely because my autonomy requires recognition (Hegel, 1979), I am obligated to promote yours as well. Autonomy is not involved in a zero-sum game.

The basic ethical concept that emerges is the concept of personal autonomy. The concept of autonomy presupposes that human beings are in some non-trivial sense possessed of free will; the possession of free will is not an obvious fact but something we come to discover about ourselves. This discovery is only possible for those who learn to control their impulses and who reject the idea that standards are external. This notion of autonomy reinforces the Oakeshottean contention that we are responsible for how we appropriate and interpret our experience.

Autonomy is the key moral concept.[23] Two important features of autonomy are worth noting. First, to govern oneself is not to be confused simply with defining oneself. Autonomy is often misrepresented by its critics (usually advocates of teleology) as a form of self-indulgence. Although it is true that advocates of autonomy deny an intrinsic teleology and recognize an enormous number of ways in which we pursue fulfillment, all of these ways avoid heteronomy and therefore any notion of imposing on others. The usual litany of counter-examples always turn out to be forms of heteronomy. Second, recognizing, pursuing, and sustaining autonomy[24] are the spiritual quests of modernity and the technological project. The ultimate rationale for the technological project is not material comfort or consumer satisfaction but the production of the means of accomplishment. *To discover that our greatest sense of fulfillment comes from freely imposing order on ourselves in order to impose a creative order on the world is perhaps the closest way of coming to know God.*

Boyle agrees that consent is the "one norm that meets the condition for being a norm of global ethics." He concedes that autonomy is one account of this norm, but that 'autonomy' has sometimes been misconstrued. For example, it is claimed that the right to refuse treatment to which one has not consented is a prelude to euthanasia or assisted suicide. To put it another way, if I consent to euthanasia or assisted suicide does that make these policies acceptable? Boyle is correct to see this as a misunderstanding of autonomy. Euthanasia and assisted suicide are forms of heteronomous behavior, defining oneself in terms of one's body rather than one's spirit.

The concept of 'autonomy' is subject to much misunderstanding. These misunderstandings have to be clarified. They are of two kinds. First, defenders of teleological conceptions of human nature frequently claim not to know what autonomy means for it seems to deny that there is a human nature. Surely something must be true about human beings in general. What they really mean is that to have a nature must mean to have a telos. This is simply not true except as a semantic point. There is a universal human condition, namely that we are free agents who act from reasons not causes. *I would maintain that after two thousand years of not being able to find any substantive empirical universal truths about human beings, the existence of alternative view of human nature is itself confirmation of the truth of autonomy as just defined.* Second, defenders of the classical view will claim that 'autonomy' has no content, like pursuing intellectual virtues or that thinking about thought is the highest good. Of course, autonomy has no content in this sense because it has no commitment to a specific telos. It establishes side-constraints on what is good but is open to infinite variety. The second objection turns out to be a disguised version of the first objection and merely shows that classical opponents of autonomy cannot think outside of their own box! As Bayertz has argued, the absence of consensus may not be a crisis but the "results of individuals now free from the power of a heteronomous morality."

Second, the concept of 'autonomy' has frequently been hi-jacked by various secular materialists (as in the previous discussion of euthanasia or assisted suicide). In rebuttal we point to Michael Oakeshott's masterful exposition of the growing historical awareness of autonomy in his book *On Human Conduct*. Human life gradually comes to be portrayed as an individual self-enactment not a passage in a cosmic process. This portrayal was greeted with confidence but also with anxiety, and revulsion. It is a condition both gratifying and burdensome. It most certainly does not mean worship of nonconformity, devotion to arbitrary self-expression, the resolution to be different at all costs, indifference to moral or prudential practices, self-gratification, or the denial of the possibility of cooperative undertaking.

What this foregoing extended argument is designed to show is that to the extent that a global consensus is possible, it will be on procedural norms and not substantive norms. Public policy cannot, therefore, be based upon a substantive ethics. We think this has important consequences for public policy in bioethics.

F. Implications of Procedural Normative Agreement

To be human is to be free; it is this fact about ourselves that defeats every coercive moral epistemology.

G. The Need for a Grand Meta-Narrative

The issue of global bioethics/politics having been raised, there is now no way to escape taking a policy position. The decision not to have a policy is always itself a kind of policy. If we want to hold and convince others to hold a policy position then we need some kind of account that can be based on some kind of consensus at some level. Otherwise what we have is no more than a fragile truce.

There are three levels of analysis that have to be clearly distinguished: (a) specific health care policies embodying bioethical principles; (b) the accounts or narrative we give of those first level principles; (c) the account we have to give (meta-narrative) of the existence of disagreement on the second or (b) level.

As a matter of empirical fact there is no consensus on (a) or policies embodying bioethical principles; as a matter of empirical fact, there is no consensus on (b) a narrative for (a). The lack of a consensus narrative (b) is not in itself a problem because *for free people, the only legitimating narrative is a personal one.* This is why authority exists only to the extent that we acquiesce in it.

So, in the end, what must be offered is a grand meta-narrative that takes the possibility of the existence of alterative narratives into account, a meta-narrative that is coherent with our understanding of human freedom (autonomy), a meta-narrative that does not rest upon or terminate in relativism, a meta-narrative that is nevertheless compatible with individuals personally holding a wide variety of metaphysical and religious positions, a meta-narrative that in the end forces us to accept responsibility for our freedom.[27]

There will probably not be agreement on a grand meta-narrative. Nevertheless, all parties to the discussion are required to present one. Failure to present one shows that (1) you have failed to understand the preceding arguments, or that (2) your lower level narrative lacks the resources to deal with conflict or that (3) you are *unwilling* to subscribe to a system of purely procedural norms for policy purposes, and therefore harbor the intent to impose your own substantive views.

If you are philosophically inclined, then not to offer a meta-narrative would be embarrassing or would show a singular lack of imagination but not incoherence; more often than not it reflects the typical inability or unwillingness to think through one's own position – perhaps a refusal to lay one's cards on the table; to refuse to do so is in the end not to be able to understand the position of others who do offer a full articulation of their position – and therefore incapacitates one for reaching a meaningful political resolution; to offer a meta-narrative that does not focus on autonomy would be to misunderstand both ourselves and the world we presently live in; to offer a meta-narrative that contravenes autonomy is to flirt with threats to liberty.

Please note that I have not (and cannot) offer a complete theoretical justification of my particular procedural consensus. What I have offered is a practical (and therefore political) justification. Within that practical justification I have offered theoretical reasons that make diversity intelligible (and not merely a surd) and that do not require the delegitimation of most moral communities (which are enterprise associations). This account preserves dignity, autonomy, identity, and encourages recognition. I take it that Tao's reformulation of Confucianism is an example of how diversity gets preserved within a larger context of mutual respect. On the other hand, I am deeply concerned about some alternative accounts for whom the modern world is an alien place or who feel threatened by diversity and autonomy.

The existence of alternative narratives does not entail moral relativism for anyone who shares my grand meta-narrative. In any case, what I have offered is such a grand meta-narrative that shows from within the perspective I outline why and how I can respect divergent narratives. It also allows for diversity in healthcare, and is therefore liberty-friendly. What we can have is a political consensus on procedural norms with the recognition that substantive moral views are housed within narratives on which there is not likely to be consensus. The only limitation on such substantive moral views is that they make provision for the fact that there is a plurality of such narratives and that agreement can only be secured on the procedural norms. This is precisely the way in which the seventeenth and eighteenth centuries resolved the religious-political question. There is no reason why that kind of resolution cannot be achieved within bioethics.

Oakeshott's distinction between civic association and enterprise association is helpful here. An enterprise association has a common/collective goal; a civic association does not. Modern states are civic associations within which we as individuals are free to voluntarily join a host of institutions that are or might be enterprise associations (e.g., the family, a religious community, etc.). It is only within a larger civic association that multiple enterprise associations can flourish.

Whatever one's substantive narrative, it cannot be a direct part of politics. There can only be a private moral and/or religious narrative; there cannot be an official moral/religious narrative. This limitation, coupled with the fact that there is no consensus moral/religious narrative, but a plurality of such narratives, means that we must tolerate all narratives that involve recognition of this point. This further entails that a definition of what constitutes an evil to be suppressed by the state cannot be defined in wholly religious terms. For example, the claim that a fetus is a person entitled from conception to the right to life is a religious doctrine, not a matter of fact.[28] This is not a compromise that religion must make with a liberal culture; it is the recognition of what religious autonomy means in a liberal culture. The same can be said of other bioethical issues such as turning-off life-support systems. Likewise, organized religions may speak out against anything they consider immoral and they should be allowed to refuse to participate in any such activity or to subsidize it.

The danger in not recognizing both the necessity for accepting agreement only on the procedural level and the necessity for providing a meta-narrative that acknowledges this is that we shall be driven to rationalize a secular morality as substantive public policy. My final claim is that the need to justify policy coupled with the inevitability of moral epistemological relativism will drive policy makers in the direction of imposing a universal secular morality. Since the only thing on which there can be agreement is procedural norms, and since procedural norms embody wholly instrumental thinking, a bio-technical instrumentalism becomes the substantive view. It can only see human beings as having physical needs like avoiding pain. By identifying people solely with their bodies, it enslaves them to their bodies and promotes a culture in which autonomy is absent. Envy is present only where autonomy is not. Instead of liberating us, it enslaves us to a materialist conception of the human predicament. We end up with Nietzsche's despised 'last man.' We would most assuredly challenge the claim that universal managed care is more consonant with freedom. Secular global bioethics too often denies any real sense of freedom.

The threat within the contemporary context is that it is one in which there might eventually be no diversity. The denial of an official religion has been transmuted into the advocacy of a secular system in which religious practices at odds with the secular agenda are denied legitimacy and funding. Militant secularism does not present itself here as one alternative but as itself a substantive view to be imposed upon all. What has emerged is a self-righteous and messianic secularism. It justifies itself by saying it is in favor of toleration and religious fundamentalists are not. In practice, secularism is too often an intolerant advocate of a reductivist and materialist way of life. Finally, state-participation in health-care is both a threat to civil association and a specific threat to religious communities.

If the resolution of these issues is ultimately political, then liberty issues move once more to the forefront. That is why it was so important to spell out the relationship between freedom (autonomy) and liberty earlier. Here it is important to remind the reader of the continuing danger of those who subscribe in one form of another to the Enlightenment Project. Adherents of Enlightenment Project scientism will not concede that there is freedom of the will. Instead they will talk about the forms of freedom worth having or "the relevant kind of freedom (or liberty),"[29] thereby revealing the refusal to distinguish between freedom and liberty.

What we are dealing with is politics and not ethics. This is the process insightfully suggested and described in Kevin Wildes' paper. Other philosophers who do not see the distinction between ethics and politics talk about this as "incompletely theorized agreement."[30] What this amounts to is that they see the formation of consensus but do not understand the process and are therefore incapable of contributing to its clarification or participating within it.

II. Practical Arguments Against Uniformity

A. Inherent Limitations of Government Sponsored Healthcare

1. Government control distorts market pricing and practices. As Bayertz and Petroni have both pointed out, in article #21 of the Bioethics Convention of the Council of Europe the commercialization of the human body or its parts is prohibited.

2. Government control undermines competition in the market and therefore undermines the necessary condition for technological innovation. The future of technological advance in healthcare is put at risk. As Petroni argues, markets properly understood are never in equilibrium; rather markets should be understood as a discovery process for the innovation of products and services. Even legal and regulatory systems should be seen as competitive rather than espousing uniformity. A super-legal and regulatory system is inconsistent with the existence of a market economy. Moreover, the EU, according to Petroni, seems to be confusing the difference between a no-risk and a low-risk strategy; consequently, in "the long run, the systematic application of the precautionary principle will lead to a less safe and a more unpredictable world" (p. 253). The Bioethics Convention, for example, promotes regulation because of its fear that without regulation scientists in one country will carry out research forbidden in other countries.

3. *When government policy is applied to practice it inevitably results in practical incoherence.* This is a point made by Petroni and exemplified within the EU. There is, for example, no hierarchy or prioritization of rights in the "Charter of Fundamental Rights of the European Union." Appeals to more than one abstraction immediately leads to conflicts. Moreover, we should not be surprised because the application even of any one abstract generalization to particular cases, as Boyle pointed out, can never be unambiguous. For example, those who hold an anti-commodification view do so as a substantive position. Not everyone shares this substantive view. Some of us would hold that it is incompatible with autonomy as well as being wrongheadedly paternalistic. Nevertheless, this becomes an example of how a prejudice becomes a policy because the process is politically driven rather than rationally driven.

4. *A rational consensus is replaced by a political consensus:* At best, government healthcare policy can only amount to a procedural consensus. As Kevin Wildes makes clear in his paper, government blue ribbon commissions only arrive at politically engineered procedural consensus. As Bayertz has

argued, a "European 'moral identity' in bioethical questions" is "the product of political construction."

5. Bureaucratization rather than moral and medical concerns become paramount. One source of pressure to move in this direction comes from self-styled 'experts' who have a vested interest in promoting the notion of national or global bioethics. These experts, the usual academic suspects,[31] are rent-seekers all too willing to accommodate the bureaucratic need to formulate uniform policies. Intellectuals are often drawn to collectivism for the following reasons: (a) they believe in a holistic good that can be grasped intellectually; (b) they perceive themselves as preeminently the persons who can engage in this apprehension; and (c) are therefore entitled to rule.

6. Such bureaucracies are inevitably captured by ideologues. All of those intellectuals who were unsuccessful in promoting some kind of collectivism within their own countries are now busily attempting to do so within the EU or the UN. Another source of pressure comes from individuals or groups with a specific ethical agenda who seek to impose their own ethical views by seizing control of the government appointed committees. This is something that Bayertz recognizes. There is a broad spectrum of such hidden agenda groups. At one end of the spectrum are secular-materialists, still holding to some version of the naturalism in the Enlightenment Project and whose goal is to promote medical practices like physician-assisted suicide and abortion. At the other end are those who seek to impose a religious agenda. As Petroni has argued, the EU seems to be aiming at creating "a leveled ideological playing field for unifying health policies of the several member states" (p. 248).

7. A politically engineered set of ethical policies is a threat to liberty. It is within a privatized system of healthcare that respect for moral diversity is most likely to flourish.[32] Moral and/or religious communities may flourish as enterprise associations within a larger civic association. In fact, the case can be made that attempting to turn the enterprise association into a crusade for uniformity threatens the integrity of the enterprise association itself. As Petroni points out with regard to the EU, the precautionary principle "corresponds to a view of society that wants to deprive individuals from their freedom of choice" (p. 253). Further, Petroni demonstrates in his discussion of healthcare in Europe that there is a natural progression from centralization to secularism to materialism to a social-collectivist conception of human welfare, "the standard social-democratic view, which consider[s] that inequalities are bad in themselves" (p. 248).

B. Public Policy Implications: Privatization

1. Privatization maximizes healthcare benefits, both materially and morally. As the previous argument indicates, the delivery of healthcare will be maximized by the private market. This is as true in healthcare as it is in

everything else. It is especially important when technological advances in healthcare are coming about at unprecedented levels. This is the argument from efficiency. Healthcare should therefore be privatized.

2. Privatization is also the policy most consistent with respect for moral diversity, autonomy, and liberty. There is no intellectual foundation or way of arriving at substantive moral agreement in general or with regard to healthcare. The practical source of attempts to arrive at such agreement is the pressure to have government subsidize or become the single payer for healthcare expenses. Government policy must inevitably practice rationing of finite resources and needs a basis for rationing decisions. It will not be able to provide one.

Privatizing healthcare is a means to preserving freedom as autonomy. The strongest and most fundamental argument for liberty is the existence of freedom as autonomy. The importance of grounding liberty is articulated in Mark Cherry's paper. All meaningful human action is to be justified as an expression human freedom or autonomy or as contributing to conditions for the exercise of such freedom and the responsibility for it. Liberty is a good thing insofar as it permits individuals to realize and exercise their freedom. Any attempt to manage the lives of responsible adults from the outside is a violation of and a denial of their freedom. It is not possible for others to make a responsible adult do or impose what is good for that adult for, by definition, what it good for an individual in the ultimate sense is that the individual has freely chosen it. Not everyone understands this, for, as Bayertz has noted, the Bioethics Convention of the Council of Europe has concluded that human dignity "excludes self-instrumentalization."

Freedom is the basis for liberty. National or global bioethics is fundamentally at odds with human freedom. Global bioethics substitutes a political process for both a market process and for the moral choices of individuals. As such it attempts to determine from the outside what is good for individuals. For that reason, malignant global bioethics is a potential threat to all forms of liberty and a denial of human freedom. Since health care is now the great item in government budgets, whoever controls healthcare expenditures has a lever for the massive reconstruction of the rest of society, a point noted by Mark Cherry.

3. If we make the mistake of allowing government control of healthcare, we still face the rationing problem. Nevertheless, rationing can be done in many ways that are compatible with or less threatening to moral diversity, e.g., stipulating the maximum amount available to any individual and permitting different moral communities to operate healthcare systems only within the limits of government 'largesse'.

Notes

1. As Solomon noted in the first draft of his paper "contemporary medical ethics is to a large extent a western invention….embedded in the particularities of a broadly technological approach to the world and too committed to a broadly liberal and

individualistic political theory..."

2. In other contexts I have identified intellectuals as those who (a) believe there is objective normative knowledge that is (b) apprehended exclusively by members of their own cognitive community and (c) which gives them legitimate claim to direct the various institutions of the world.
3. See Arendt (1958), Capaldi (1998), Sandel (1984), Manent (1998), Neuhaus (1986), Habermas (1973), Maritain (1951), Novak (1993), Oakeshott (1991), Rorty (1990), Voegelin (1987), and West (1997).
4. John Rawls (1971), pages 7-22, 60-67, 277-280, 302-303, 440, 541-548; Robert Nozick (1977), pp. 26-35, 149-164; Berlin (1990); Charles Taylor (1992) Chapter 2, "The Self in Moral Space, pp. 25-52; and pp. 499-521; Michael Oakeshott (1991), pp. 5-42; Michael Oakeshott (1996), Chapter II, pp. 108-184; John Gray (1991); Jurgen Habermas (1996); Richard Rorty (1990
5. Alasdair MacIntyre (1981, p. 6).
6. Fernando Rielo (2000, p. 125).
7. The full implications of this are that moral diversity will have to be accepted by default. Other grounds will be the difficulty of applying general principles to particular cases and prudence for effective governance.
8. See N. Capaldi (1998). MacIntyre, in his enormously important and influential book, *After Virtue* (1981), identifies the 'Enlightenment Project' as the "project of an independent rational justification of morality" (p. 38). While we use the same expression as MacIntyre, namely 'Enlightenment Project', and while we agree that part of that project was to establish the authority of Judeo-Christian morality by reason alone, that is to secularize morality, we give a more systematic account of that project. We further suggest that the attempt to secularize morality antedates the Enlightenment; finally we would disagree with MacIntyre's analysis of specific figures such as Hume and Kant. MacIntyre's own agenda to defend an Aristotelianized version of Christianity obscures important differences between the *philosophes* and their critics. Nevertheless, what is important here is our agreement with MacIntyre's recognition that contemporary moral discussion is rooted in something we can all identify as the 'Enlightenment Project'. See also Adorno and Horkheimer (1990). Proponents of the Enlightenment Project are secularists. See Solomon. There are secularists who claim not to be proponents of the Enlightenment Project. The problem with such 'secularists' is that they never articulate a full blown moral theory with all of its metaphysical and epistemological roots on view. At the very least, advocates of the Enlightenment Project do so forthrightly and therefore it is possible to engage them in conversation. Secularism without explicit foundations is no more than a collection of 'private' moral intuitions. In the end one cannot have a serious philosophical conversation with such people. One can only engage them rhetorically.
9. See Becker (1962), Chapter Four, for an exposition of the position that the dream of a technological utopia is the common inheritance of liberals, socialists, and Marxists.
10. Habermas' refusal to embrace the full Kantian position including freedom of the will allows him to arrive at similar conclusions even though he rejects the positivism of analytic philosophy.
11. The politicization of Enlightenment Project (and analytic) ethics is noted by Solomon in his discussion of Rawls.

12. See Rorty (1979), Margolis (1995), and Capaldi (1998).
13. See Engelhardt (2000), Chapter One, for the definitive expression of this point and its application to bioethics.
14. The most that Kant can accomplish, says Delkeskamp, is a meta-morality that captures what we shall call procedural norms.
15. This is a point made by Frege and heavily emphasized by Wittgenstein.
16. The following argument is inspired by the works of Hegel, Kojève, and Fukuyama (1992). I take it that I am dealing with what Solomon has insightfully called the "export problem". I also run the risk of what he has aptly identified as "triumphalism". I think I am innocent of these potential dangers but the manner in which I do this, if successful, may reflect more fundamental disagreements. I DO NOT CLAIM TO HAVE AN ARGUMENT WHICH BY APPEAL TO REASON WILL PERSUADE PEOPLE TO ADOPT MY VERSION OF GLOBALISM. The status of my claim is (a) that as a matter of empirical fact economic practice is moving in a global direction and this will be (may be) followed by greater homogenization in other areas (e.g., politics) but not total homogenization. That is, it will be compatible with diversity, especially in health care. (b) Reflection on this practice will lead to further consensus in theory both ethical and political, but (c) not necessarily in terms of our personal narratives. The real level of disagreement has to do with the relationship of theory to practice. I take theory to be a reflection of practice, not vice versa. Theory, for me, does not access an independent structure from which to judge practice. I suspect that Solomon is much closer to traditional epistemological realism than I am. In the end, I maintain that reason has to be supplemented by narrative.
17. The Technological Project has so far been described in simple fashion. A detailed account of the Project would have to take seriously questions and criticisms about the viability of the project and some of the serious ethical questions embedded within it. While this is not the place to respond to all of those legitimate concerns, a few things are worth mentioning. First, I do not understand the technological project in simplistic material terms. On the contrary, I see the project as the spiritual quest of modernity, or as an expression human autonomy. The spiritual quest is already articulated by Descartes who insisted upon a fundamental metaphysical dualism within which our minds are free; the argument from autonomy is already present in Hegel's exposition. Hegel distinguishes between consciousness and self-consciousness. He is concerned with how we become self-conscious, specifically conscious of our freedom. Self-consciousness is neither innate (introspectively apprehended) nor externally induced. There is an aspect of consciousness, however, that we project outward, namely the will. To be apprehended, the will must give itself content by putting itself into something outside itself. Labor is an example of how we gain insight into our own agency or subjectivity. There is a second source, namely recognition by another conscious will. In assembling these two perspectives, we become fully self-conscious. The technological project, in short, does not connote a crude reductive materialism or determinism. On the contrary, as Descartes, Kant, and Hegel stress the project only makes senses as a fundamental expression of human freedom and dignity.
18. 'Liberty' is the absence of arbitrary external constraint. To have political liberty is to be able to restrain or limit the government. 'Freedom' (hereafter, autonomy) is an inner condition, the condition of imposing order on oneself. Liberty is a means

to freedom. Liberty degenerates into license only when it is not in the service of freedom.

19. For a variety of reasons I would like to avoid or do away with "rights" talk altogether. It appears as if this can be best done by absorbing what I want to say about "rights" into the discussion of the rule of law, especially as formulated by Hayek and Oakeshott.
20. "Rights" change their meaning completely when understood in terms of the determinism and reductivism of the Enlightenment Project.
21. A. Sen (1970).
22. One of the reasons I insist upon using this concept is that it is an example of how the evolution of a concept deepens our understanding of its meaning. The ancients found the locus of autonomy in the Polis. It was the Polis that was to be free by governing itself. It is part of the glory of Christianity that it transferred the locus of freedom from the Polis to the individual. It is not an accident that Christianity is a significant contributor in the history of liberty.
23. We must distinguish between "ethics" and "morals." Ethics applies, strictly speaking, only to teleological systems; moral philosophy (deontology) denies the existence of teleology. From Kant onward, however, a number of theorists including Hegel and Mill combine both by making autonomy our ultimate "end."
24. We have in the main body of the work treated autonomy in a purely formal way. We do not believe this is a wholly adequate treatment anymore than Kant's categorical imperative is satisfactory when left without content. Autonomy, we would argue, has to be seen within the context of a life-narrative. I do not think that any narrative, either personal or communal, is self-explanatory; what makes a narrative meaningful is its incorporation into an account of God's revelation. 'Biblical" narrative, so to speak, is the only meaningful narrative.
25. Michael Oakeshott (1996), pp. 234-42.
26. Bayertz refers to this as a "unity-in-diversity" (2006, pp. 216, 217, 220).
27. Consider the following statements from Butterfield (1949): "When we have reconstructed the whole of mundane history it does not form a self-explanatory system, and our attitude to it, our whole relationship to the human drama, is a larger affair altogether—it is a matter not of scholarship but of religion" (p. 22); "Ultimately our interpretation of the whole human drama depends on an intimately personal decision concerning the part we mean to play in it" (p. 86).
28. I do not want to deny that there are some difficult legal issues here, but I do want to assert that attempts to resolve them by democratic means constitutes a greater threat to the integrity of religion than living in a sinful world. For the record, I want to state that I oppose abortion from a religious perspective, but I also oppose its criminalization. Criminalizing abortion is one of a number of policies that constitute a serious threat to the viability of religion. Conscientious objectors are an analogous category.
29. This was a comment on a previous commentary of this paper made by Janet Radcliffe-Richards. I think there is something intellectually dishonest about this, specifically, a refusal to say outright that they deny freedom of the will. The inability of philosophers so committed is a reflection of their notorious inability to make sense of such a denial.
30. As I indicated earlier, the collapsing of the distinction between ethics and politics is symptomatic of the Enlightenment Project. There are many analytic philosophers

who simply do not see the basis of their own position. They prefer instead to claim that they are non-ideological and simply hold a basketful of positions. There is a strange inability or unwillingness to examine the basket apart from the contents.

31. Solomon points out that some of these people have achieved the status of public intellectuals.
32. Kurt Bayertz has called attention to Gilbert Hottois, who in "A Philosophical and Critical Analysis of the European Convention of Bioethics," *Journal of Medicine and Philosophy* Vol. 25 (2000), has maintained that the Convention is in tension with the human rights tradition.

References

Adorno, T.W. & Horkheimer, M. (1990) *Dialectic of the Enlightenment.* (J. Cumming, Trans.). New York: Continuum.

Arendt, H. (1958). 'What was authority?' in *Nomos I*: Authority. Cambridge, MA: Harvard University Press.

Becker, C.L. (1962) [1932] *The Heavenly City of the Eighteenth Century Philosophers.* New York: Yale University Press.

Berlin, I. (1990). 'Two concepts of liberty' in *Four Essays on Liberty.* Oxford: Oxford University Press.

Butterfield, H. (1949). *Christianity and History.* New York: Scribners.

Capaldi, N. (1998). *The Enlightenment Project in the Analytic Conversation.* Dordrecht: Kluwer.

Engelhardt, H.T. (2000). *The Foundations of Christian Bioethics.* Lisse: Swets & Zeitlinger.

Fukuyama, F. (1992). *The End of History and the Last Man.* New York: Free Press.

Gray, J. (1991). 'Postscript: After Liberalism,' in *Liberalisms.* pp. 239-266 London: Routledge.

Habermas, J. (1973). *Legitimation Crisis.* Boston: Beacon Press.

Habermas, J. (1996). "A discourse-theoretic justification of basic rights," (pp. 118-131) and "Citizenship and national identity," (pp. 491-515) from *Between Facts and Norms.* Cambridge, MA: MIT Press.

Hegel, G.W.F. (1979). *Phenomenology of Spirit,* (A.V. Miller, Trans.). Oxford: Oxford University Press.

Huntington, S. P. (1993). "The clash of civilizations," *Foreign Affairs* 72: 22-49.

Huntington, S. P. (1996). *The Clash of Civilizations and the Remaking of the World Order.* New York: Simon and Schuster.

Kojeve, A. (2000). *Introduction to the Reading of Hegel.* New York: Basic Books.

MacIntyre, A. (1981). *After Virtue.* Notre Dame, IN: University of Notre Dame Press.

Manent, P. (1998). *City of Man.* Princeton: Princeton University Press.

Margolis, J. (1995). *Historied Thought, Constructed World: A Conceptual Primer for the Turn of the Millenium.* Berkeley: University of California Press.

Maritain, J. (1951). *Man and State.* Chicago: University of Chicago Press.

Neuhaus, R. J. (1986). *Naked Public Square.* Grand Rapids, MI: Wm. B. Eerdmans Publishing Company.

Novak, M. (1993). *Spirit of Democratic Capitalism.* Glencoe: Free Press.

Nozick, R. (1977). *Anarchy, State, and Utopia.* New York: Basic Books.

Oakeshott, M. (1991). *Rationalism in Politics and Other Essays.* Indianapolis: Liberty Press.

Oakeshott, M. (1996). *On Human Conduct.* Oxford: Clarendon Press.

Rawls, J. (1971). *A Theory of Justice.* Cambridge, MA: Harvard University Press.

Rielo, F. (2000). *A Dialogue with Three Voices,* (D. Murray, Trans.). Madrid: Fernando Rielo Foundation.

Rorty, R. (1979). *Philosophy and the Mirror of Nature.* Princeton: Princeton University Press.

Rorty, R. (1990). 'The priority of democracy to philosophy,' in A. Malachowski (Ed.), *Reading Rorty,* pp. 279-302. Oxford: Basil Blackwell.

Rorty, R. (1997). *Achieving Our Country—Leftist Thought in Twentieth Century America.* Cambridge, MA: Harvard University Press.

Sandel, M. (Ed.). (1984). *Liberalism and Its Critics.* New York: New York University Press.

Scruton, R. (2002). *The West and the Rest.* Wilmington, DE: ISI Press.

Sen, A. K. (1970). 'The impossibility of a Paretian liberal,' *The Journal of Political Economy,* 78: 152-157.

Taylor, C. (1992). *Sources of the Self.* Cambridge, MA: Harvard University Press.

Voegelin, E. (1952). *The New Science of Politics.* Chicago: University of Chicago Press.

West, T. G. (1997). *Vindicating the Founders.* Totowa, NJ: Rowman and Littfield.

A Confucian Approach to a "Shared Family Decision Model" in Health Care: Reflections on Moral Pluralism

Julia Tao Lai Po-wah

I. Introduction: The Problem of Many Voices

A central question in contemporary bio-medical ethics is that given the rich moral resources we have, which standards for action and what reasons for justification should we adopt for the care of individual patients. What basic moral premises should guide us? Whose rules of moral evidence should be definitive? Whose voice should have priority in making treatment decisions? How should the moral authority of these different voices be weighed? In order to search for answers, this paper anchors abstract theorizing in concrete discussions and examines one particular bioethical problem: that of the principles according to which critical or end-of –life treatment decisions should be made. It examines different accounts of regional or particular solutions to this problem. From these particular solutions, the paper reflects on what we can learn from them to help us understand and find approaches to the decision-making problem on the one hand, and what we can say about the claims of moral universalism and moral particularism on the other hand.

H.T. Engelhardt, Jr. (ed), *Global Bioethics* (pp. 154–179).

In terms of substantive content, the paper describes and analyzes three distinct traditions (or "models") for the treatment decision process, each anchored in a different source of authority and a different value orientation. They are the physician-centered model, the patient-centered model, and the family-centered model. At the end the paper considers a fourth model, the shared decision model based on the Confucian notion of human agency. It argues that the fourth model has certain advantages over the other three by emphasizing connectedness, engagement and interdependence among the family, patient, and physician. It is able to provide a better balance among these three elements in the decision process by avoiding the excesses of familism, individualism, and paternalism.

The intention of the paper however, is not to recommend a globally applicable standard. These are four distinct models, representing different cultures, traditions, and foundational principles. These four models imply not only surface standard disagreement, but deep disagreement over fundamental principles as well. They cannot be regarded as variations of a single universal standard of patient autonomy where disagreement or difference is merely a matter of degree. Instead, their disagreement shows substantial incommensurable difference. Worse yet, critical reason alone lacks the capacity to allow us to determine when we know what the correct moral account is. To acknowledge this state of affairs is not to embrace a moral relativism but to recognize the unavoidable limits of rationality, the limits of philosophy itself. Nor do we have a perspective outside of any particular perspective in terms of which we can judge sub specie aeternitatis which approach to bioethics best recognizes and balances the importance of individual autonomy, the authority of physicians, or the importance of families. The weighing of these and other moral considerations is always determined within the specific context.

This paper thus begins with the acknowledgement that different regions, cultures, traditions and societies do share a set of common values. The phenomenology of our moral context reveals a robust pluralism of moral perspective. In each particular case, we find particular models for decision-making, understandings of the values of family, and appreciations of the authority and importance of individuals. In this essay's exploration of medical decision-making, all of the models addressed share values in common, although they do not share a single criterion by which to rank and weigh these common values. We do not have a single value, perspective, or principle by which the advantages and disadvantages of the different models and treatment approaches are prioritized. What is being supported is that we offer the specific context, practice, and history of each tradition and each society. Different countries have different social structures, and differ in the relative importance they give to these three elements, resulting in different countries having different laws and professional standards to reflect the priorities in their own societies. What the paper recommends however is that although the prioritization will have to be local and particular, the method and procedure of bioethics should be universal and global. This universalism of methodology is the method of rational enquiry and the procedure of public justification. Yet this methodology cannot deliver content or resolve the controversies separating different moral visions and narratives without already presuming a particular moral account, such as the revised Confucian account which I will develop. The paper argues for the moral point of view that although we cannot have global ethics in terms of universal contents, we should strive to promote global ethics in terms of universalism of method and procedure based upon critical reflection and rational justification. Nevertheless, we will need to acknowledge our unavoidable dependence on non-rational sources of moral content. We will need to recognize the limits of rationality, the limits of philosophy itself.

II. Models of Medical Decision Making

Generally speaking, one can identify three different models of decision making with regard to end-of-life and other critical treatment decisions. They endorse different modes of involvement of the patient, the family and the physician in the decision process. These three models are (1) patient-centered; (2) family-centered; and (3) physician-centered models. In the patient-centered model, the guiding value is patient autonomy. In the family-centered model, the guiding value is family relationship. In the physician-centered model, the guiding value is medical beneficence. In terms of practical outcome, individual patient decision prevails in the first model; in the second model, family decision prevails; and in the third model, physician decision prevails.

A. Patient-centered Decision Model

Under this model, the physician is required to disclose medical information to the patient directly so as to enable her to make judgments and to give her informed consent to a health-care procedure or to withhold it. This model entitles a competent patient to weigh the benefits and burdens of alternative treatments according to his or her own values, to refuse any treatment and to select from among available alternative treatments (see for example, Brock, 1998; Childress & Fletcher, 1994; Wear et al., 1993; Faden & Beauchamp, 1986; Katz, 1984). If, however, the patient is incompetent, a surrogate will have to decide for the patient. Surrogate decision-making is guided by three principles which seek to extend the patient's personal autonomy into a future time (Brock, 1998, p. 233). First is the principle of advance directives which requires the surrogate to follow any instructions or preferences relevant to the treatment choice in the patient's advance directive if one exists. Second is the principle of substitute judgment which requires the surrogate, in the absence of an advance directive, to use her knowledge of the patient to attempt to make the decision that the patient would have made in the circumstances that then obtain, if the patient were competent. Third is the principle of the best interest which will be adopted only if the surrogate has little or no relevant knowledge of the patient's concerns and values. One then looks to what most reasonable persons would want in the circumstances.

This model is justified by the principle of patient autonomy which gives patients the right to make choices about their own medical treatment. It is the principal legal and moral basis which grounds the requirement of informed consent of the individual patient in health care, particularly in countries where there is a strong emphasis on individualism and self-determination such as the United States (Brennan, 2000). Under this model, the individual is the sole source of authority of consent to treatment decisions. It is committed to upholding individual self-determination. It is also very clear that individual interests count primarily in this model.

B. Physician-centered Decision Model

Under this second model, physician authority in making treatment decisions is emphasized. Treatment decisions are conceived primarily as clinical decisions. Physicians are the principal decision-makers because of their superior knowledge, training, and experience. It is recognized that under the imperative of the so-called Hippocratic principle, the physician has the duty to act so as to benefit the patient and keep the patient from harm according to the physician's ability and judgment (see for example, Veatch, 2000; Beauchamp & Childress, 1994; Engelhardt, 1986). What best serves the patient's well-being depends on which alternative treatment, including the alternative of no treatment, best furthers the patient's overall values and plans of life. Identifying the patient's best interest should be left to the physician.

In practice, there are some variations. In countries such as England and other common-law countries, the basic attitude is that patients are better served by relying on physicians' recognized duty to provide only that treatment to an incompetent patient that is both reasonable and in the best interest of the patient. But in cases where patients are competent, the principle of individual self-determination still prevails. However, in societies like Hong Kong and Japan, physician paternalism commands much wider acceptance (see for example, Code of Practice, Hong Kong Medical Council, 2001; Hoshino, 1997). In the issue of withholding or withdrawing life support for the terminally ill and in the issue of in-hospital resuscitation intervention regarding patients who may or may not be competent, codes of practice unambiguously indicate that decisions are the responsibility of physicians. Some of these codes and guidelines require physicians to have open communication and discussion with patients (if competent) and their family members. Physicians are also required to take the life goals, values, and preferences of patients into account. Where mentally incompetent patients are involved, they are to apply the best interest principle to arrive at a treatment decision. But patient best interests are generally determined in a paternalistic way by the profession, as recommended in the Walton Report: "In determining the patient's best interests, the doctor should act in accordance with a responsible and competent body of relevant professional opinion." (Keown, 1995, p. 100) Under this model, there is no ambiguity that physicians are the principal decision-makers, and that life-and-death treatment decisions are to be made by physicians who are required to seek support and acceptance, rather than consent, from the patient and/or her family.

C. Family-Centered Decision Model

Under this model, the family is the legitimate decision-maker. It is also the authority for giving consent to treatment procedures (see for example, Hui, 1999; Yamazaki, 1997; Ohara, 2000). Physicians have the duty to inform families of the diagnosis, prognosis, and available treatment alternatives. But they would leave it to the judgment of the family to decide how much and when and by what means to share the information with the patient herself. This practice applies to all treatment procedures even if the patient is competent. The central idea is that patients come attached to families. Families are also places where people are cherished. They are networks of mutual giving and taking. They are also the locus of responsibility to look after and to protect the patient whose dependency for support and assistance at such a critical stage should be fully recognized and affirmed. Under this mode, decisional authority is unambiguously vested with the family.

The model is dominant in countries such as mainland China and Japan where there is strong emphasis on the family. In these cultures, the family is the principal decision-maker, the authority for consent, and the designated recipient of medical information (see for example, Yamada, 1999, Hui, 1999; Yamazaki, 1997). Physicians are required to take families seriously by treating the family as the unit of communication, negotiation and participation in medical decisions, instead of the isolated individual patient. The model gives the family the authority to determine whether and when to inform the patient throughout the treatment processes.

In real life practice, the rules, procedures, and practices for medical treatment decision making in different societies reflect different degrees of influence of these three decision models. They raise fundamental questions about what values should guide us to determine the proper roles of the three parties to these decisions, namely the patient, the physician, and the family. Given the ascending importance of the value of Respect for Patient Autonomy in many western societies, is it able to provide a universal ethical framework to guide treatment decision-making across cultures and societies? Will progress in bioethics bring about some kind of convergence in the creation of a global bioethics, independent of the norms and practices of any particular culture? Unfortunately, the end of these reflections will bring us to the conclusion that a global bioethics cannot be rationally justified and that free and responsible individuals will need to devise strategies to live in the face of intractable moral pluralism.

III. Patient-Autonomy as a Universal Standard: Conceptual and Practical Problems

In many societies, the bioethical revolution of the last twenty years has largely consisted of a shift in the way medical decisions are made by the physician, acting on the principle of beneficence, to respect for the patient's right to decide these matters for himself or herself. Emphasizing autonomy in terms of patient self-determination provides a corrective to the excesses of medical paternalism in the past centuries (Brock, 1988; Childress, 1982; Dworkin, 1971). Increasingly, it appears that health care ethics in different countries and societies are converging on an ethics of respect for patient autonomy which can develop into a unifying framework for a global bioethics.

However, an ethos of patient autonomy also brings thorny problems of a practical and a theoretical nature, which it cannot resolve. The question then arises of the perspective from which one should resolve such controversies. On the practical level, it cannot offer help to guide us to make adequate responses to questions such as, "Should there be limits to patient autonomy?" Within a particular perspective, we can ask and answer such questions as: on what grounds may heath care professionals legitimately say "no" to patient requests or demands? May health care professionals say "no" because, for example, their personal or professional integrity would be violated, because the treatment would be expensive, or because they feel the treatment would not be in the best interest of the patient? An ethos of patient autonomy is also unable to help answer the question, "How much say should family members have?" If a decision is likely to have a profound impact on the life of a family member or relative, should that family member or relative not have a say in the decision? How should they participate in the decision-making process? Should their participation be restricted to a family conference with the health care team, or should they be allowed a more extensive role in the decision process? Are they to be involved as care-givers, providers of support, or are they to be treated as co-authors of shared decisions which have significant meaning for their individual as well as collective identity? Particular answers to these questions require particular contexts. In what follows, the reader is offered a geography of possible approaches to criticizing these three models so as to lead the reader to affirming a model of shared decision-making.

On the conceptual level, there is also increasing recognition that there can be more than one conception of the notion of autonomy, more than one way of interpreting what constitutes the core idea of autonomy. There are also different ways of weighing the value of respect for patient autonomy in health care decision- making in different cultures and societies. As pointed out in the earlier analysis, the notion of patient autonomy has much less moral force in some countries than others. All in all, these different conceptions and considerations raise questions about the fundamental meaning of respect for patient autonomy and about the foundational value of patient autonomy in contemporary medical decision making.

IV. Reflections on the Notion of Respect for Autonomy

There are different notions of respect for autonomy, based upon different philosophical justifications. The two common notions are autonomy as individual self-determination and autonomy as capacity for critical self-reflection.

A. Autonomy as the Right to Individual Self-Determination

Personal autonomy is important because it is generally considered to be foundational to our moral agency. A popular contemporary understanding of autonomy is self-determination. Kant (1959) and Mill (1972) are often cited as philosophical sources for a justification of this notion of autonomy. Kant's view supports the claim that rational beings are always to be treated as ends and never as means, and contrasts autonomy, the ability to be self-legislating with heteronomy, being subject to the laws of another. Although the central idea in Kant's concept is the autonomy of the will, contemporary interpretations tend to focus more narrowly on the Kantian notion of self-legislation to justify the claim of autonomy as self- determination. Mill, on the other hand, claims that individuals should be free to shape their lives in accordance with their own views in order to actualize their individuality within the limits of not harming others and not harming one's own ability to make free choices. This capacity to control and direct our lives is the central basis of the moral requirement of respect for persons and is the source of human dignity. It defines our humanity. Self-determination in this sense is equated with self-control and self-direction.

On this understanding of autonomy as self-determination, the essential conditions for autonomy are: rational capacity for self-legislation and individual freedom through non-interference by others. By the exercise of self-determination, we can have substantial control over our lives and the kind of person we become, and thereby take responsibility for our lives. This notion of autonomy is foundational to the concept of a patient's right to autonomy which Bruce Miller (1981, p. 24) explains in this way, "the right to autonomy is the right to make one's own choices, and ... respect for autonomy is the obligation not to interfere with the choice of another and to treat another as being capable of choosing." It has led to an understanding of patient autonomy in terms of patient self-determination in treatment decision-making, expressed through the legal and moral requirement of informed consent.

But there are increasing concerns raised about this conception of patient autonomy. One of the central criticisms, in the words of John Hardwig, is that it creates a kind of "individualistic fantasy" (1998, p. 57). According to Hardwig, this has several important consequences for contemporary health care ethics. First, it puts forth a false picture of human life as separate and unconnected. It implies that I would have no duty to consider the impact of my life on others. This has led much bioethical discussion to approach issues of life or death as if the only person affected is the one who lives or dies, and fails to recognize that what happens to us and the choices we make can dramatically affect the lives of family members and intimate others.

Second, it creates a misconception that self-sufficiency is a necessary condition of autonomy, understood as independence of or from others. This in turn has two implications. It can demand too much of us by failing to recognize that we are finite beings with limited capacities (O'Neill, 1989). It can further lead to a general denial of human need, contempt for human dependency, and hostility towards our helpers (Pullman, 1999). The other implication is the illusion that we can think about our choice outside the web of relationships that surround us. It fails to recognize that responsibility in a family is not a one-way street and that the sick, the infirm, and the dying also have obligations to their families and close ones. The myth of self-sufficiency can cause us to ignore the fact that in making treatment decisions in these circumstances, we are searching for the best ending, not only for the patient, but for everyone concerned in the family relationship network of mutual giving and receiving.

Third, an emphasis on patient autonomy does not give sufficient moral attention to the significance of family relationships in medical decision- making. Family relationships are often recognized only for their instrumental function to provide options and support to the patient in order to enable her to exercise the right to autonomy and make choices about her medical treatment. The intrinsic value of family relationships in creating shared meaning tends to be neglected, and family members are brought into these decision processes as objects, rather than subjects, as instruments, rather than co-authors, of patient choice and autonomy. Patient autonomy and the requirement of informed consent furnish the means for people to express their wishes, but they provide no help in thinking about what those wishes should be, nor in understanding the clinical realities of the dying process for various diseases. For such assistance, people must continue to rely on health care professionals who take care of them and on the family members and others who care for them. For most patients, a death which is remote, isolated, and disconnected from the relationships that give meaning to life is not a good death. A good death would need to involve the family.

B. Autonomy as the Capacity for Critical Self-Reflection

The individualistic conception of patient autonomy discussed in the earlier section is a reflection of the traditional ethics of medicine, which shares with the more general traditions of ethics a primary concern with individuals as it has developed in western liberalism (Veatch, 1997; Engelhardt, 2002). The view that health belongs to the individual is in keeping with the individualistic tradition of the reigning liberal political ideology in countries such as the United States. But questions of who should decide and what constitutes patient autonomy continue to be debated in the broader context of cross cultural medical decision- making and remains the central challenge to bioethics in the contemporary world of pluralistic societies.

Ezekiel Emanuel and Linda Emanuel in 1992 (p. 2225) put forth a deliberative model of decision- making grounded in a modified interpretation of the notion of patient autonomy which downplays some of its individualism. On this interpretation, critical assessment and reflection are conceived as the essence of autonomy. Such a conception of autonomy endorses a more positive role for the doctor by emphasizing the decision process as a joint deliberative process between patient and doctor. They argue that:

> Freedom and control over medical decisions alone do not constitute patient autonomy. Autonomy requires that individuals critically assess their own values and preferences; determine whether they are desirable; affirm, upon reflection, these values as ones that should justify their actions; and then be free to initiate action to realize the values. The process of deliberation integral to the deliberative model is essential for realizing patient autonomy understood in this way. (Emanuel & Emanuel, 1992, p. 2225)

Under the deliberative model, physicians do not simply defer to the requests or decisions patients make, as a simple-minded notion of patient autonomy could suggest. Rather, they collaborate with their patients and prompt them to reflect on what decisions are best for them. This model emphasizes a joint deliberative process involving doctor and patient as the essential condition for the realization of patient autonomy.

Gerald Dworkin (1997) made a similar attempt to re-work the notion of autonomy to steer it away from the strong interpretation of individual self-determination. He proposes a weak and content-less notion of autonomy which can legitimate greater involvement by the doctor in treatment decision-making, and which can also endorse some exceptions to the requirement of informed consent in real-life practice. On this view, autonomy is conceived as the capacity for critical reflection. It denotes "a second order capacity of persons to reflect critically upon their first order preferences, desires, wishes and so forth and the capacity to accept or attempt to change these in light of higher order preferences and values" (Dworkin, 1997, p. 20). The capacity to engage in this kind of critical reflection is a distinctively human capacity. It is this capacity for critical reflection on one's desires and preferences and to make judgment on these desires and preferences which is (partly) constitutive of what it is to be an agent. In pursuing autonomy, one shapes one's life, one constructs its meaning.

But because people can give meaning to their lives in innumerable ways, there is no particular way of giving shape or meaning to a life. Such a weak notion of autonomy entails a procedural rather than a substantive independence from others. Because it has no particular content, it also allows for the possibility of a patient granting complete authority to a doctor. Respect for autonomy in this sense is important and fundamental, but not supreme. It is not absolute either and there can be exceptions to the requirement of informed consent which Dworkin identifies to include emergency, incompetence, waiver, and therapeutic privilege.

Notwithstanding these attempts to develop a weaker notion of autonomy and to admit a more active role of the physician, the central idea remains that health belongs to the individual and that autonomy is invariably an individual good which defines human agency. It is therefore not surprising that health care ethics in western liberal societies do not emphasize the place and role of the family in medical decision-making. There is also little commitment to make more practical and conceptual room for family values in health care decisions (Nelson & Nelson, 1995). Such a perspective is in strong contrast to cultures where people are convinced that health cannot be understood outside the context of family relationships:

> Health has family and social aspects for every individual within the Chinese cultural context. When we were young, we were taught that you have to take care of your body, because when you take care of your body you are doing good for your parents…. When we were young, every time our parents asked us to put on lots of clothes when we went out, they would say, "take care of your body and you will do good to your parents and you will be a good kid."
>
> In this aspect, the motivation to keep oneself healthy is a family obligation….Another aspect to being healthy is the informal care among the family. The family has 100% obligation to care for other members in certain kinds of illness or trouble… so we have a very heavy sense that we have to take care of our family members if someone gets sick (Anderson & Kirkham, 1999, p. 59).

In cultures such as the Chinese, health does not belong to the individual alone. The sick individual is to be relieved of a large share of personal responsibility, including most of the decision-making process of her own medical care, even though the patient may be rational and competent. Family members are expected to take over that responsibility and assume the various roles of being caregiver, protector, and surrogate decision-maker. All these practices are carried out on the basis of respect, rather than disrespect, for the sick patient. This is even more so in the case of elderly patients because of the moral imperative of filial piety. Deeply ingrained in the

Chinese mindset is this saying from *The Book on Filial Piety* which still commands great moral force today, "The body, including our hair and skin, we receive from our parents. We dare not cause any injury to it, and this is the beginning of filial piety" (quoted by Hui, 1999, p.134). There is no question of loss of dignity for a Chinese elderly sick parent in being dependent on her children. She is fully entitled to this kind of dependency. The moral imperative of the doctrine of filial piety also legitimates, if not also requires, that dying elderly patients be protected from the terrible news of their illness which may add harm to the patient.

V. Ethics and Bioethics in the Confucian Tradition

In contrast to western liberal medical ethics, Chinese medical ethics focuses on sustaining the patient's connectedness and interdependence with her physician and her family in the health care process, instead of focusing on safeguarding or extending the patient's autonomy, understood as freedom from interference and capacity for choice- making independent of and from others. There is no notion of this idea of patient autonomy in traditional Chinese medical ethics. Nor is there a strong patient autonomy ethos in many contemporary Chinese societies. This is because an individualistic notion of autonomy cannot sit well with the Confucian moral tradition which has been, and still is, a major moral and intellectual resource for the development of medical ethics in Chinese societies. Nor does it square with the strong Chinese family culture supported by Confucian tradition where there is absence of any notion of autonomy as self-determination.

The dominant discourses on patient autonomy emphasize the independent nature of human choice and individuality. They reflect an individualistic understanding of the moral agent, and give little attention to the interpersonal dimension of choice and moral agency. They tend to view human rationality as a given, rather than as an achievement which requires for its development, sustainability, and realization, family relations and social contexts.

A. Human Relationships and Moral Character

In contrast to western liberal individualism, Confucian moral philosophy offers a very different self-understanding of the moral agent. It presupposes human relatedness, rather than separation of persons, as the essence of human existence (Tao, 1999, p. 578). For Confucius, being a human being is essentially relational. To the Confucian Chinese, what differentiates humans from animals is the capacity for forming human relationships and for following morality Mencius, an important Confucian scholar, explains the distinction between humans and animals in this way:

> Slight is the difference between man and brutes. The common person loses this distinguishing feature, while the gentleman (moral person) retains it. Shun (sage king) understood the ways of things and had a keen insight into human relationships. He followed the path of morality (Mencius, 4A:19).

This is very different from the emphasis on a capacity for autonomy understood as self-determination or rationality as the essence of humanity which characterizes mainstream western liberal moral philosophy. From the Confucian perspective, human relationships are morally significant because they are both identity-conferring and meaning-conferring. In other words, forming, developing, and sustaining human relationships are the distinctive functions that a human being as a human being must have. Human relationship is the distinct mark, the end, which constitutes the essence of a human being, instead of, for example, rational activity as presupposed by liberal individualism. Possessing this self-conscious keen interest in human relationships and so "by nature" following "the path of morality," are ways to reach the final destination which is to exhibit the perfect human relations of the ancient sages (Hui, 2000, p. 105). Fulfillment of this distinctively human function by humans is compared by Mencius to the fulfillment of the function to produce perfect circles and squares by a carpenter's compass and square in this way:

> The [carpenter's] compass and square produce perfect circles and squares. By the sages, the human relations are perfectly exhibited (Mencius 4A2).

Human relationship is the human good. What is distinctive about human beings is not only the capacity for exercising autonomy but also the capacity for making relationships marked by value. The development of relationships depends upon the development of virtues, understood as a kind of excellence of ethical character. In order to exhibit perfect human relations to realize the human good, human beings must cultivate their moral character through developing virtues. Cultivation of the moral virtues is essential to achieving excellence in human relationships. Because of its emphasis on the role of moral virtues and self-cultivation, Confucian moral philosophy is often characterized as a virtue-centered ethics explicitly directed to human relationships (Wong, 1986, pp. 153-155). It is predicated on an important claim of "equal moral worth" posited by Confucius who conceives of human worth in terms of moral perfectibility or personhood (Tao, 1998, p. 606). On this claim, the source of our human worth is located in our potentials for moral virtue which is in our innate human nature. Mencius compares these potentials for moral virtues to the sprouts or seeds of the grains of a plant in this way:

> The heart of compassions is the sprout of benevolence; the heart of shame, of dutifulness; the heart of courtesy and modesty, of observance of the rites; the heart of right and wrong, of wisdom. Man has these four sprouts just as he has four limbs. For a man possessing these four sprouts to deny his own potentialities is for him to cripple himself (Mencius 2A6).

He argues that "A Sage and I are of the same kind," and that "Anybody can become a Yao or a Shun (Sage kings of the past) (Mencius 6A7).

Cultivation of the four sports to develop *jen* as disposition of character is the moral responsibility of humans. However, development of *jen* or humanity is not a natural process. Development of our potentials and transformation of our human nature can only take place through practical activity in the context of our social relationships and in the fulfillment of our roles according to virtues. Natural relationships within a family are the roots of morality. On the Confucian conception, "Filial piety and brotherly love are the roots of *jen*" (*Analects,* 1:2). Given that *Jen* or humanity is in fact rooted in family love, the achievement of *jen* is the expansion of this root of family love. A person of *jen* starts from loving his parents, and then gradually expands the circle of the love. Parental love is the root and other forms of love are extensions from this root. It is an important teaching of Confucius that "the young should behave with filial piety at home, and with brotherly love abroad" (*Analects,* 1:6); so that eventually "all within the Four Seas are his brothers" (*Analects,* 12:5).

Not surprisingly, human relations in the Confucian society are highly valued and are governed by clear and distinct moral virtues in this way:

The father is righteous and protective;
The mother is loving and caring;
The elder brother is fraternal;
The younger brother is respectful;
and the son is filial.

The process of expanding one's family love is a long process of self-cultivation. More importantly, it is also a process which depends on one's own motivation and voluntary commitment, and not on others as Confucius reminds us that "*Jen* can only come from the self, how could it come from others" (*Analects,* 12:1). Through self-cultivation, "A person of *jen* extends his love from those he loves to those he does not love" (*Mencius,* 7B:1). Thus there is no assumption of any notion of the human subject being prior to, and independent of, experience as a necessary requirement of moral agency presupposed by western liberal individualism. Instead, Confucian practical humanism teaches that human beings are what they make of themselves through moral learning in the social context to achieve self- perfection and transformation through exhibiting virtues in human relationships. Differences in learning, experience and personal efforts account for differences in individual practices and achievements. The extent to which we are able to achieve virtues and display "perfect" human relations is a matter of individual strivings. This explains why Confucius makes the point that "people by nature are close to one another, and by daily practice [or by custom] diverge from one another" (*Analects,* 17:2).

B. Moral Learning and Practical Reason

It is therefore not surprising that Confucian moral philosophy emphasizes moral learning and moral experience as being essential to the development of moral virtues and human relationships. As Confucius himself reminds us, "One who is fond of *jen* without being fond of learning is liable to lead to foolishness" (*Analects,* 17:8; cf. also 8:2). Given our human nature, the Confucian ideal is to realize our human good, our humanity or virtue (*jen*). But it is not claimed that human behaviors are completely determined. What is valued in a Confucian agent is not a capacity of intuition either, but a judgmental capacity perfected by learning and thinking. Contrary to the popular belief that Confucian ethics is a conservative moral doctrine because it emphasizes habituation and does not have any conception of practical reason, Confucian moral philosophy, in fact attaches great moral autonomy to the individual self because of its belief that the individual is an active self capable of achieving a state of humanity (*jen*) and developing virtues through learning and experience.

Ethical virtue in the Confucian conception is in some sense similar to Aristotle's conception of practical reason. Practical reason, according to Aristotle, is associated with the function of a person as a social being. It is concerned with action about what is good or bad for a human being (1140b4-6). It involves evaluations of conceptions of what ends are really good. In a similar vein, the Confucian ideal of the person of virtue is someone who "in dealing with the world is not for or against anything. He follows righteousness as the standard" *Analects,* 4:10. The Chinese character for "righteousness" is the word "*yi,*" meaning appropriateness. The virtuous person is therefore someone who, in handling the practical affairs of the world, is able to exercise independent judgment based upon the requirement of appropriateness, and not personal or material desires alone. And Confucius has also once said of himself, "I have no preoccupation about the permissible and the impermissible" (*Analects,* 18:8). A person of virtue can employ reason to evaluate actions and situations independently of any preconceived ideas or biases. He is able to modify his viewpoint and position based upon his independent judgment according to the principle of appropriateness.

Because of this emphasis on moral learning and practical reasoning, Confucian moral philosophy places great importance on developing capacities for independent judgment, self-examination, critical evaluation, and directing the will, which are considered to be the core of moral cultivation. Confucius himself reminds us that "He who learns but does not think is lost, he who thinks but does not learn is in danger" (*Analects,* 2:15). The importance of self-examination for moral learning is illustrated in this way:

> Tseng-tzu said, "everyday I examine myself on three points: whether in counseling others I have not been loyal; whether in intercourse with my friends I have not been faithful, and whether I have not repeated again and again and practiced the instructions of my teacher (*Analects,* 1:4).

In addition to the capacity for self-examination, a virtuous person possesses the disposition to judge correctly. The independence of the mind in making judgments free from the mere gratification of material desires is underscored by Mencius when he identifies the innate mind seeking the virtues of benevolence, righteousness, courtesy, and wisdom. Through the ability to evaluate and to choose values which transcend the demands of our desires, the mind is able to direct its own course of action.

The conception of the will also has an important place in the Confucian account of agency. Its pivotal role can be seen in Confucius's autobiographical note, "At fifteen, I set my will on learning. At thirty I took my stand..." (*Analects*, 2:4). The notion of will implies self-direction and self-identity of the moral agent. It also entails choice, voluntary strivings, and practical rationality as essential elements of moral agency.

Although all human beings are born with the potential for virtues, to realize virtues requires capacities for critical reflection, self-examination, independent judgment, will-setting, and sustained engagement in goal-directed activities in social relationships. It is in the context of these relationships that we acquire the moral and intellectual virtues that make it possible for us to achieve the transition from the infantile exercise of animal intelligence to the exercise of independent practical reasoning. We continue to the end of our lives to need others to sustain us in our practical reasoning. This explains why on the Confucian account, a person is always a person-in-relation. Moral learning and self cultivation is a life long process that can only be carried out in a social context and through the fulfilling of mutual responsibility. The ability that humans have to detach themselves from the immediacy of their own desires, their capacity to imagine realistic alternative futures, and their disposition to recognize and to make true practical judgments concerning a variety of kinds of goods constitute a distinctively human form pf practical reasoning.

In many ways, one can find much resonance between the Confucian account of moral agency and Gerald Dworkin's idea of critical self-reflection. What is missing in Dworkin's formulation is an account of the essential conditions for the development of our human capacity for critical self-reflection. The Confucian thesis provides important insights into the requirements of natural and social relationships as the necessary conditions for the development and realization of our practical rationality, and our capacity for moral autonomy.

To some extent, the Confucian thesis concerning moral learning is also echoed by MacIntyre (1999) who, in his critique of liberal individualism, argues that to be an effective independent practical reasoner is an achievement, and it is always an achievement to which others have made essential contributions. The central thesis in MacIntyre's view is that our reflective capacities do not involve the deployment of some rarefied culture-free faculty of Reason. Neither is the reflective disposition self-made or a gift of the gods. All are developments of our natural capacities, things we learn to be and to do, not transcendental capacities we simply have. Moreover, it is only as participants in a social network of giving and receiving that we are able to develop our capacity for critical reflection. The transition entails a sequel of three movements from merely having reasons for action, to being able to evaluate our reasons, to making judgments about the goodness of our reasons. MacIntyre argues in concert with the Confucian tradition, that what we need from others, if we are not only to exercise our initial animal capacities, but also to develop the capacities of independent practical reasoners, are those relationships necessary for fostering the ability to evaluate, modify, or reject our own practical judgments, and to ask whether what we take to be good reasons for action are really sufficiently good reasons.

Under the influence of the Confucian moral tradition, it is not surprising that the notion of respect for an individual's right to self-determination is a weak notion in Chinese culture. As Hui observes (1999, p. 132), "its emphasis on familial and social relations challenges the assumption in western health care ethics that the patient is the one to be told of the diagnosis and prognosis and to make medical decisions." For the same reason, whereas family input is usually not determinative in the west, in the Chinese culture, it is decisive. In recent cross-cultural research concerning informed consent (Fan. *et al,* 2001), we learn that even in mainland China, the common practice is that patients are not expected to be told the news of a terminal illness. Furthermore, within the Chinese culture, physicians traditionally command a respect equivalent to that of parents in the family because they are expected to act caringly and knowledgeably as parents do, under the common saying, "physicians have the heart of parents." Therefore, it is not uncommon that patients and their family find it quite natural to submit to the opinion of their physician (Hui, ibid). Such a practice is certainly at odds with the notion of full disclosure of relevant information to the patient, making the requirement of patient informed consent hardly enforceable. This has led to the issue of a management decree issued by the Chinese Ministry of Health in 2002, requiring all medical professionals to inform patients about their illness and about the treatment risks to which they might be exposed
(http://www.moh.gov.cn/wsflfg/fl/1200207260012.htm).

There is also an increasing concern on the part of some that withholding information from the patients can compromise the patient's agency by excluding her from any real engagement or full participation in an important social situation to which she is a key part of, especially where her own life and death are at stake. Putting material information and decisions under the exclusive control of the family or the physician, and excluding the patient from processes of deliberation and evaluation, do not seem to square with the demands of independent judgment, practical reasoning, and voluntary strivings emphasized in Confucian moral agency.

VI. Shared Decision Model

The analysis in the earlier sections shows that each of the three medical decision models, the patient-centered model, the physician-centered model and the family-centered model, can be viewed as problematic. They can be seen as posing problems of excessive individualism, unjustified paternalism, and oppressive familism which can erode solidarity, limit freedom, and stifle agency. The coordinal questions remains: how can one in a principled fashion, balance respect for different philosophical values and beliefs? Can one show how one ought to harmonize the roles of different decision makers in treatment decisions? This continues to be the central challenge for bioethics across different societies in the new century.

Confucian philosophical insights on human self-understanding and moral agency provide valuable intellectual and moral resources for constructing an alternative model of "shared family- decision" to meet this challenge. Such a model draws on the Confucian conception of the relational nature of human existence and the pivotal role of family relationships in nurturing human agency as its philosophical foundation. It is guided by the central concern that if a patient loses the support of her social relationships, she is in danger of losing the conditions for human agency.

A "shared decision model" is thus focused on creating engagement, supporting sharing, and sustaining deliberations among family members, including the patient herself, to arrive at a joint decision under the assistance of the doctor. It takes as its starting point the perspective that the patient is always "a patient- in-the-family." A patient and her family are co-authors of the life which they share, and the individual identity which they each have acquired. Such co-authorship of their shared life and individual identity constitutes the basis of their solidarity and mutual responsibility. Medical decisions taken as family-decisions both express and sustain solidarity and mutual responsibility which are the important sources of meaning and social being. Doctors are assigned a pivotal role in this model, because of the special duty they owe to patients, to oversee their welfare and to seek cooperation with their family.

Under this decision model, the physician is vested with the responsibility of first breaking the news about the patient's illness to the family with the objective of seeking an alignment of expectations and building a cooperative relationship before embarking on the second stage of informing the patient. Depending on the outcome of his discussion with the family, the doctor may decide to entrust the family with communicating the information to the patient in a manner deemed by the family to be most fitting the patient's personality, style of coping, and emotional state was to help her accept the reality of her illness. Alternatively, the doctor may decide, with the agreement of the family, to communicate directly with the patient herself, either in the presence or absence of the family.

Having the doctor first break the news to the family instead of to the patient is based upon respect for the doctor's overall responsibility to the patient to protect her well-being in virtue of the doctor-patient relationship. It is also based upon respect for the special place of the family in the life of the patient. The approach is grounded on *"justified paternalism."* The assumption is that the family is normally most concerned about the patient's welfare and is also most knowledgeable about the patient's personality and preference. Their input and assistance will facilitate the doctor to help the patient learn about her illness in a way that will cause her the least harm. Informing the family will also enable the doctor to establish a cooperative relationship with the family, while at the same time, strengthening the connectedness between the patient and the family.

The process of deliberating on treatment procedures will begin on the basis of this cooperative relationship, involving all three parties. This is justified on the basis of *"human solidarity"*. The assumption is that illness is not an individual affair. Deciding on treatment procedures is not a matter of seeking solutions to satisfying individual preferences, wishes, or desires. In fact, when being confronted with human illness and treatment decision making, we become more aware of the cooperative value of human activities and the interconnected nature of human lives. Exceptions are accepted only where the patient makes an expressed a wish to give the decision authority to the physician or to the family. They are justified in terms of the value of *"recognized human dependency"* under which a patient's wish to claim diminished social responsibility is given due respect and recognition.

For cases where the doctor is confronted by the family's objection to informing the patient about the nature of the patient's illness and where the patient has not made any request for information, the doctor will continue to discuss and negotiate with the family until the family is successfully persuaded to give up its objection to inform the patient. However, if negotiation with the family is unsuccessful and the patient has asked for information from the doctor about her illness, the doctor will be obliged by his duty to the patient to inform her about her illness, and in the presence of the family, if possible. This is justified in terms of the doctor's duty to honor the value of *"trust in the doctor-patient relationship."*

Treatment deliberations, which involve all three parties, namely the patient, the family and the doctor, should focus on seeking concurrence of views, agreement of expectations, and acceptance of reality. The patient should have the freedom to choose which family members to involve in the deliberation. Treatment decisions should be justified on the ground of *"common good and mutual responsibility"*. The assumption is that by being closely interconnected in the lives of one another through their relationships, the family is making decisions which will affect them all and not just the individual patient. Decisions should therefore pay due regard to both the individual good and the common good of the family. They should also take into full account the mutual responsibility that family members owe to one another for the development of their individual good. The deliberation process will be a process of repeated negotiations, re-interpretations, and re-alignments of expectations until a family decision is finally reached. What is being achieved, which is of value, is not only consensus in a treatment decision, but a new chapter added to the shared narrative which they have co-authored.

In this model, the family is also the authorized decision maker by default if the patient is incompetent and if there are no advance directives. In the circumstances where surrogate decisions are to be made, whether by the family (by default), or by the physician (by authority from the patient), the decision should be grounded on *"reasonableness and appropriateness."* Instead of taking the patient's wishes as sovereign, or accepting the patient's sole interests as overriding, this approach emphasizes decisions which are reasonable and appropriate. This would mean taking into account what the reasonable person would want, as well as what would be appropriate to the particular circumstances of the family and appropriate to the particular realities of the broader health care context of the community.

In case of conflicts, such as where there is lack of agreement on a family decision even after long processes of deliberation, and where the patient's interest is at stake, the doctor should seek decision or approval from an independent body, such as the ethics committee, the court, or a guardian appointed by the guardian board by acting on *"justified paternalism."* The difficulties go much deeper than an ethics committee, court, or guardian can adjudicate, if that guardian is forced to make decisions from nowhere: outside of any particular cultural and moral context. It is only within a particular cultural and moral context that one finds available an understanding of such cardinal concepts as reasonableness, sense of moral appropriateness, and reasonable person. It is only then that such concepts can provide concrete guidance. We are once again returned to where we began, faced with a plurality of moral accounts justifying different models of medical decision-making at the end of life. If the narrative just given has brought the reader to accept particular crucial understandings of virtue, connectedness, and sharing, then one can come to appreciate the one-sidedness of the patient-centered decision model, the physician-centered decision model, and the family-centered decision model. If one has entered into the narrative developed by this essay, then one will have come to accept without foundational grounding or justification a particular moral perspective in terms of which the family-centered decision model can be revised to take into account materials affirmed within the other two models. Responsible action is always within a context in terms of concrete commitments. Free individuals appear constrained to enter into a particular perspective if they are actually going to act concretely, to have real relationships with other particular persons.

VII. Shared Decision Model: What Difference Does It Make?

The essential feature of such a "shared decision model" is that it is oriented from the very beginning to creating sharing, cooperation and interdependence among the patient, the family, and the doctor. It is less bound by, and therefore less obsessed with, discharging negative duties, such as guaranteeing non-interference, protecting individual interests, and safeguarding separation of agents. It is more focused on the positive functions of creating engagement and sharing interdependence which are essential virtues for promoting practical reasoning for making hard choices in highly complex and difficult circumstances. Non-interference, separation, and exclusion are negative virtues which do have their role and significance in concrete human relationships and human development. Their place and contribution should no doubt be duly recognized. But they do not bespeak all the content of our moral experience or all that constitutes the human good.

Admittedly, the model legitimates a pro-active role for the physician who is vested with overall responsibility for initiating and sustaining the deliberation and decision-making processes. This authority is in a large sense derived from the trust vested by patients in the doctor-patient relationship. The pro-active role is considered to be a justified paternalism. This is consistent also with the caring role of the doctor emphasized in the Confucian medical tradition. Under this model, justified paternalism is also balanced against other important values in the deliberation process to reduce the threat of excessive paternalism. Thus, although it endorses justified paternalism, the model does not legitimate full-scale paternalism as in the case of the traditional "physician-centered decision model". The ultimate authority for decision making is not vested in the doctor although his input is integral to the deliberative process.

Unlike the patient-centered model, this model is committed to the perspective of the patient as "the patient-in-the-family" rather than an isolated, unconnected individual. Medical decisions involving critically ill, long–term care, or dying patients are family decisions, not individual decisions. However, it differs importantly from the family-centered model by ensuring the non-exclusion of patients who wish to be involved, and by making information accessible to patients who wish to be informed. In this way, it is concerned with upholding the agency of the patient by not denying her knowledge of herself, and by not depriving her of opportunities to participate, while a family decision is being made regarding her illness. As a member of the family, she has a right and obligation to participate. The model also guarantees non-coercion, rather than non-interference, of the patient by respecting her freedom to choose which family members to include in the family-decision process.

The patient's involuntary deprivation of knowledge and exclusion from decisions are not acceptable because they undermine, rather than, enhance family solidarity and mutual responsibility which are core to the Confucian system of ethics. They also go against the Confucian notion of human agency which underscores the importance of independent judgment and voluntary strivings for achieving moral well-being. Under this model, the patient is the one who authorizes the family decision, but she does not determine the content of the family decision.

A shared decision model allows the space for patients and their family members to bring their own resources of meaning and caring to bear on the task of understanding and responding to human illness and human vulnerability. It sustains patients and their family to continue to be co-authors of the life which they share and the separate identities which they possess, until they reach the finishing point of that co-authorship, and together bring it to a meaningful close. Yet the progress to this finishing point will only make sense if one has entered into the moral narrative just developed and in the process accepted foundational moral premises and rules of moral inference. Although the process through the narrative is conducted in terms of reasoning, rational discourse, and critical assessment, the content to which reason turns has come in "beyond reason" from the content of the narrative. The concrete force of the narrative, which appears to be driven by critical moral rationality, is in fact acquired outside of the rational field of vision.

VIII. Conclusion: Liberty and Responsibility in a World of Multiple Narratives

Where does this set of reflections lead us? On the first level, we are provided with a concrete set of moral reflections that form the philosophical plot of a moral narrative leading the reader from three alternative models of medical decision-making to an account of shared decision affirmed within this narrative. Yet, on a global field of multiple narratives, it is but one narrative among others. There is the heuristic benefit of being provided with an account in concrete. Narratives like human life are not lived in the abstract. They are tied to particular moral questions, quandaries, and conflicts. One must approach such problems up to one's armpits in the concreteness of the debates.

The paper describes three distinct "models" of end-of-life and critical treatment decision-making, finds problems with each, and proposes an alternative, with implied contrast with liberal ideas of moral autonomy and understandings of practical reasoning. The discussion shows that we do have common values, but no single universal principle to prioritize values. There may even be some values that we do not all share. It is enough for our intractable moral pluralism that we have no way of ordering even the values we do share. We are left without a global bioethics, without a universal moral vision that can be justified in terms of rationality itself. This does not lead to a relativism in the sense of any thing goes, and there are no rational rules. These four models share similar values, although there is no agreement on a single principle or criterion for ordering, weighing, and prioritizing these shared values. They give rise to and coalesce to form different models or traditions because of different practice, culture, context and history. The challenge is that one cannot show where the narrative should go, that is, which content critical rationality should affirm, without already conceding at the outset, or at least along the way, particular crucial understandings of moral reasonableness, appropriate reasonableness, and acceptable moral action.

Indeed, as this paper shows, for any ethical problems in the real world, we are pressed to recognize at least three levels of moral reflection. The first is the context within which all real moral controversies arise: particular problems with particular people within particular human relationships set within particular social and cultural contexts. Second, we should require all moralities of each culture and tradition to be justified by the same standard tests of rationalism—public debate, free enquiry, and rational justification, i.e. appeals to reason and justified by reasoning. But finally, we are pressed to an even further level of reflection within which we are confronted with the challenge that no general structure can be discerned in moral reality by appeal to which we might justify present judgments and determine how we must judge in the future. What moral pluralism recognizes is that there is a plurality of moral points of view and affirms that, among the many moral points of view, no one is clearly superior to another. Thus it seems that we are confronted with a situation where moral reality is capricious, moral claims groundless, and moral disagreement irresolvable.

It is true that particularism in this sense supports a kind of reason holism, a claim that reasons are sensitive to context, contrary to universalists who hold the view that reasons are atomistic, i.e. insensitive to context. But this does not mean that particularists cannot admit the possibility of invariant reasons. Neither does it mean that particularists have to embrace a strong and wide "no-rules/no universal" position. What is being argued for in this paper thus far is an increasing appreciation of the "situatedness" of moral obligation. This implies accepting that the structure of moral reality is not best captured by systems of moral principles and that moral judgment involves a sensitivity to context which outruns anything moral rules can establish. The important recognition is that in some particular case, certain morally relevant features will be "salient". These salient features jointly constitute the "shape" of the situation and to grasp this shape is to see what one has reason to do, since "to see a feature as salient is to see it as making a difference to what one should do in the case before one".

But we can also try to further enrich the particularist's position at our third level of reflection. Instead of embracing the view that no property has moral relevance independently of its relation to other properties, particularists can support some account of general relevance on the basis that human beings are situated in a shared background which has both biological and social roots. It is because we share so much biology and psychology that accounts for the great overlap in our cultures, despite their vast differences, as well as for our shared biologically and psychologically grounded sentiments and ways of seeing the world, in spite of our many disagreements.

It is this commonality of form of life, or of life-world, which underlies all possibility of agreement, and hence of discourse and peaceable collaboration itself. It enjoins particularists to employ a broader notion of moral significance in understanding the salient features of a moral situation than what has been acknowledged so far. This broader notion of significance requires us to admit that features may be "salient," in the sense that their presence is something no morally sensitive agent could ignore, even where they have no bearing on the agent's reasons. Features are "salient" in this sense because of their enduring moral significance, derived from our shared biologically and psychologically grounded sentiments and ways of seeing. They include features such as suffering, compassion, and justice which possess enduring moral significance because of the fact that they are an appropriate object of moral concern and a source of moral commitment. A special regard for their properties is fundamental to our sense of morality. Such concerns and commitments are crucial to our understanding of ourselves as moral agents. They justify the limits of morality defined by deontological constraints such as "Do not cause unnecessary suffering," "Do not kill innocent," "Do not exploit your fellow human beings," or "Do not do unto others what you do not want done unto you". These constraints can be true for the particularist in the sense of fixing a default position about killing, causing suffering, exploiting humans, or dehumanizing others, etc. But only attention to particular cases will determine whether some act of killing, or causing of suffering, or exploiting, or dehumanizing, etc. is justified.

Moral progress does not have to imply moral convergence. Although we cannot have moral universalism in terms of content, this does not have to imply moral skepticism or moral relativism. The argument that we ought to respect equally, or at least allow, fundamentally different moral systems in different parts of the world is itself giving universal status to one particular moral view. Upholding particularism does not imply abandonment of reason or the substitution of open public debate with merely private claims. Even if there is no agreement about the content of moral rationality, there are still judgments to be made of quality and worth for those who are living a certain way, and there are assessments about whether we should try to adopt certain ways of being that are not at present our own.

In this context of irresolvable moral pluralism, the charge of free and responsible individuals will be first to acknowledge moral diversity as well as its irreducibility. Recognizing the limits of reason will require, at least at the third level of philosophical reflection noted above, relying on the peaceable collaboration of individuals embedded within competing moral narratives. Philosophy has a special role in debates on bioethical dilemmas and principles in a world of moral pluralism, since the enterprise of philosophy is founded on reason and reasoning, not legitimation by the method of majority voting, nor colonization. The contribution of philosophy is to uphold reason to support rational enquiry and public debate of bioethical issues, both to clarify and examine concepts or examine and challenge arguments, and to uphold critical self-reflection for self-correction and self-improvement.

In the new world of moral diversity, there are many moral voices. Yet, as this paper argues, there is in our moral diversity an underlying commonality. Neither the diversity nor the commonality should be denied. Nor should we fall from awareness of the importance and depth of our shared background of moral concerns and ways of engagement with the world, which are crucial to our understanding of ourselves as moral agents. The particularist, in order to countenance the full context of particular moral judgment, must also include the agent's attempt to live a certain kind of life which is disposed to view certain properties as of enduring moral significance, but without compromising at the same time her holistic vision of the constitution of moral reasons in particular cases.

Note

Unless otherwise indicated, all translations of Analects and Mencius quoted in this paper are by Professor D.C. Lau.

References

Anderson, J., & Kirkham, S.R. (1999). 'Discourses on health: a critical perspective,' in H. Coward & Ratanakul, P. (Eds.). *A Cross-Cultural Dialogue on Health Care Ethics* (pp. 47-67). Waterloo, Ontario: Wilfrid Laurier University Press.

Aristotle. (1915). *Ethica Nichomachea,* (Trans., W.D. Ross). London: Oxford University Press.

Beauchamp, T. L. & Childress, J.F. (1994). *Principles of Biomedical Ethics.* New York: Oxford University Press.

Brennan, T.A. (2000). 'Just doctoring: medical ethics in the liberal state,' in R. Veatch (Ed.), *Cross–Cultural Perspectives in Medical Ethics,* 2nd Ed. (pp. 137-147). Sudbury, MA: Jones and Bartlett Publishers.

Brock, D.W. (1988). Paternalism and Autonomy, *Ethics,* 98, 550-566

Brock, D.W. (1998). 'Medical decisions at the end of life,' in H. Kuhse & Singer, P. (Eds.), *A Companion to Bioethics* (pp. 231-241). Oxford: Blackwell.

Childress, J. F. (1982). *Who Should Decide? Paternalism in Health Care.* New York:

Oxford University Press.
Childress, J.F. and Fletcher, J.C. (1994). 'Respect for autonomy,' *Hastings Center Report,* 24(3), 33-35.
Chinese Ministry of Health (2001. Retrieved 25 August 2005 from theWorld Wide Web:
中華人民共和國執業醫師法
http://www.moh.gov.cn/wsflfg/fl/1200207260012.htm
Dworkin, G. (1971). 'Paternalism,' in R.A. Wasserstrom (Ed.), *Morality and the Law* (pp. 107-126). Belmont, CA: Wadsworth.
Dworkin, G. (1997). *The Theory and Practice of Autonomy.* New York: Cambridge University Press.
Emanuel, E.J., & Emanuel, L.L. (1992). 'Four models of the physician-patient relationship,' *Journal of American Medical Association,* 267, 2221-2226
Engelhardt, H. T., Jr. (1986). *The Foundations of Bioethics.* New York: Oxford University Press.
Engelhardt, H. T., Jr. (2002). 'Morality, universality, and particularity: rethinking the role of community in the foundations of bioethics,' in J. Tao (Ed.), *Community and Society: Reflections on the (Im)Possibility of Global Bioethics* (pp. 19-38). Dordrecht: Kluwer.
Faden, R. R. & Beauchamp, T.L. (1986). *A History and Theory of Informed Consent.* New York: Oxford University Press.
Fan R.P., Tao, J. & Chan H.M. (2001).The Principle of Informed Consent and Chinese Familialism in Health Care, a research project funded by the Research Grants Council of the University Grants Committee of Hong Kong.
Hardwig, J. (1998). 'Dying at the right time: reflections on (un)assisted suicide,' in H. LaFollette (Ed.), *Ethics in Practice: An Anthology* (pp. 53-65). London: Blackwell.
Hong Kong Medical Council. (2001). Medical Code of Practice.
Hoshino, K. (1997). 'Bioethics in the light of Japanese sentiments,' in K. Hoshino (Ed.), *Japanese and Western Bioethics* (pp. 13-24). Dordrecht: Kluwer.
Hui, E. (1999). 'Chinese health care ethics,' in H. Coward & Ratanakul, P. (Eds.), *A Cross-Cultural Dialogue on Health Care Ethics,* (pp. 128-138). Waterloo, Ontario: Wilfrid Laurier University Press.
Hui, E. (2000). '*Jen* and perichoresis: the Confucian and Christian bases of the relational person,' in G.K. Becker (Ed.), *The Moral Status of Persons: Perspectives on Bioethics* (pp. 95-118). Atlanta: Rodopi.
Kant, I. (Trans. 1959). *Foundations of the Metaphysics of Morals,* (Trans., L.W. Beck). Indianapolis: The Bobbs-Merrill Company, Inc.
Katz, J. (1984). *The Silent World of Doctor and Patient.* New York: The Free Press.
Keown, J. (Ed.). (1995). *Euthanasia Examined: Ethical, Clinical and Legal Perspecitves.* New York: Cambridge University Press.
Lau, D.C. (Trans.). (1979). *Confucius, The Analects.* London: Penguin.
Lau, D.C. (Trans.). (1984), *Mencius,* New York: Penguin.
Legge, J. (1960). The Works of Mencius. *The Chinese Classics,* Vol. II. Hong Kong: Hong Kong University Press.
MacIntyre, A. (1999). *Dependent Rational Animals.* La Salle: Open Court.
Mill, J. S. (1972). On Liberty. *Three Essays.* Oxford: Oxford University Press.
Miller, B. L. (1981). 'Autonomy and the refusal of lifesaving treatment,' *The Hastings Centre Report,* 22(9), 24.

Nelson, H. L. & Nelson, J. L. (1995). *The Patient in the Family: An Ethics of Medicine and Families.* New York: Routledge.

O'Neill, O. (1989). *Constructions of Reason: Explorations of Kant's Practical Philosophy.* New York: Cambridge University Press.

Ohara, S. (2000). 'We-consciousness and terminal patients: some biomedical reflections on Japanese civil religion,' in G.K. Becker (Ed.), *The Moral Status of Persons: Perspectives on Bioethics* (pp.119-128). Atlanta/Amsterdam: Rodopi.

Pullman, D. (1999). 'The ethics of autonomy and dignity in long-term care,' *Canadian Journal on Aging,* 18(1), 26-46.

Tao, J. (1998). 'Confucianism,' in R. Chadwick (Ed.), *Encyclopedia of Applied Ethics,* Vol.1 (pp. 597-608). San Diego: Academic Press.

Tao, J. (1999). 'Does it really care? The Harvard report on health care reform for Hong Kong,' *The Journal of Medicine and Philosophy,* 24(6), 571-590.

Veatch, R. M. (1997). *Case Studies in Allied Health Ethics.* Upper Saddle River, N.J.: Prentice Hall.

Veatch, R. M. (2000). *Cross-cultural Perspectives in Medical Ethics.* Sudbury, MA: Jones and Bartlett.

Wong, D. (1986). *Moral Relativity.* Los Angeles: University of California Press

Yamada, T. (1999). 'Recent Development of Bioethics in Japanese Style,' paper presented at the *International Conference on Bioethics: Individual, Community and Society: Bioethics in the Third Millennium,* Centre for Comparative Public Management and Social Policy, City University of Hong Kong

Yamazaki, F. (1997). 'A thought on terminal care in Japan,' in K. Hoshino (Ed.), *Japanese and Western Bioethics,* (pp. 131-134). Dordrecht: Kluwer.

Lost in Translation—Bridging Gaps through Procedural Norms:
Comments on the Papers of Capaldi and Tao

Kurt W. Schmidt

Translated by Christiane Hearne and Sarah L. Kirkby

In the 2004 Oscar winning movie *Lost in Translation* (USA/Japan 2003) the American movie star Bob Harris (played by Bill Murray) is invited to Tokyo to shoot a commercial for whiskey. During a marvellous scene of the film Harris tries to follow the excited explanations of the Japanese director who was not satisfied with the first take and now instructs him in Japanese, over a long period of time, how to act in front of the camera. With an unvarying smile the translator is saying: "He wants more intensity!" What, wonders Harris, confused, is that all the director has said? The whole meaning of this lengthy stream of words? The rest is *Lost in Translation*. Even translations cannot bridge the cultural gaps.

The film deals in a subtle manner with the problems of communication in a global world. It points to an important recognition concerning the link between the USA and Asia which is also apparent in Capaldi's and Tao's papers: the greater the knowledge about other cultures and the greater the

H.T. Engelhardt, Jr. (ed), *Global Bioethics* (pp. 180–206).

range of experiences with different value concepts, the less likely will be the attempt to establish a system of global ethics. In his *manifesto* Capaldi therefore rejects the idea of assigning any specific content to national or global ethics. The only conceivable and possible solution would be an agreement on *procedural norms* (Capaldi, 2006, p. 142).

Capaldi's paper fascinates by its radical and uncompromising approach. For Tao's position, it is equally true that she does not try to set up a system of *global ethics*, instead she presents a strictly context-related harmonization proposal by including the family into the medical decision-making process. Although the two papers are very different, there are common points in their general orientation.

One of the strengths of Capaldi's contribution is that his analysis of the global situation does not lead to resignation or ethical *relativism*, but points to a clear direction: "To the extent that a global consensus is possible, it will be on procedural norms and not substantive norms" (Capaldi, 2006, p. 142). In concrete terms, he believes that human freedom and liberty are most readily promoted in the free market. In line with his radical attitude, he does not plead for "a bit more market" within an existing system, but for a "free market" using the health system as an example. For advocates of the classic welfare state, this may well send their blood pressure soaring.

Capaldi maintains that healthcare should be privatized because privatization maximizes healthcare benefits, and privatization is the policy most consistent with respect to moral diversity, autonomy and liberty. "Privatizing healthcare is a means to preserving freedom as autonomy" and within a privatized system of healthcare the "respect for moral diversity is most likely to flourish" (Capaldi, 2006, p. 148ff).

The trend to introduce greater market influence into the health service sector is noticeable throughout Europe and gaining ever greater momentum against the background of the cost explosion in this sector and the general crisis of the welfare state. Economic criteria have always been a basis of health care. It is however hotly debated whether the market and privatization in the health sector should now govern *everything*, especially because critics deny that the market is able to achieve the very goal formulated by Capaldi ("a means to preserving freedom as autonomy" (Capaldi, 2006, p. 148). They believe it to be a fatal misconception that the experiences and arguments from other sectors of the national economy can be transferred to the structure of the health sector. It is proposed, instead, to allow the market *limited* access to the health sector in order to strengthen freedom and autonomy.[1] Capaldi has a number of strong arguments showing that the opponents of the market system are in many cases concerned with retaining concrete values which they do not want to be sacrificed on the altar of the market economy. However—according to Capaldi—these values are not legitimized by all parts of the pluralistic society. Two aspects are mentioned in particular:

1. Organizing the health sector along market lines means degrading human beings to the *homo oeconomicus* level (Dahrendorf, 1977). The individual human being represents more than can be expressed in economic terms. This criticism is not intended as a general condemnation of economics, but as an objection to giving it an *omnipotent role.* The laws of economics are in danger of exceeding their boundaries and becoming the standard for man's entire social existence if economic dictates are set above the functions of society as a whole. Under the rule of capital, market and competition, society will be reduced to the construct of a *market society* (Deppe, 2004, p. 9).
2. One of the sharpest German critics, social medicine specialist Hans-Ulrich Deppe (2004) from Frankfurt, objects that health and sickness in general cannot have the character of marketable goods. *Worldwide there is no single health care system that is organized completely on the basis of market economy rules.* Deppe gives the following reasons for this:
   - Health is a practical value essential to life. It is a collective and public good, similar to clean air for breathing or drinking water.
   - It is not possible to decide against sickness in the way one can reject consumer goods.
   - The patient does not know when or why he/she becomes ill, nor does he know the type of illness. As a rule, the patient will not be able to determine the availability, type, time and extent of the service. His position as a "customer" who can freely choose, reject or delay matters, is thus greatly restricted.
   - Due to illness, the patient is in a state of uncertainty, weakness, dependence and need coupled with fear and embarrassment.

These descriptions of the market/customer and patient conditions indicate to Deppe that it is necessary here to "exercise *public protective functions*" (Deppe, 2004, p. 10). Since Deppe considers that comprehensive care during sickness cannot be regulated by the mechanism of supply and demand, the health sector is seen by him as an example of the theory of market failure. The results that the distribution forces of the market could produce are insufficient in the health sector because the market is a blind power. "It is without direction and requires fixed objectives. Therefore the state, the democratic community, has an important duty here. And any decisions affecting the direction must be made on a political level" (Deppe, 2004, p. 10). It is precisely this *setting of objectives* that is sharply criticized by Capaldi. However, if we leave the objectives of the health sector entirely to the market then—the analysis goes on—we would be experiencing nothing less than a radical cultural turnaround in Europe. This also explains why the debate about the power of the market in the field of health care is conducted in such a heated fashion: certain values which have up until now played a role in the

European tradition (or more precisely, in individual European countries) could now be pushed aside and cause a crisis of identity (also in the political parties [!]), although Bayertz (2006) and Petroni (2006) quite rightly point out that these "European values" are standing on a thin political foundation. To support individual values, efforts are being made in the different countries as well as jointly through resolutions of the European Parliament. This is illustrated by four examples:

A. Sale of Human Tissue and Organs

In Chapter VII, Article 21, the European *Convention on Human Rights and Biomedicine* ("Bioethics Convention") of 1997 prohibits financial gains from the human body and its parts. The current Directive of the European Parliament concerning human tissue and cells upholds this approach and prohibits potential donors any such sale. However, the main intention here is to protect the citizens against the risk of transmittable diseases by introducing a safety standard.[2] "Patients can now be sure that human tissues and cells derived from donations in another Member State nonetheless carry the same guarantees as those in their own country" (European Commission, 2004). Additionally, the text adopted by the Council clarifies "that payment for human tissues or cells is not acceptable in Europe." "Offering human cells for large amounts of money on the Internet, for instance, to provide bone marrow or egg cells must not be allowed in Europe in the future," explains Peter Liese, a CDU member of the European Parliament (Liese, 2004). Human cells and tissue must, on principle, only be obtainable on a non-commercial basis. "The trade with cells and tissue can only take place if they are processed as part of medical products, e.g., medicines. Cells and tissue as such must not be trade objects" (Liese, 2004).

However, it will still need to be examined whether the "market rules" have not found their way into this Directive after all. The last draft of December 16, 2003, Amendment 69 (Article 12, paragraph 1, subparagraph 1) proposed the following changes compared with the previous draft (here in italics): "Member States shall *endeavour to ensure* voluntary and unpaid donations of tissues and cells. *Donors may receive compensation, which is strictly limited to making good the expenses and inconveniences related to the donation. In that case, Member States define the conditions under which compensation may be granted.*" (European Parliament, 2003) It remains to be seen how these exceptions will be described, or rather formulated in detail by the Member States. So far everything indicates that the aim here is to avoid regarding the human body or parts of the body as a "merchandise". This is an area where the application of the laws of the market is unwanted. Apart from guarding against these market influences (which has however not been completely successful), the other reason given is that (as in the case of blood donations) payment would increase the safety risk for the recipient because it would attract donors from certain risk groups. Mark Cherry has subjected this entire issue to a critical analysis and puts forward arguments why, especially in the case of human tissue and organ donations, the market could bring about the greatest advantages (Cherry, 2004). However, the refusal to consider the body as a merchandise seems to many members of the European Parliament an important part of European identity: it is against human dignity.

B. Euthanasia

After the Netherlands, Belgium and Switzerland amended their criminal law so that physicians in these countries are now enabled to participate in euthanasia measures without legal prosecution, a motion was tabled in the European Parliament to discuss this subject within the European community. If one discusses it from a market perspective and takes account of opinion polls conducted to explore the population's attitude to active euthanasia, one could imagine that some countries will have both hospices for palliative medicine and hospices for active euthanasia because this is what "the market" requires. The reactions to putting this subject on the EU agenda have shown that this is an issue that presents an extreme challenge to the "cultural identity" of some countries. From the point of view of the market, it seems only a question of time before there is a demand for the introduction of such measures. At the same time, there are many opponents in Europe who do not want to see their "moral and cultural achievements" destroyed by the requirements of the market.

C. "Body Worlds" Exhibition

Since 1997, there has been a passionate and controversial discussion in Germany whether the exhibition of dead bodies ("Body Worlds") by Gunter von Hagen, an anatomist from Heidelberg, should be allowed at all. To an extent hitherto unknown Hagen has succeeded in utilizing the laws of the market (supply and demand) in different parts of the world to create an enterprise worth millions of Euros. The question whether it is ethically and legally permissible to plastinate dead human beings and to present them in an "artistic manner" at public exhibitions, has been the subject of heated debate which has not diminished in intensity over the years (Wetz & Tag, 2001). This contentious issue shows quite clearly how the "market orientation" as a process of cultural change is being perceived within German society. While one side accepts that the market orientation pervades all aspects of human life, others protest against the loss of values resulting from complete market orientation which does not even hesitate to "infringe on human dignity" (Körtner, 2001).

D. Malaria Medicines

The globalization of the market leads to an ever greater concentration of the pharmaceutical industry. The takeovers and mergers during the past years show that the industry is clearly focusing on certain (profitable) production areas. Accordingly, unprofitable areas, such as the research on new malaria medicines, have been abandoned with disastrous effects for those suffering from the disease in Africa. The unrestrained market forces therefore not only produce "losers", but can literally have deadly consequences for which no-one feels any longer responsible.

I. The Free Market

Questions like distributive justice leads people in Europe to take notice of their own wealth and to reflect critically upon the free market and economic conditions. From an economic standpoint global society may be perceived as a "three-entity problem":

> Very large sections of global society have a *premodern* lifestyle; this of course refers to the Third World, to which the permanent problems of migration and fundamentalism may be attributed. Where single nation states try to control their society with taxes, the people have a *modern* lifestyle. And in all the places which are home to the knowledge society, where global economic players have control and 'smart cities' are springing up, the world is *postmodern*. It is impossible to predict how these three entities will influence each other—and in truly mathematical terms this renders the development of global society incalculable (Bolz, 2002, p. 11).

Defenders of the free market as a remedy to combat this *incalculability* can currently be certain of significant support but they must also expect strong opposition and hefty criticism, especially when the influence of the state is restrained in favor of the free market and (classic) *market liberalism* is propounded. It is not only the globalization opponents, but also representatives from the most diverse parties and groups, who fear that if market liberalism is ultimately victorious over the *welfare state,* the social divide between rich and poor will widen even further, with devastating consequences for society. Following the collapse of Communism, these two models are seen as the only ones remaining for the preservation of internal order within highly developed societies.

Critics of market liberalism stress that the marketplace alone cannot, as proposed since the 1960s by theoreticists like Milton Friedman (1982),[3] steer the system towards a satisfactorily socially balanced society (Ulrich, 2002). They also, to cite one of their most uncompromising and harshest verdicts, state that "the neoclassical theory is an interesting theoretical model, but lacking in any real analytical value" (Altvater & Mahnkopf, 2002, p. 465).

A trump card which market liberals like to play when faced with such provocation is the argument that no country has ever really tried to find out how a society would develop if left *solely* to the conditions of the marketplace. Where attempts have been tentatively made, the state has always intervened far too quickly, undermining developments decreed (by the state) to be "sociopolitically problematic" and therefore unacceptable. The market liberals believe far more "staying power" to be needed, however, since difficult developments of this nature are to be foreseen and need to be weathered if the free market is to have a chance of redressing the balance and ultimately creating happiness for all. This, counter their opponents, is highly unlikely and, even if it were otherwise, could only be achieved on the backs of a large group of interim "losers", for which there could be no moral justification.

The "effects of the market system on civilization" also need to be taken into account, since history has taught us at least the following: *no democracy without a market system!* (Bolz, 2002, p. 14).[4] The conclusion to be drawn from this is not a cynical recommendation to replace morality with the mechanism of the marketplace. It is far more a case of recognizing the importance of cooperation: "It is intelligent to be nice. But anybody trying to be successful by exploiting the stupidity of others destroys the very environment in which he could be successful. The more complex an economic system is, the more one's own success depends on the success of others" (Bolz, 2002, p. 14). According to Bolz, this realization has direct consequences for efforts to create a global ethics: "People with this attitude will stop attempting to export the Western universalist view of human rights and instead infect the 'high-risk states' with the consumerist virus. This is why economic relations should also be maintained with those countries not meeting our ethical standards. Pragmatic cosmopolitism is but consumerism. We therefore plead... in favor of the traders and not the heroes—in other words: in favor of middle-class consumerism" (Bolz, 2002, p. 14). Karl Marx was early to recognize the power of the market. 150 years ago he wrote of the middle classes: "The inexpensive prices of their wares are their heavy artillery with which to shoot down all the Great Walls of China there are..." (2004, p. 66). For Bolz the Western world has only one hope remaining after the horrible experience of 9/11, and that is: market peace! Since the market is based on money economy, only one lifestyle is viable for a mass democracy: consumerism. It is almost as though Karl Marx' *Communist Manifesto* were being replaced by a new, more promising *Consumerist Manifesto*! Bolz advocates recognition of the strengths within the weaknesses of this system. The crucial issue here will be whether this vision could succeed, whilst at the same time not losing sight of the "losers" (for example of globalization) and facilitating the intervention of the welfare state. In contrast to Capaldi, for the European critics market *and* freedom are not possible at the same time; we have to priorizise: freedom *before* market. Therefore we have to finish the work of the Englightenment in regard of the market: the *Entzauberung of the market*, the market has to lose its magic (Ulrich, 2002). The human life has not been put under the "laws and the logic of the market"; the market has to be incorporated in the good life of the people.

One of the basic problems underlying this debate is that over the years it has developed into a battle between two alternatives: market liberalism *or* the welfare state (Mayer, 2001). A quotation often supplied in this context stems from the scientific works of F. A. von Hayek, namely that "social market economy" is *not* market economy at all, but far more an economy of state coercion. This often leads straight to the assertion that between state "planned economy" (in the form of whichever social or welfare state model) and liberal market economy there is nothing. One has to opt for one or the other.

And yet this is not necessary at all, attributing to the marketplace as it does an "oddly irresponsible role" (Daeubler-Gmelin, 1996, p. 92). Just the methodical process alone of defining market economy in this way and repressing social responsibility at an early stage, if not denying its existence altogether, rules out the very possibility of responsibility and thus further options being acknowledged. "Those blind to social responsibility and such further options rip the economy out of its settings as if it could survive in isolation on a desert island. And yet it obviously cannot: firms depend on the very stability of the society surrounding them..." (Daeubler-Gmelin, 1996, p. 93).

II. Medical Decision Making

No firm can act alone, no firm is an island, no firm could face the future with a single business partner without taking those around it into account. This provides us with an—admittedly somewhat tenuous—link to Julia Tao's text, which could be paraphrased thus: no patient is an island; we all live *from* social relationships, *in* social relationships and *for* future relationships. This is one reason why the Western model of patient autonomy has recently come in for increasing criticism, or at least when it is reduced to an individual's right to decide according to his "free" will, ignoring those around him.

For the psychiatrist Klaus Doerner, the naked physician-patient relationship does have the potential for profound intimacy and trust, like all other relationships between two people, and yet it is neither binding nor effective when it takes place outside the social context. In addition, the proximity-distance balance of this dyadic relationship can easily fail: either a symbiotic melting takes place or both sides retreat into their autistic or narcissistic shells. In Doerner's view, good and helpful medicine therefore has to be "trialogic" and involve third parties (next-of-kin), has to take place in a physician-patient-family context (Doerner, 2001, p. 155).

The interconnections between the patient and his (genetic) family are made particularly transparent by the field of molecular genetic diagnostics:

> Take, for example, Mrs. X, who undergoes genetic testing for hereditary breast cancer. Unfortunately the result is positive and she tells her family about it, horrified. In so doing, however, she informs her daughter about the fact that she too is at an increased risk of contracting this disease. The problem being that her daughter had previously had no idea about this risk, maybe not want-

> ing to have been informed. By exercising her right to know, Mrs. X simultaneously violates the right of her daughter not to know. How are the 'autonomies' of the different persons involved—synchronously and diachronously—to be weighted when the field of diagnostics ceases to be limited to individuals? (Bayertz & Schmidt, 2005).

Although the question about global vs. regional bioethics is a meta-level one, Julia Tao opts to base her arguments on a specific moral question. To this end she takes a situation which is just as relevant to China as to the USA, Gambia or Greenland: who should be involved and to what extent when diagnoses are explained and therapies selected?

A. The Classic Models

Tao describes three "classic" basic models for the physician-patient relationship frequently referred to in the bioethical literature: *physician-centered, patient-centered* and *family-centered.* The strengths of the different models cannot hide the fact that all of them have deficits regarding mediation among the "entities" physician-patient-family. In order to relieve this tension, Tao introduces a fourth model, the "shared decision model based on Confucian notion of human agency" (Tao, 2006, p. 155). Flouting expectations, this model does not serve to present a globally applicable standard, however, its strength instead lying in the provision of a better balance among the three elements in the decision-making process: physician-patient-family. It is based on the belief that we should adopt an approach to bioethics that recognizes the importance of families and physicians as well as patient autonomy.

B. The Shared Decison Model

Tao shows that the three common medical decision models, the *patient-centered,* the *physician-centered* and the *family-centered model* are problematic in their own ways. "They can be seen as posing problems of excessive individualism, unjustified paternalism and oppressive control which can erode solidarity, limit freedom and stifle agency." (Tao, 2006, p. 170) Indeed, how to harmonize the roles of different decision makers in treatment decisions will continue to be the central challenge for bioethics across different societies in the new century.

As a solution on the road to harmonization, Tao proposes a *shared decision model* "focused on creating engagement, supporting sharing and sustaining deliberations among family members, including the patient herself, modern to arrive at a joint decision under the assistance of the doctor" (Tao, 2006, p. 170). It takes as its starting point the perspective that the patient is always "a patient-in-the-family." Its foundations lie in the Confucian concept of the "relational nature of human existence and the pivotal role of family relationships in nurturing human agency as its philosophical foundation. It is guided by the central concern that if a patient loses the support of her social relationships, she is in danger of losing the conditions for human agency" (Tao, 2006, p. 170).

In each of the three classic models Tao describes, two "chief protagonists" are face-to-face and must reach a decision: in two models these are the physician and the patient (in one the physician has the leading role, in the other the patient), and in the third model they are the patient and the family (which includes the patient). In contrast, the "shared decision model" emphasizes the *process character* inherent to all shared decision models: not unique interventions and talks, but a continual exchange which shapes the protagonists step-by-step and gradually leads to a convergence.[5]

In bioethical literature, many authors have so far concentrated on the physician-patient relationship and their arguments typically revolved around the physician's obligations to patients. It is only since the 1990s that increased attention has been given to the family and its role in medical decision-making, but the importance of the family in clinical practice still seems to be much greater than one would assume on the basis of some the ethical reflections in the literature. Against this background, Tao's contribution is all the more important.

Tao points out that her model of *shared decision making* must always be related to a specific context: moral controversies arise with particular people within particular human relationships and within particular social and cultural contexts. This means that in China and Hong Kong, as elsewhere, the values of the particular patient, the actual family and the individual physician have to be continually re-examined. Furthermore, even where this appears to be clarified for a particular region, it will still be necessary to take account of the *intracultural* variability (of family structures, but also of, e.g., religious communities).

Tao does not want her contribution to be understood as a globally applicable model. Nevertheless, when she describes the significance of the family in a society with a Confucian tradition, the reader wonders how these values of the family could be respected in an *intercultural* setting. We could imagine the case of a German physician treating an Asian female patient in a hospital of a large German city. Could Tao's concept not lead to a "global solution" after all? It is certainly true that Tao draws out attention to a conflict that may arise during the intercultural communication between the physician and the patient.

If we widen our perspective as proposed here, then Taos suggestion—from a Western vantage point—looks like an effort to protect the high value accorded to the family in Asia against the "destructive" influence of Western values (above all autonomy and confidentiality). However, in Western countries it is precisely the principles of autonomy and confidentiality that are designed to protect the patient against "harmful outside influences", including those possible from the family. This does not mean that the patient in Western countries is regarded as an individual detached from all relationships. In Europe and the USA, the family plays a central, if not *the* central role in the structure of the society. However, it is clear, even in the legislative systems, that the rights of the individual take first place. In Germany, for example, the protection of the family did not form part of the classic liberal basic rights of the 19th century (Schwab in Begisheva, 2004). It was not until the Weimar Constitution of 1919 that the family was given special protection by the state.[6] The family itself, so critics say, is only trusted by the state to a limited extent when it concerns the family's protective function in relation to the well-being of an individual family member. If an adult in Germany is incapable of decision (for example, because of prolonged loss of consciousness resulting from an illness), the other members of the family cannot automatically act for the patient.[7] A person incapable of decision will be assigned a guardian legally appointed by government authorities. This guardian will usually be a family member but under the supervision of the court.

At the same time, the great emphasis placed on autonomy in Western countries has led to considerable uncertainty in recent years. It is being realized more and more that the patient very much depends on his or her family and social environment. This attitude is reinforced by the considerable crisis that the welfare state is experiencing at present: in countries with a highly developed social welfare system where the citizens now have to take cuts in the services and benefits available, the question of the individual's responsibility towards other family members needs to be asked (particularly with regard to the acceptance of costs for health and social services). Already in medieval times, this question had led to an ethical distinction between *ordinary* and *extraordinary means* and the discussion today should help relatives to determine the moral limits of their (financial) duty to assist. Consequently, there are *external factors* involved which justify a critical look at the basis for arriving at a "free decision" on the part of the individual patient or the family members (see below).

Tao describes the process of *shared decision making* using the example of breaking bad news. According to the fundamental principle proposed by her, the physician first informs the family and then agrees any further measures with them. This approach is grounded for Tao in "justified paternalism". Her assumption is that the family is normally most concerned about the patient's welfare and is also most knowledgeable about the patient's personality and preferences (Tao, 2006, p. 171). While this approach may function very well in Hong Kong, the first step, i.e., the first discussion with the family, would be quite difficult in a European or, more precisely, German context. This does not mean that it is inconceivable that the physician would first talk with the family (within Europe there are considerable differences with respect to the behaviour towards the family, particularly when it is a question of communicating a negative prognosis), the problem is more that such a procedure would violate the principles of self-determination and confidentiality, and in legal terms the physician would act contrary to the law governing professional secrecy as long as the (presumable) agreement of the patient has not been obtained.

How could the physician know whether the hypothetical female patient from Asia would agree to his approach, considering that her particular set of values is completely unknown to him? The physician could *first* speak to the patient to obtain her agreement to talk with the family (or specific family members). Such an agreement by the patient would remove the ethical and legal obstacles from a "Western" point of view. The course of events could be as follows:

C. Case

Mrs. A, born in Pakistan, has been living in Germany with her husband, her children and her extended family for the past 5 years. She is admitted to hospital in a large city because of stomach pains. The German physician does not know the patient, nor the family, but he has heard that in Pakistan the physician is traditionally expected to keep bad news away from the patient and discuss matters with the family (Moazam, 2000). However, since Mrs. A has been living in Germany for some time, the physician is unsure about the patient's concept of values; he does not know to what extent the patient has preserved traditional attitudes and to what extent she may already have adopted European ideas. With the help of a Pakistani hospital nurse, he is able to communicate easily with her so that he can ask her directly how she wishes all further matters to be discussed before and after the examinations. Mrs. A tells the physician that he should discuss everything with her husband and the oldest son, as traditional in her environment.

A clear answer and a clear agreement. We should therefore be able to overcome our ethical and legal reservations about talking matters over with the family. Technically speaking this is correct, but closer examination reveals a number of questions that show the true complexity of such a case:

Free consent

The patient's decision should be based on *free* consent. She should not be intimidated by physical violence, threats of any kind, fear of punishment or coercive action, but should instead be able to make her own independent decision. Can the physician be sure, in the given situation, that the patient actually has this freedom? How far should he go to ascertain this?

Authenticity

On the basis of his experience, the physician may recognize that the patient is under a threat and afraid to speak freely and that she is in fact not giving her "free consent". He may find ways to build up a trusting relationship with the patient and enable her to make her own decision. However, what would be the case if the family structure for generations has been such that the patient has never been able or allowed to express her will freely in the context of a physician-patient relationship? Let us assume that Mrs A.

lives in a family environment where she, as a woman, has no right to free expression and has never experienced this freedom. Would she then be able to understand the physician's explanation that she has a *free choice* between making her decision on her own, delegating this to the family or discussing it together with members of the family?

The fact that a patient complies, without voicing objections, with the values within the family and the family tradition, does not at all mean that the patient is acting *autonomously* in such a situation. Hyun (2002) has stipulated that the criterion of "authenticity" must be satisfied. Authenticity "is not a matter of what a person *does,* but a matter of the *social context* in which she comes to have her values" (Hyun, 2002, p. 17). For Hyun "a person's values will fail the authenticity condition if she accepted them and holds them because she has suffered serious deprivations of legitimate alternatives and goods that remain open to others in her social milieu. Her values will be authentic only if they lack a causalhistory in this respect." (Hyun, 2002, p. 17). Accordingly, the patient's decision must not only be made by her, it must also be *authentic.* However, is it realistic to expect the physician to determine whether the patient has really made an *authentic* decision?

III. I-dentity Versus We-dentity

When Tao underlines the Confucian significance of the family in medical and therapeutic decision-making, this initially sounds exotic. In Asian countries the family comes over as having a different status and basis than it has in Europe or North America. The differences between Western and Asian societies have been explained using the contrasts individualism vs. collectivism and have been summarized in the play on words "I-dentity" vs. "We-dentity" (also see below: Kaessmann, 2000). And yet doubt is growing as to whether these extremes are appropriate, failing as they do to take the heterogeneities of the individual societies sufficiently into account; China, for example, cannot be clearly categorized as a collectivist society.

Similarly, there are doubts as to whether the importance of the family and a comprehension of We-dentity are really so alien to the citizens of the Western world as to be contrastable. Maybe Tao's remarks could be more global than intended. After all, Confucius has been pictured in the American Supreme Court in Washington, D.C. alongside Western philosophers as a man significantly capable of settling differences between disputing factions. Tao's interesting text leaves one inspired to subject the role and significance of the family in routine decision-making inside the hospitals of Western industrial nations to a renewed critical analysis.

A. Who Belongs to the "Family"?

Let us imagine a situation where Mr. A—53 years old, married with three grown-up children—is facing a difficult operation. Mr. A has told his physician in confidence that he has a 33-year old lifetime companion, and he does not want his wife to know anything about this. The question is now whether the lifetime companion counts as part of the "family"? Should the physician actively involve her, as desired by the patient? At the same time, any such talks must not come to the knowledge of the wife. This type of request would offend the values held by a number of medical colleagues and nursing staff.

The example shows that the hospital environment may uncover "family problems" that are evaded or deliberately left unresolved in everyday life, but suddenly need to be confronted when an illness occurs. In Germany, the unclear "family boundaries" are particularly noticeable with patients from Mediterranean countries. Since it is often a moral duty of the relatives to visit the patient, the problem arises how this wish of the "family", which may sometimes number 20-30 persons all wanting to visit the patient, can fit in with the routine of the hospital. Apart from the problem of space (small rooms), there is a constant conflict with the interests of fellow patients who may feel irritated by the visits of these extended families that speak in a foreign language and sometimes bring their own cooked food with them.

So what exactly is a "family"? It is interesting to note that the German Civil Code does not define what constitutes a family. Although Article 6 of Germany's Basic Law stipulates that marriage and family are under the special protection of the state, it does not explain what is really understood by "family", who belongs to the family, against whom the family should be protected, and what the special protection of the family consists of. Since the German constitutional law is not allowed to adopt any specific religious or ideological interpretation of the family, one may assume that it is the *social* function of the family that is meant to be protected (Pirson, 1987, p. 650f.). The family is protected because it creates the essential conditions that enable the individual to take advantage of the given opportunities and become integrated in his or her social environment.

In Tao's shared decision model, the physician therefore carries out a *social function* by deliberately linking the three elements *physician-patient-family*; his behaviour as a moderator actually contributes to the stabilization of society! However, assigning such a specific meaning to the role of the physician, will continue to be disputed in the medical fraternity worldwide.

B. Christian Context

The fact that sickness affects not only individuals but also those around them has shaped Christian culture. In Europe and Asia Minor, the emergence of medical treatment and the spreading of hospitals for the healing and care of the sick is intrinsically linked to the Christian body of thought. "And whether one member suffer", remarked Paul the Apostle about the Christian community, "all the members suffer with it" (I. Cor. 12:26). In her speech to the Lower Saxonian Medical Council about the forthcoming challenges to healthcare in the 3rd millennium, Bishop Kaessmann, the Head of the Protestant Church in Lower Saxony, Germany, said: "Christians are unable to look away uncaringly when other people are forced to suffer" (Kaessmann, 2000) and went on to emphasize a point of orientation which Christian health ethics has to offer, namely our fellow men, *others*.

> We live in an age with a disturbed balance between I(dentity) and We(dentity). Emanuel Lévinas' philosophy, with its orientation to *others* as a basic ontological category, shows that this diagnosis is also possible without reference to Christian theology. [...] In order for a modern post-industrial society to function effectively, the all-encompassing positive version of the Golden Rule is paramount: "Do unto others as you would have them do unto you." (Matt. 7:12)... The social coherence of our society depends on there being enough people who orientate their comprehension of solidarity to this form of ethics directed at others (Kaessmann, 2000).

IV. Truth Telling

> "The moral imperative of the doctrine of filial piety also legitimates, if not also requires, that dying elderly patients be protected from the terrible news of their illness which may add harm to the patient" (Tao, 2006, p. 164).

This view was also practiced in the Western world for a long time. Thomas Percival, whose work *Medical Ethics* was first published in 1803, remarked in this context that for a patient "who makes inquiries which, if faithfully answered, might prove fatal to him, it would be a gross and unfeeling wrong to tell the truth" (Radovsky, 1985). Even into the 1960s the majority of physicians in the USA, for example, were convinced it was better *not* to tell a patient the whole truth about his disease (cancer) if the patient did not give the appearance of being able to bear it.

In a European study, Thomsen, Ostergaard, Wulff, Martin and Singer (1993) investigated the behavior of European gastroenterologists when diagnosing cancer. Gasteroenterologists in all parts of Europe were asked to consider a case of colonic cancer and to state what they would tell the patient and the patient's spouse. A North-South divide became clearly apparent: In Northern Europe gastroenterologists usually reveal the diagnosis to both the patient and the patient's spouse, in Southern and Eastern Europe they usually conceal the diagnosis from the patient, in many cases even when the patient has asked to be told the truth. Most would tell the spouse the full truth about both diagnosis and prognosis. "The variation probably reflects differences in both doctors' attitudes and patients' expectations." (Thomsen *et al.*, 1993, p. 473)

What has increasingly manifested itself in Western Medical Ethics textbooks since the 1960s, namely a demand for patients to be told the truth and their autonomy thus respected, has not really become established throughout the Western world in practise, although great changes have undoubtedly been seen. Cultural differences can still be seen between the individual countries today (Akabayashi, Fetters & Elwyn, 1999, Thomsen *et al.*, 1993).

This finding can also be interpreted as an indication of secularization: in the Christian religion it is traditionally important to prepare oneself for death, i.e. to make one's peace with God and one's fellow mortals first. With regard to spiritual salvation, it is therefore irresponsible not to inform a Christian of his approaching death. For an Orthodox Christian priest it is important whether a patient has shown remorse and entered into a pius and prayerful relationship with God (Joseph, 1998, p. 277; Engelhardt, 2000). Robbing an Orthodox Christian of the opportunity to do so would amount to a violation of his spiritual salvation. This view is bedded in traditional Catholicism and still noticeable in Martin Luther's *Sermon on preparing for death* from 1519. In both cases, individuals are responsible prior to death for their transition to the next life. This responsibility cannot be wholly transferred to another.

Addressing the family first and deciding with the next-of-kin whether and to what extent a patient should be informed is decidedly problematic (Schmidt & Wolfslast, 2002). How is a physician to know whether the opinion of the next-of-kin is really in line with the best interests of the patient? Or whether the next-of-kin, when desiring the truth to be withheld, are not really just trying to protect themselves from further problems and existing fears? In a case study, White and Fletcher (1990) have summed up the paradoxical nature of such situations in their very apt title: The Story of Mr. and Mrs. Doe: "You can't tell my husband he's dying; it will kill him". It is not the patient himself who is unable to take the truth about his fatal disease, but his wife. She is the one in primary need of help with coming to terms with the truth.

Truth Telling in the Literature

There have been repeated descriptions in the literature of the physician's conflict when revealing diagnoses between his obligation to tell the truth to patients, his desire to count on the family and his worries about the damage which informing a patient could cause. The literature is thus a mirror of society's struggle with the priorities of different values.

In his play 'Professor Bernhardi' from 1912, the Austrian physician and writer Arthur Schnitzler (1862-1931) permits the main character Dr. Bernhardi, a Jew and Senior Physician, to refuse a Catholic priest the right to visit a dying patient. Her life cannot be saved, but in a last fit of euphoria she thinks she is going to get better. Professor Bernhardi does not wish to take this feeling of happiness away from her. He believes one of his obligations as a physician to be: "...if I no longer have the power to do any more, then at least to allow my patients to die as happily as possible."

Bernhardi refuses the priest the right to visit the patient because just the sight of him could reveal to the patient that she is about to die. As a physician who is totally focussed on life on earth, he does not want to take her hopes away; the priest, on the other hand, has obligations to her spiritual salvation and does not wish to be stopped. For an Orthodox Christian priest, the physician's actions are totally unacceptable because care for the soul is ultimately far more important than any (medical) care of earthly matters.

In Tennessee Williams' play *The Cat on a Hot Tin Roof*, a physician opts, in agreement with the family, not to tell the plantation owner Big Daddy on his 65th birthday that he has an incurable form of cancer. The power which can lie in withholding such a truth and the shock a person can suffer when he later finds out he has been lied to have rarely been portrayed so drastically. Whereas the family had previously represented a safe haven to the patient, in his disillusion he now sees it as a den of deceit.

These literary examples demonstrate how, in *Dr. Bernhardi,* family support could have been helpful to the patient; in Big Daddy's case in *The Cat on the Hot Tin Roof* it ultimately led to a catastrophe.

V. The Role of the Family

If we take the Enlightenment to be a process which has critically questioned *all traditions,* passed-down interpretations of the world and social lifestyles in order to expose situations in which people have *not been allowed to speak for themselves,* then this process should also include the institution of the family (and the free market, as seen above). Regarding the medical ethical and legal development and codes of the last few decades against this background of increasing liberation from guardianship and a strengthening of free, autonomous decisions, the impression is created that *in theory* the influence of the family has been increasingly excluded from the physician-patient relationship. This is not surprising, as the family has always *partly* been a source of repression.

For the field of medical care, liberation from the tradition of guardianship meant protecting every adult from being subjected to the actions of third parties. Patients should be able to make their own decisions and, for this reason, the family should remain excluded from the physician-patient relationship until the patient decides to grant it access. The only gatekeeper to further measures should be the patient himself. Just as the physician has to inform the patient about all planned interventions and measures so that the patient has a chance to reject them, the patient has to have the power to decide which information is passed on to his family in order to prevent them from deciding anything for him. Currently at the peak of this development in the Western world, we are witnessing an ethical and legal situation in which patients are informed by their physicians of potential interventions almost as offers which they may reject, even if to do so would be detrimental to their health. Even though in some European countries individual issues still remain vague and in need of clarification (e.g., the regulation of passive euthanasia), we can establish that in the Western theoretical debate on medical ethical and legal issues, consensus has largely been reached that the patient is central to all decisions.

And yet if we take a look at hospital routines in practise, the family has far more importance than the theoretical debate would lead us to believe. Many studies and investigations have shown that patient autonomy is consistently flouted. Sometimes spouses and relatives are informed first, without the consent of the patient and permission to operate is given—illegally—by the next-of-kin,[8] the question arise: has Europe misunderstood the Enlightenment? What is really surprising in this context is the silence of the patients being ignored. What if the family were a constellation in which healthcare matters were removed from the strict idea of autonomy, even in Europe? Tao's text challenges us to take a fundamental look at the role of the family within the Western industrial nations as far as the informing of patients and decisions for or against therapy are concerned.[9]

A. Is a "YES" really a "YES"?

From a Western point of view, the opportunity to exercise one's free will is a basic precondition. However, the existence of the "free will" of human beings has often been questioned in the past, both in fundamental respects and in concrete situations. This challenge comes mainly from four different quarters:

1. In the field of *natural science,* brain researchers doubt the very existence of the free will and believe it to be an illusion (Singer, 2003).
2. Contrary to this, the *philosophical argument* claims that human freedom, or lack of freedom, lies outside the scope of brain research and is thus not subject to any scientific proof. Human freedom is so deeply interwoven with our daily practice of communication and moral judgement that, as a fundamental element, it cannot seriously be called into question (Nida-Rümelin, 2004).
3. In *psychology,* the existence of the free will is basically not doubted, but it is questioned whether human beings are capable of making a free decision under certain circumstances, e.g., during an illness or before an important operation. Since the concept of *informed consent* assumes a healthy person as a point of reference, it has to be inquired individually whether the sick person is perhaps at the time restricted in his or her freedom due to fear, pain, external constraints, etc. (Grisso & Appelbaum, 1998).
4. Considering in particular that the lives of human beings are structured by relationships on which they "depend", the influence that the social environment has on the patient must be critically examined.

This situation is exemplified by the following four constellations:

Situation 1: *The patient says "yes"*

The patient agrees to a course of chemotherapy proposed by the physician. Later on during the conversation the patient mentions casually that he himself is against chemotherapy, but that he is doing this to oblige his wife. How should the physician react? What is his duty? Preserving the life of the patient? Pretending not to hear the patient's remark? Praise the patient for his altruistic attitude? Or should the physician try to strengthen the patient's autonomy to enable him to make a "free decision"?

Situation 2: *The patient says "no"*

A cancer patient does not agree to the dialysis ordered by the physician and is aware that he will die within the next few weeks as a result of this decision. The physician will want to check whether the patient has really understood the severe consequences of this decision. He will provide the patient with further information since the physician has a duty, both in ethical and legal terms, to convince the patient to accept the life-saving treatment, although he will finally have to respect the patient's refusal. As the physician probes into the background, the patient admits that he would really have accepted dialysis but that he does not want to cause any more problems for his family who has apparently already suffered a great deal because of him. Is it the task (duty of care) of the physician to oppose this decision by the patient? Should he strengthen the patient's autonomy by not respecting this decision at this point?

Situation 3: *The patient says "yes" (against the will of the family)*

The patient wants to go home after his operation and rejects the idea of going into a nursing home. In view of her age, his wife feels that she does not have the strength to look after him. The costs for home nursing services would only be partly paid for by health insurance. The family would have to get into considerable debt, not least because the house or rather the patient's room would require alteration work. In addition, the son has just started his own business and taken up a large loan, so that this plan would not be financially feasible. A place in a nursing home would be possible, but the patient is against this. Should the physician try to convince the patient to "give up his own will"?

Situation 4: *The patient says "no" (but the family wants it and puts pressure on the physician)*

The physician informs the patient about a new type of procedure which is much less risky and has better chances of success than the conventional method of operation. It would, however, have to be paid for privately. The patient rejects this proposal because he doesn't have the financial resources and doesn't want to burden his children. Should the physician discuss this with the family?

These examples are not discussed any further in the present context (helpful ideas are provided by Mappes and Zembaty, 1994), but they show that, on the one hand, the family can mean constraints for the patient, and on the other it can also be a foundation for making a free decision. In this sense, the *shared decision model* fulfils an important function by allowing all involved a greater degree of freedom and responsibility.

B. Example: Organ Donation

In 1997, after a spate of prolonged and hefty debates, a transplantation law was finally passed in Germany. Particularly controversial was the type of consent to be practiced, the ultimate agreement being to a so-called "extended consent solution", i.e. the surgeon may remove organs following the occurrence of whole brain death provided he has *either* the written consent of the brain-dead patient or the consent of the next-of-kin. It was (ethically and legally) indisputable, even before the law came into force, that removal was permissible if a valid organ donor card existed. In practice the next-of-kin were always informed prior to the planned organ removal. If the next-of-kin then requested that organ removal not be performed because they did not consider themselves be able to cope with it emotionally or otherwise, the organ removal was not carried out. Today nothing has changed regarding this readiness to accept a veto from the next-of-kin. And yet this practice—especially in our context here—raises some fundamental questions: Why are the next-of-kin informed at all? And even if they are informed, what gives them the right to contradict the obvious desire of a patient to donate his organs? Why does the physician not see himself as champion to the *explicit will of the patient* and defend this will against the family? Why does the physician bow to a veto by the family, especially taking into account the fact that, in the light of the present shortage of donor organs, each organ not removed amounts to a lost chance to save the life or improve the quality of life of a potential recipient?

Even though, legally and ethically, the issue of organ removal centers around the will of the patient, in practise the *family* ultimately makes the final decision. On closer observation, however, the reason why the family is given such power is not to guarantee it a life free of additional trauma or emotional stress, but because physicians are afraid that families could turn in outrage to the public/media and cast an unfavorable light on the intervention so desired by the brain-dead patient, describing it as e.g., "insensitive butchering" which coldly ignored the feelings of the grieving relatives. Since in a liberal democracy the entire transplantation system is based on public acceptance (altruistic donors), and since organ transplants cannot be performed without public cooperation, the high level of sensitivity shown in this field is understandable (Schmidt, 2000). Family peace is only held in such high regard because a negative public view would ultimately be disadvantageous for the entire transplantation system which, after all, is founded on voluntary, unpaid donations. The will of the individual (donor) is sacrificed to the good of the overall system. It should be mentioned here that nobody has a *right* to have his organs explanted and transplanted, and yet in our context it is significant that individual cases are always considered with the overall system in mind. Negative coverage affects not only the hospital or country concerned, but reaches far beyond national boundaries to affect the rest of Europe and ultimately the entire transplantation medicine zone (e.g. EURO-TRANSPLANT).[10] A family veto is paid so much attention due to its "global significance".

If we take a look at these aspects against the background of the big three *Market, Freedom* and *Family,* then we see that within the European system the family does not exactly protect the autonomous and free decision of the individual, but far more represents a threat to it. It will be an exciting discussion with Capaldi and others to determine whether the introduction of a market system to organ donation and the establishment of a "organ market" would lead to the will of patients being more readily acknowledged.

VI. Market, Freedom and the Family

Looking back to the history of Western medicine, the health market can be seen as the possibility to create the independence of the physician-patient relationship. In the battle of words which takes place in Plato's *Politeia* between Socrates and Thrasymachos, the view is expressed that an individual good can only be determined by taking public interest into account. For the judiciary and for medical science this means that both professional groups tend to be beneficiaries of a society which has failed in its efforts to educate. Judges and physicians appear (falsely) as "healers" in a society which has lost or not yet achieved its absolute state (Kersting, 1999, p. 130ff.). And yet they will never be able to eliminate the deficits as long as they continue merely to cure the symptoms. From Plato's point of view, it is therefore not in the public's best interest to care for the chronically sick (and in so doing, only to prolong their miserable existence anyway) or to look after the weak and dying. The only justification for physicians is their promotion of mentally and physically fit citizens for the benefit of the State. Physicians "believe they do not have to care for people incapable of living in the circles familiar to them because it would help neither themselves nor the State to do so" (*Politeia,* p. 407e).

Against this background, the development which has taken place in the Western world over centuries, from the Ancient view of the physician as a *civil servant* to the modern *private service for the sick,* achieves enormous significance (Weizsäcker, 1975, p. 214). Medical practice has increasingly compacted to become a doctor-patient relationship which is primarily bound to the patient. Patients' complaints are concealed from "curious eyes", medical secrecy (the Hippocratic Oath!) is also drawn upon to protect the patient privacy. The political and social side of physicians is increasingly becoming a personal and psychological sphere, turning the occupation of physician into an occupation—to a degree market-orientated—where patients are fundamentally "free" to choose their own doctors. Medical discretion is legally safeguarded and the resulting guaranteed intimacy represents "psychologically speaking, an existential issue of modern man" (Weizsäcker, 1975, p. 214). "The sociological effects of competition, price fixing, liability, boycott etc. are also moving medical practise closer to free production and free trade—not despite the medical ideal of being solely personal, but precisely *because* of it" (Weizsäcker, 1975, p. 215; original italics). Precisely because the patient is the primary concern here, the occupational freedom of physicians and the protection of such are not questioned by public bodies. If the medical profession is criticised, it is on the stage or in other media, but this criticism never refers to the freedom of the profession as such, because this is unavoidably connected to the protection of patient privacy.

These comments by the German physician Viktor von Weizsäcker from 1927 describe the development of the medical profession in Germany from Plato to the 20th century. It was almost impossible to contemplate the severe setback it was to suffer during the period of National Socialism or that the task of the physician should once again become linked to (eugenic) State goals. The terrible experience of medicine under Nazi rule has led to the private relationship between physician and patient being protected in the Nuremberg Code and close attention being paid to ensuring that diagnostic explanations and therapeutic options are kept as free from outside influences as possible.

Autonomy Enhancement by Including Family

Over the past few years, several authors have spoken out in favor of the family being taken into greater consideration in the therapeutic decision-making process. In his provocative text "What about the family", John Hardwig (1990) questioned the patient-centered ethos, whilst Jeffrey Blustein (1998) continued by pleading for what he called "a communitarian account of the role of the family in acute care decision making" (Blustein, 1998, p. 81). In his opinion, "the locus of decisional authority should remain the individual patient, but ...family members, by virtue of their closeness to and intimate knowledge of the patient, are often uniquely well qualified to shore up the patient's vulnerable autonomy and assist him or her in the exercise of autonomous decision making. Families, in other words, can be an important resource for patients in helping them to make better decisions about their care. Recognition of this fact leads to a broader understanding of the duty to respect patient autonomy than currently prevails in acute care medicine" (Blustein 1998, p. 82).

However important and correct the theoretical considerations surrounding patient autonomy may be, clinical routines show that many patients, influenced by their diseases, "are not ideally autonomous agents but anxious, fearful, depressed, often confused, and subject to ill-considered and mistaken ideas" (Blustein, 1998, p. 89). Patients' capacity for autonomy can be enhanced by conversations with other family members! The important point here, however, is that family members "have no veto power over a patient's decision and would have to honor the choice ultimately made, no matter how foolish or idiosyncratic." But in an open discussion with family members the patient could better understand what a particular treatment decision would cost other family members and might give the patient a compelling reason to alter an initial choice. "For the physician, the duty to respect patient autonomy has as its corollary a duty to engage in conversation with patients and to encourage and facilitate conversation between patients and other persons to whom they are close" (Blustein, 1998, p. 90). If the physician is to treat "the patient in the family" appropriately, the physician must be cognizant of the "family in the patient." Family communication may assist patients in making autonomous decisions about how or whether to treat their illness. The family is an important factor in most people's lifes, for better or for worse. This means that the health of individuals is influenced by family relationships "and that such relationships can play a vital role in restoring the autonomous functioning that illness undermines" (Blustein, 1998, p. 90). Like the free market has to be tied in the good life of the free citizen, the family has to be tied in the good life of the patient.

Notes

1. There are numerous examples of the way the German health sector is opening up to the market. The statutory health insurance companies, for example, have recently started to offer bonus schemes where points are awarded for the participation in fitness programmes, periodic preventive medical check-ups and other preventive measures. These points can then be exchanged for goods or financial bonuses. The patient also has the option to reduce his health insurance contribution by agreeing to pay a certain amount himself (own-risk clause).
2. The Council of Ministers adopted a Directive setting high quality and safety standards for dealing with human tissues and cells throughout the EU. Health and Consumer Protection Commissioner David Byrne welcoming the adoption by the Council said "We now have rules in place with comprehensive and binding requirements for the safety and quality of cells and tissues from donor to patient. This is positive news for hundreds of thousands of patients in Europe who every year, undergo some form of therapeutic treatment based on the use of human tissues and cells. Patients can now be sure that human tissues and cells derived from donations in another Member State nonetheless carry the same guarantees as those in their own country" (European Commission 2004).
3. In the preface to the second German edition, appearing 40 years after the initial publication of the original, Horst Siebert, President of the Institute for World Economy in Kiel (Germany), stresses that Friedman's book may be a "classic", and yet its analyses of the significance of "economic freedom" for individuals

and for society are not at all worn-out or old-fashioned, but still of great interest today (Siebert, 2002, p. 11).

4. See the political reforms for more democracy of the Peoples' National Congress in China in March 2004, especially the protection of private property (P.K. 2004).
5. The American *President's Commission* (1982) also emphasized that ethically valid consent to a medical intervention represents a "process of shared decision-making". The primary focus here is on the fact that a patient's decision cannot be said to occur at a single moment in time, with the legal consequence (e.g., in Germany) that the informing of patients about medical interventions is not understood as a unique act, but as a process, and that informative talks are to be repeated if necessary (Schmidt & Wolfslast 2002). In their influential book *Principles of Biomedical Ethics,* Beauchamp and Childress describe the stepwise guiding of patients towards informed consent as a model with seven stages: assuming the fundamental prerequisites (1) competence and (2) voluntariness, they describe the process as (3) disclosure, (4) recommendation, (5) understanding, (6) decision and finally (7) authorization (Beauchamp & Childress 1994, p. 145).
6. Critics maintain that the well-being of single persons or childless couples is today still promoted to a greater extent than the well-being of parents with children (reduced professional chances, lack of day nurseries, etc.).
7. Even where the citizen has previously designated his or her own proxy, the court often has to be asked to approve this action. The fact that a new draft law now proposes to assign proxy power to family members automatically must be regarded, quite simply, as a measure to reduce costs.
8. German law decrees that a patient who is unconscious for a longer period of time due to an accident or as a result of severe disease and who requires medical treatment is allocated a supervisor to represent his will in healthcare matters. The legal practise in many US states, e.g., Texas, whereby potential decision-makers are listed hierarchically (first the spouse, then the children, then the parents, etc.) would be unthinkable from a German point of view. The family is strictly rejected as a naturally legitimate advocate since it is impossible to guarantee with the necessary certainty that they will act according to the patient's interests and will. Tellingly, a suggestion published in the German journal *Der Anaesthesist* that the Texan model of automatic representation through close family members for patients no longer able to make their own decisions could also be adopted in Germany (Schmidt & Sold 2001) met with hefty criticism (Scharf, Edwin, Staetling & Bartmann, 2001).
9. A study in North Germany reached the conclusion that numerous interventions are carried out in patients without their consent, without the involvement of the—legally responsible—German court for matters of guardianship, and without the nomination of a legal supervisor to represent the will of the patient and officially give consent (Scharf *et al.* 2001). The workgroup was led to assume that the German system of courts for guardianship would collapse under the pressure if all physicians were to obey the law and apply for legal consent before performing medical interventions in patients unable to make their own decisions.
10. The population of Western Europe, for example, reacts very sensitively to reports about organ trade and sales in Asia Minor and Iraq, as well as the removal of organs from executed persons in China.

References

Akabayashi, A., Fetters, M.D., & Elwyn, T.S. (1999). 'Family consent, communication, and advance directives for cancer disclosure: a Japanese case and discussion.' *Journal of Medical Ethics*, 25, 296-301.

Altvater, E., & Mahnkopf, B. (2002). *Grenzen der Globalisierung. Ökonomie, Ökologie und Politik in der Welktgesellschaft*, (5th ed). Münster: Westfälisches Dampfboot.

Bayertz, K. (2006). 'Struggling for consensus and living without it,' in H..T. Engelhardt, Jr., *Global Bioethics: The Collapse of Consensus*, pp. 207-237.

Bayertz, K., & Schmidt, K.W. (2005). 'Testing Genes and Constructing Humans – Ethics and Genetics,' in G. Khushf (Ed.), *Handbook of the Philosophy of Medicine*, Vol.I. Dordrecht: Kluwer Academic Publishers.

Beauchamp, T., & Childress, J. (1994). *Principles of Biomedical Ethics* (4th ed). Oxford: Oxford University Press.

Begisheva, A. (2004, 10 March). 'Kein Mutterland,' *Frankfurter Rundschau*, 59, 31.

Blustein, J. (1998). 'The Family in Medical Decisionmaking,' in J. F. Monagle & Thomasma, D.C. (Eds.), *Health Care Ethics.* Gaithersburg: Aspen Publications.

Bolz, N. (2002). *Das konsumistische Manifest.* München: Wilhelm Fink.

Capaldi, N. (2003). Manifesto: Moral Diversity in Health Care Ethics. *Conference paper.*

Capaldi, N. (1998). 'Was stimmt nicht mit der Solidarität?' in K. Bayertz (Ed.), *Solidarität. Begriff und Problem* (pp. 86-110). Frankfurt: Suhrkamp.

Cherry, M. (2004). 'Global bioethics: preserving the possibility for liberty in health care,' in this volume.

Däubler-Gmelin, H. (1996). 'Menschenwürde in der Marktgesellschaft. Aufgabe der Politik und Erwartungen an die Kirch, in R. Weth (Ed.), *Totaler Markt und Menscehnwürde* (pp. 89-109). Neukirchen-Vluyn: Neukirchener Verlag.

Dahrendorf, R. (1977). *Homo sociologicus* (15th ed). Opladen: Westdeutscher Verlag.

Deppe, H.U. (2004). 'Kulturwende in der Medizin,' in G. Ulshöfer *et al* (Eds.), *Ökonomisierung der Diakonie* (pp. 9-21). Frankfurt: Arnoldsheimer Texte, Haag & Herchen.

Doerner, K. (2001). *Der gute Arzt. Lehrbuch der ärztlichen Grundhaltung.* Stuttgart/ New York: Schattauer.

Engelhardt, H. T. Jr. (2000). *The Foundations of Christian Bioethics.* Lisse: Swets & Zeitlinger.

European Commission. (2004). *European Commission welcomes new rules to guarantee safety and quality of human cells and tissues.* Brussels, March 2, 2004. [Online]. Available: http://europa.eu.int/rapid/start/cgi/guesten.ksh?p_action.gettxt=gt&doc=IP/04/288|0|RAPID&lg=EN&display=

European Convention. (1997). 'Convention for the protection of human rights and dignity of the human being with regard to the application of biology and medicine: convention on human rights and biomedicine.' *The Journal of Medicine and Philosophy*, 25(2) 2000, pp. 259-266.

European Parliament. (2003). *European Parliament legislative resolution on the Council common position adopting a European Parliament and Council directive on setting standards of quality and safety for the donation, procurement, testing, processing, preservation, storage and distribution of human tissues and cells* [Online]. Available: http://www3.europarl.eu.int/omk/omnsapir.so/pv2?PRG=CALDOC&TPV=PROV&FILE=20031216&TXTLST=1&POS=1&LASTCHAP=20&SDOCTA=18&Type_Doc=FIRST&LANGUE=EN

Freedman, B. (2000). 'The roles and responsibilities of the ethics consultant,' in Baylis (Ed.), *A Retrospective Analysis of Cases.* Hagerstown, Maryland: University Publishing Group.
Friedman, M. (1982). *Capitalism and Freedom* (2nd ed). Chicago: University of Chicago Press.
Grisso, T., & Appelbaum, P.S. (1998). *Assessing Competence to Consent to Treatment.* New York: Oxford University Press.
Hardwig, J. (1990). 'What about the family?' *Hastings Center Report,* 10(2), 5-10.
Hyun, I. (2002). 'Waiver of informed consent, cultural sensitivity, and the problem of unjust families and traditions.' *Hastings Center Report,* 32(5), 14-22.
Joseph, Rev. Father T. (1998). 'Secular vs. Orthodox Christianity: taking the kingdom of heaven seriously.' *Christian Bioethics,* 4 (3), 276-278.
Kant, Immanuel. (1797). 'Über ein vermeintliches Recht, aus Menschenliebe zu lügen,' in W. Weischedel (Ed.), *Werke in zehn Bänden,* (7, pp. 637-643). Darmstadt: Wissenschaftliche Buchgesellschaft.
Kaessmann, M. (2000, January 19). 'Gesundheitsethik für das Kommende Jahrhundert aus Christlicher Sicht' Rede beim Neujahrsempfang der Ärztekammer Niedersachsen, Hannover.
Kersting, W. (1999). *Platons Staat.* Darmstadt: Wissenschaftliche Buchgesellschaft.
Körtner, U.H.J. (2001). 'Der unbezähmbare Tod,' in F.J. Wetz & Tagg, B. (Eds.), *Schöne neue Körperwelten. Der Streit um die Ausstellun* (pp. 241-265). Stuttgart: Klett-Cotta.
Liese, P. (2004). *Ministerrat nimmt Einigung mit Parlament zu Qualität und Sicherheit von Zellen und Geweben formal an.* [Online]. Available: http://www.euro-liese.de/get.php4?bereich=0&id=466
Lost in Translation (USA/Japan 2003) Director and Script: Sofia Coppola.
Luther, M. (1519). 'Ein Sermon von der Bereitung zum Sterben,' in O. Clemen (Ed.), *Luthers Werke* (6th ed, pp. 161-173). Berlin: de Gruyter.
Mappes, T.A., & Zembaty, J.S. (1994). 'Patient choices, family interests, and physician obligations.' *Kennedy Institute of Ethics Journal,* 4(1), 27-46.
Marx, K. & Engels, F. (2004). *The Communist Manifesto,* L.M. Findlay (ed.). Orchard Park, NY: Broadview Press.
Mayer, K.U. (Ed.) (2001). *Die Beste aller Welten? Marktliberalismus versus Wohlfahrtsstaat.* Frankfurt: Campus.
Moazam, F. (2000). 'Families, patients, and physicians in medical decisionmaking: a Pakistani perspective.' *Hastings Center Report,* 30(6), 28-37.
Nelson, J.L. (1992). 'Taking families seriously.' *Hastings Center Report,* 22(4), 6-12.
Nida-Rümelin, J. (2004, March 2). 'Tief in Unserer Lebenswelt Verwurzelt.' *Frankfurter Rundschau.*
Petroni, A.M. (2006). 'Perspectives for Freedom of Choice in Bioethics and Health Care in Europe,' in this volume.
Pirson, D. (1987). 'Ehe und Familie als Gegenstand rechtlicher Ordnun, ' in R. Herzog (Ed.), *Evangelisches Staatslexikon I* (3rd ed., pp. 650-658). Stuttgart: Kreuz.
Plato. (1986). 'Politeia,' in E. Grassi (Ed.), *Sämtliche Werke,* Vol. 3. Hamburg: Rowohlt.
President's Commission. (1982). *President's Commission for the Study of Ethical Problems in Medicine and Biomedical and Behavioral Research. Making Health Care Decisions: The Ethical and Legal Implications of Informed Consent in the Patient-Practitioner Relationship.* Washington D.C: U.S. Government Printing Office.

Radovsky, S.S. (1985). 'Bearing the News.' *The New England Journal of Medicine,* 313(9), 586-588.

Scharf, V.E., Straetling, M., & Bartmann, F.J. (2001). *Stellvertreterentscheidungen in Gesundheitsfragen und Patintenverfügungen.* Special Publication.

Schmidt, K.W. (2000). 'Ethische Problemfelder der Organtransplantation,' in E.M. Engels, Badura-Lotter, G. & Schicktanz, S. (Eds.), Neue Perspektiven der Transplantationsmedizin im interdisziplinären Dialog, (pp. 35-55). Baden-Baden: Nomos Verlagsgesellschaft.

Schmidt, K.W., & Sold, M. (2001). 'Stellvertreterentscheidungen in Gesundheitsfragen und Vorausverfügungen von Patienten.' *Anaesthesist,* 50, 200-201.

Schmidt, K.W., & Wolfslast, G. (2002). 'Patientenaufklärung. Ethische und rechtliche Aspekte.' *Deutsche Medizinische Wochenschrift,* 127, 634-637.

Schnitzler, A. (1912). ,Professor Bernhardi. Komödie in fünf Akten,' in A. Schnitzler (Ed.) *Das weite Land. Dramen* 1909-1912, 7th ed, (pp. 149-294). Frankfurt: S. Fischer.

Siebert, H. (2002). 'Geleitwort,' in M. Friedman (Ed.), Kapitalismus und Freiheit (2nd ed., pp. 11-14). Frankfurt: Eichborn.

Singer, W. (2003). *Ein neues Menschenbild?* Frankfurt: Suhrkamp.

Stephan, R. (1986). *Beck'scher Ratgeber Recht* (2nd ed.), München: C.H. Beck.

Tao, L. J. (2004). 'A Confucian approach to a "shared decision model" in health care: reflection on moral pluralism,' in this volume.

Thomsen, O.O.,Wulff, H.R., Martin, A., & Singer, P.A. (1993). 'What do gastroenterologists in Europe tell cancer patients?' *Lancet,* 341(8843), 473-476.

Ulrich, P. (2002). Der entzauberte Markt. *Eine wirtschaftsethische Orientierung.* Freiburg: Herder.

Weizsäcker, V. (1975). ,Der Arzt und der Kranke,' in K. Rothschuh (Ed.), *Was ist Krankheit?* (pp. 214-232). Wege der Forschung CCCLXII. Darmstadt: Wissenschaftliche Buchgesellschaft.

Wetz, F.J., & Tag, B. (2001) Schöne neue Körperwelten. Der Streit um die Ausstellung. Stuttgart: Klett-Cotta.

White, M.L., & Fletcher, J.C. (1990). 'The story of Mr. and Mrs. Doe: "You can't tell my husband he's dying; it will kill him.' *Journal of Clinical Ethics,* 1(1), 59-62.

Struggling for Consensus and Living Without It: The Construction of a Common European Bioethics

Kurt Bayertz

On Tuesday 19th December 2000, the British House of Commons passed a bill extending the grounds for research using early human embryos and allowing the creation of embryos by a new cell nuclear replacement technique ("therapeutic cloning") for a wider range of research purposes. One month later, on 23rd January 2001, the House of Lords agreed to this bill. – What might be seen as a domestic parliamentary decision caused excited reactions in some other European countries. In Summer 2000 the European Parliament had already passed a Resolution (advisory only) demanding that the British Government withdraw all plans to allow human embryos to be cloned for research. The European Parliament, as stated in the text,

> considers that therapeutic cloning poses a profound ethical dilemma, irreversibly crosses a boundary in research norms and is contrary to public policy; calls on the United Kingdom Parliament members to reject the proposal to permit research using embryos created by cell nuclear transfer; repeats its call to each Member State to enact binding legislation prohibiting all research into any kind of human cloning within its territory and to provide criminal penalties for any breach... (House of Commons, 2000, p. 32)

H.T. Engelhardt, Jr. (ed), *Global Bioethics* (pp. 207–237).

Two months after the British decision (but without mentioning it) the French President Jacques Chirac declared that he opposed the therapeutic cloning of human beings and warned against "a utilitarian conception of the human being which would call into question the very foundations of our civilization"[1] (2001). In Germany some Christian politicians even went further and demanded sanctions against Great Britain by the European institutions; for them, the British decision amounted to a revocation of membership in occidental culture or to a splitting of Europe and its moral identity.

These reactions illuminate two important things. On the one hand, there is a strong appeal to a specific European cultural and moral identity. "Europe" is not used as a mere geographical term, referring to the western appendage of the Asian continent, beginning with the Ural and ending with the Portuguese Atlantic coast, or to a number of states which are accidentally located in close neighbourhood. Instead, "Europe" is seen as a part of the world with a genuine historical and cultural identity, including a common set of values. Beyond its geographic meaning, the term "Europe", therefore, refers to a historically grown model of society and civilization, a way of life, different from other ways of life in other parts of the world. On the other hand, it is by no means clear which elements are included in this cultural and moral identity, how they are to be interpreted, or what their respective weight is. There are many disagreements and passionate debates about this. The Members of the British House of Commons presumably did not intend to violate European morality or to depart from the occidental culture, but were convinced that their decision was in accordance with this morality and culture. Since the British decision concerning therapeutic cloning is not the only example of such a disagreement, it is fair to state that there is a tension between the *supposition* that there is such a thing as a common European morality and the *fact* that this common morality is neither well defined nor undisputed.

The aim of this paper is to address this tension in the field of bioethical questions, as well as to explain its background and its implications. My aim, therefore, is mainly analytical, not evaluative. I will not ask "who is right" or "what is right", but "what is going on" with bioethics in Europe and try to give some explanations. The premise of this approach is that bioethics is presently undergoing a change in function.[2] At least parts of it are extending beyond the academic world and beginning to play a public, a political or a legal role. Bioethics has become the ideological basis of *biopolitics;* some have spoken of a passage "from bioethics to biolaw"[3] (Mazzoni, 1998). This means: in this paper I will refer by "bioethics" not (at least not in the first instance) to the respective academic endeavours and debates, but to the "official" decisions and documents which regulate professional action in the field of medicine, medical research and health care.

In the *first* section I will deal with how a European moral identity may be understood and what its major elements in the field of bioethics may be. *Then*

I will discuss some of the limitations of this identity and show that there is a lot of difference and divergence among different European countries. And *finally* I will focus on the fact that the "official" type of bioethics I am dealing with in this paper is the result of a political construction and venture some speculations about what the prospects of such constructions may be.

1. Struggling for Consensus in Europe

There have been many attempts[4] to describe or define what the "European identity" might be; and, more specifically, what the cultural and moral elements of this identity might be. I would like to start with a rough distinction between two different approaches to this endeavour. This first is *positive* and *substantial*. It consists in identifying one crucial idea, principle or value, or several ideas, principles or values, which are constitutive of the European identity. There are three main candidates which have been mentioned again and again from antiquity to the present times: *freedom, individuality* and *rationality*. To mention only one example of this positive, substantial approach I quote from Georg Wilhelm Friedrich Hegel's *Encyclopaedia*:

> The principle of the European mind is, therefore, self-conscious Reason which is confident that for it there can be no insuperable barrier and which therefore takes an interest in everything in order to become present to itself therein. The European mind opposes the world to itself, makes itself free of it, but in turn annuls this opposition, takes its Other, the manifold, back into itself, into its unitary nature. In Europe, therefore, there prevails this infinite thirst for knowledge which is alien to other races. The European is interested in the world, he wants to know it, to make this Other confronting him his own, to bring to view the genus, law, universal, thought, the inner rationality, in the particular forms of the world (Hegel, 1845, § 393Z).

Usually, such ideas, principles or values like freedom, individuality, and rationality are traced back to one or more of the main epochs or traditions which have shaped European history. There are three of them which play an important role here: (a) Greek and Roman antiquity, with their emphasis on the rational approach to reality and on political liberty; (b) Christianity as the origin of the idea of an unalienable value of each human being and consequently of equality and dignity; and (c) the Enlightenment as the source of important moral and political values like toleration, human rights, and democracy. This positive, substantial approach, irrespective of the merits it may have, faces two problems. The first is that each idea, principle or value which is declared as constitutive of the European identity has a broad variety of meanings; two people speaking of freedom, individuality or rationality can connect very different ideas with these concepts and draw very different conclusions from them. When, for example, Max Weber (1920, pp. 1-16) in the preface to his collected essays on the sociology of religion underlined "rationality" as the main feature of European culture, he had in mind something very different from Hegel's concept of Reason. It is at least an open question if concepts like rationality have enough determinate content to provide the intellectual basis of a European identity. And, moreover, what about the important theories and movements which have, in one way or another, criticized the ideas of freedom, individuality, and rationality? Are they not (or not truly) "European"? The second problem is that these ideas have spread all over the world and have developed deep roots in major parts of it. If freedom, individuality and rationality are constitutive of the European identity, then at least North America and Australia have long become "European". It is hard to see how a distinctive European identity could be based on such ideas or values.

More promising, therefore, seems the second approach. It is *negative* in that it does not primarily try to identify some substantial content constitutive for the European identity, but draws a distinction between "Europe" and something else, preferably a threat or an enemy. And it is *functional* in that it does not only allude to an existing European identity but invokes and postulates such an identity as necessary. The advantage of this functional, i.e., programmatic and constructive, approach lies in the fact that broad concepts like "freedom", "individuality", and "rationality" take shape and gain more content when they are used as means of demarcation from something which is (supposedly) not "free", not "individual(istic)" and not "rational". If we go back into history, we will see very easily that the idea of a European identity has mostly had this negative and functional character. It regularly came into play as a reaction to a threat and was intended as a means to overcome this threat. This should be no surprise because it is quite a common phenomenon that identities become more important and stronger the more they are in danger. The idea of Europe has developed historically in demarcation from and in confrontation with other parts of the world: especially "the East". This began very early. In his *History*, Herodotus starts with a report of the origins of the enmity between "Greeks" and "Barbarians" and gives a detailed description of the war with the Persians (Herodotus, I, 3/4). The sharp line drawn here between the oriental and the occidental world continued to exist in a new form after the splitting of the Roman Empire in 395 and became even deeper when in the following centuries Islam developed and became a strong political and military force, conquering Spain in the 8th century and besieging Vienna in the 17th century. At the beginning of the 20th century, the dualism between "Europe" and "the East" changed again, when the Soviet Union originated and spread its influence over a third of the world.

What does this mean for the topic of this paper? When in recent times the cultural and moral European identity has increasingly been invoked and when there are intensive activities to formulate a common European bioethics, then we have to conclude from the previous considerations about the negative and functional character of this concept that there is (or is perceived) some kind of threat to it. But where could this threat come from? Obviously, it cannot be "the East", because there is no Soviet imperium any more and it is hard to see how the Islamic world should be a threat in bioethical questions. The answer is that the threat for what is seen as the common European bioethical identity does not come any more from the outside; instead it comes from within. There are two main developments which form this threat.

The first is the rapidly increasing progress of biotechnology during the last decades. The permanent revolution of medical technology and biotechnology in general (especially of gene technology) and the new options for all subjects involved has for years been observed with suspicion by many people, including many politicians. Such concerns have not only led to public debates in several countries, but have triggered political activities at a transnational level, too. In the 1970s the *Council of Europe* already began to occupy itself with the new developments in biomedicine and biotechnology[5]. In 1982 the *Parliamentary Assembly of the Council of Europe* passed Recommendation 934 on genetic engineering, which in its first sentence alludes to "public concerns about the use of new scientific techniques for artificially recombining genetic material from living organisms" and then explicitly links some of the questions raised by this technology to the guarantee of human rights:

> The rights to life and to human dignity protected by Articles 2 and 3 of the European Convention on Human Rights imply the right to inherit a genetic pattern which has not been artificially changed (Council of Europe, 1982, §4.i).

The text further recommends that the Committee of Ministers:

> provide for explicit recognition in the European Convention on Human Rights of a right to a genetic inheritance which has not been artificially interfered with, except in accordance with certain principles which are recognised as being fully compatible with respect for human rights (as, for example, in the field of therapeutic applications) (Council of Europe, 1982, §7.b)

This line of argument was continued during the 1990s when the European "Bioethics Convention" was drafted, publicly discussed and then ratified.[6] The full title of this convention makes it explicit that the ethical and social problems of modern biomedicine are interpreted as human rights problems: *Convention for the Protection of Human Rights and Dignity of the Human Being With Regard to the Application of Biology and Medicine.* It is then only consistent that this Convention was issued by the *European Council* which—facing the splitting of Europe into two blocks—in 1950 had agreed upon the *Convention for the Protection of Human Rights and Fundamental Freedom.* Then the threat to human rights and dignity had been a political one; now, since the 1990s, it is a scientific and technological one.

The second development is the ubiquitous process of *globalization*. What is meant here is not a specific and narrowly conceived economic change, like the origin of transnational companies and the internationalisation of markets, but a pervasive social evolution which touches all parts of society and moulds all levels of human life. This is so because the economic changes coincide with strong neoliberal ideology, and with powerful scientific and technological achievements. "Globalization" will bring about a model of society which Jürgen Habermas (2001) has polemically characterised as having four features: (a) the anthropological image of the human being as a rationally deciding businessman who exploits his own labour power; (b) the political image of a post-egalitarian society which accepts the marginalisation and exclusion of certain individuals; (c) the economic image of a democracy which reduces citizens to the status of members of a free-market society and redefines the state as a service enterprise for clients and customers; and (d) by the strategic thought that there is no better policy than that which runs by itself. According to Habermas, the neo-liberal world-view and the corresponding model of society does not fit the normative self-understanding of Europeans.[7]

But how and why may globalization be seen as challenge to the European culture and morality and, more specifically, as a threat to the European *bioethical* identity? There are two different, but connected answers to this: (a) The economic development and the scientific-technological progress both lead to an erosion of traditional political and social structures and institutions. An important example in the biomedical field is the fact that medical actions increasingly take place outside the established medical system; the physician-patient relationship is going to be replaced by a provider-consumer relationship. This is important because the classical structures and institutions are not seen as mere social facts, but as embodiments of values. European medical ethics always focused on the physician-patient relationship as a special moral relationship; and the values inherent in this relationship cannot be upheld when medical action is increasingly determined by free market mechanisms and instrumental reasoning. The laws of supply and demand take the place of moral laws; scientific expertise and technological imperatives take the place of compassion and care. Nothing could be more misled, from this perspective, than the idea that the free market provides the appropriate model for dealing with moral problems of health care. For an influential group of bioethicists in the US, exactly this is the case. In Engelhardt's vision of the future, the general practice of moral stranger's resolving controversies will have a character illustrated by the free market:

> Each participant can bring a quite different understanding of successful market transactions, the purposes of the market, and the goods it supports. However, each can also recognize a practice that all can understand as justified simply and barely through the permission of those who enter it. The

> authority of the endeavour depends not on any particular ranking of goods, moral narrative, or ordering of right-making principles. Across moral communities the authority of the market can be regarded neutrally as drawn simply from the permission of those who engage it (Engelhardt, 1996, p. 114f).

The idea here is of a common European morality as a counter-design to this market-model; its premise being the conviction that there is nothing neutral with the market. Quite the contrary, the market-model has to be seen as the epitome of a specific and particular moral vision—one which eliminates all cultural diversities and moral pluralism.

(b) It can be argued that the modern type of economy and the modern type of technology converge in their common tendency to erode the traditional, value-based *way of thinking*. What they foster is not a type of content-full reason, which Hegel had in mind, but an instrumental kind of rationality which has been analysed by Max Weber. But while Weber soberly tried to balance the gains and losses of the "Occidental rationality" many accounts today stress the losses and deplore the erosion of values. In former times, this mainly negative view of the rationalisation and modernisation of society was prominent on the right side of the political spectrum; during the last three decades of the 20th century it spread to the other parts, including the political left (the movement of the Greens is the most obvious, but not the only example). This holds especially with respect to the recent scientific and technological developments in the area of biology and medicine. Many religious believers, conservative politicians, Green or feminist activists, and remained socialists agree with the statement that some of the most fundamental European values are endangered by an increasing pressure (i) not only by the market imperatives of a globalized economy, but also (ii) by a naturalistic image of the human being, provided by the advances of biomedical science, and (iii) by the recent biotechnological achievements with their tendency to more or less subtle forms of instrumentalisation, and reification of human beings.

But what are these fundamental European values? The most important one is *human dignity*. There can be not doubt that during the last decades human dignity has emerged as the central and most important value or principle of the project of a common European bioethical framework. This concept can be traced back to the three main elements of European identity which have just been mentioned. We find this concept in parts of Greek and Roman philosophy, especially in Stoicism; it is a substantial element of Judeo-Christian anthropology, which views the human being as "imago dei"; and it has been philosophically elaborated by Enlightenment philosophers like Immanuel Kant. Moreover, this value plays a key role in the constitutional law of many European countries: Belgium, Czech Republic, Denmark, Finland, France, Germany, Greece, Ireland, Lithuania, Poland, Russia, Spain, Sweden and Switzerland. It is not by accident, therefore, that European international documents concerning bioethical questions rely heavily on this value. This is especially true for the important "Bioethics Convention" of the *Council of Europe*. The concept of human dignity not only appears in the official title of this convention but is at the center of its Article 1 which defines the purpose and object of the convention:

> Parties to this Convention shall protect the dignity and identity of all human beings and guarantee everyone, without discrimination, respect for their integrity and other rights and fundamental freedoms with regard to the application of biology and medicine (de Wachter, 1997, p. 15).

The *Explanatory Report* accompanying the convention underlines this central role by confirming that human dignity "constitutes the essential value to be upheld" and explaining that it "is at the basis of most of the values emphasised in the Convention" (Council of Europe, 1997b, §9). Unfortunately, the *Explanatory Report* does not say what the term "human dignity" means, nor what follows from the moral principle, which prescribes the protection of human dignity. There is a lot of debate about the correct interpretation of this key term and it is impossible to go into the details of this discussion here (Bayertz, 1996; the bibliographies by Haferkamp, 1996; and Center for Ethics and Law, 1999). But there is a widespread inclination to a "substantialist" interpretation of this term, which includes a more or less fixed image of the human being. This results in a tension between the concept or principle of human dignity on the one hand, and the concept or principle of autonomy on the other. Whereas the concept of autonomy did not play a central role in traditional European medical ethics, it has become fundamental during the last two decades, in part because of the strong reception which has greeted US American bioethics. The "Bioethics Convention" is very clear about this central role; the chapter on "consent" is the first after "general provisions" and Article 5 states as a general rule:

> An intervention in the health field may only be carried out after the person concerned has given free and informed consent to it. This person shall beforehand be given appropriate information as to the purpose and nature of the intervention as well as on its consequences and risks. The person concerned may freely withdraw consent at any time (de Wachter, 1997, p. 20).

But according at least to some influential line of bioethical thought, informed consent is seen as a necessary rather than a sufficient condition for a medical intervention to be morally legitimate. If there is the above mentioned substantial image of the human being and its integrity, which must not be violated (human dignity), then there are limits to what a competent human subject is allowed to do, even if no other person is affected. There are certain limits to autonomous human self-determination, which becomes obvious when we look at the "appropriate" reasons justifying medical or biotechnological interventions in human beings. Such interventions are legitimised mainly or even exclusively by their medical—i.e., in the last instance, by their therapeutic—goal. The French Law *Concerning the Human Body* of 1994 prohibits any intervention in the integrity of the human body unless there is a "therapeutic necessity for the person."[8] Human reproductive technologies are a good example: whereas in the US the use of such technologies is often justified by the right to a free choice of reproductive options, the justification in Europe is primarily medical: as a therapy for unwanted childlessness. It is only consistent, therefore, that in its Article 12 the "Bioethics Convention" confines predictive genetic tests to a medical framework:

> Tests which are predictive of genetic diseases or which serve either to identify the subject as a carrier of a gene responsible for a disease or to detect a genetic predisposition or susceptibility to a disease may be performed only for health purposes or for scientific research linked to health purposes, and subject to appropriate genetic counselling (de Wachter, 1997, p. 21).

In most cases of everyday medicine this special way of legitimizing medical interventions makes only a philosophical but not a practical difference. But there are at least some areas where there are practical differences, too. Maybe most important is the question of commercialisation. Whereas many bioethicists in the US do not see major moral problems in the commercialisation of human organs and tissue, Article 21 of the Convention prohibits any financial gain from the human body or its parts. The same holds for the legal systems of many European states (like France and Great Britain), which do not consider individuals as "owners" of their bodies; other countries (like Germany and the Netherlands) at least limit individuals severely in their free disposition over their bodies. This excludes the legal possibility of selling organs or tissues, including blood (ten Have & Welie, 1998). Likewise, contracts between parents and surrogate mothers would not be enforceable by law. Such limitations to the disposal of individuals over their own bodies are justified by the principle or value of human dignity, which is meant to exclude not only the instrumentalisation of other people, but self-instrumentalisation, too.

Another important element of European bioethics besides human dignity is the principle of *equitable access to health care.* There is a widespread consensus in Europe that everyone who needs medical help should receive it, independent of individual financial background. From a US-American point of view, Europe is a "socialist" continent where each person is thought to have a legitimate claim to every treatment which is medically necessary. Although there are intense (and controversial) discussions about how this claim can be upheld in an era of rapidly increasing costs, only very few people dare principally to call into question what is stated in Article 3 of the "Bioethics Convention":

> Parties, taking into account health needs and available resources, shall take appropriate measure with a view to providing, within their jurisdiction, equitable access to health care of appropriate quality (de Wachter, 1997, p. 19).

This right to health care on the side of the recipient has its necessary counterpart in the principle of solidarity on the side of the community (or state), providing this help and paying for it. Solidarity implies the idea that there are certain social obligations human individuals have towards each other. In contrast to the US health care system, all European countries ensure (almost) universal health care coverage for their citizens.

II. Living Without Consensus in Europe

Thus far the *idea* of a common European bioethics. Once we move from the theoretical program to the practical reality we will soon notice that "European bioethics" is one thing, and bioethics in Europe quite another. It is one of the main theses of the present paper that the common European outlook in matters of medicine and health care is but narrow; and that all political attempts to construct and implement a common outlook will be of only very limited success. To lend this claim plausibility, let us step back from bioethics for a moment and take into consideration European culture on a more general level.

Any idea of Europe having a uniform tradition and monolithic culture is far from the historical as well as the contemporary reality. Why this is so becomes immediately clear on a closer look at the abovementioned roots and/or elements of European identity. These roots or elements are heterogeneous and in—sometimes latent, sometimes open—conflict with each other: in some respects the pagan world-view of Greek and Roman antiquity is hard to reconcile with Christian religion; and the Enlightenment has (in part) developed as a counter-movement to Christianity. If Europe has ever been a unity at all, it has always been a unity-in-diversity, or even a unity-in-controversy. Looking back, therefore, we do not find only unity and agreement, but also divergence and controversy at different levels. What has been characteristic for Europe—at least during its history after the Middle Ages—is its ability to develop ways of living with dissensus rather than reaching consensus. One important example is the idea of toleration which emerged when the religious homogeneity of Europe collapsed after the Reformation. At first, this idea was by no means welcomed by everybody; and it took some hundred years to convince the Catholic Church that there is no reasonable alternative to the freedom of religion. But finally this insight gained the upper hand, formulated impressively by John Locke in his *Letter Concerning Toleration:*

> It is not the diversity of opinions, which cannot be avoided; but the refusal of toleration to those that are of different opinions, which might have been granted, that has produced all the bustles and wars, that have been in the Christian world, upon account of religion (Locke, 1667, p. 53).

As a second example one might add the recognition of political pluralism in the 19th century; it had become clear after the French Revolution that the rival coexistence of different political parties was no temporary fact, but a structural feature of modern societies. Again, there was a lot of reluctance concerning this insight, but finally the idea of political pluralism and the implementation of democratic institutions were widely accepted. In both cases the "solution" to the problem had not been to re-establish consensus, but to find ways of *living peacefully with dissensus.* And in both cases what was first allowed only reluctantly, was later increasingly welcomed as a value in its own right: toleration of pluralism.

With cultural pluralism things are somewhat different, in that this has always been regarded as an achievement. The assessment has always prevailed that the diversity of art styles and of ways of life in the different European countries—and the competition between them—has been one of the strengths of European culture. And exactly this diversity and competition seems to be threatened today to a degree previously unknown in history. Engelhardt has described this threat as follows:

> [T]here is a global market ethos directed at the satisfaction of needs, inclinations, and drives that is powerfully refashioning tastes. To sell effectively to the largest market, one harnesses the most basic human concerns, passions, and interests. Mass marketing focuses drives that support mass culture. The result is a cultural homogenization: one encounters McDonald's, Coca-Cola, Kentucky Fried Chicken, and Microsoft from Buenos Aires to Cape Town, Madrid to Kyoto. Fashions in music, clothes, and television are becoming global. All of us are invited to pursue self-satisfaction and self-realization, as this can be facilitated within a global market set within an evolving cluster of common global images of human well-being, satisfaction, and flourishing (Engelhardt, 2003, p. 27).

Many artists, philosophers, intellectuals and politicians also believe that the specific humanistic culture which has developed in Europe over the many centuries since the end of the Middle Ages has to be defended against this threat of the global market, its economic imperatives and its instrumental way of thinking. The increased invocation of the European cultural and moral identity, the repeated appeals to be reminiscent of this identity and to strengthen it have to be interpreted as a reaction to the challenge of triumphant capitalism and its uniforming power.

The decisive point for the present context is that all this holds for morality, too. The cultural pluralism characteristic of Europe includes a plurality of moral convictions and ethical approaches. There is no monolithic "European morality" and there has never been one (or at least not during the last centuries). In cultural as well as in moral matters, Europe is and has been a unity-in-diversity, too. Any aspiration, therefore, to construct a European "moral identity" as a homogeneous system of values, principles or ideals, which would (or at least could) function as the basis for a comprehensive moral consensus, is without historical precedent and basis.

If we return to the contemporary field of bioethics, we will have reason to expect considerable diversity within Europe in dealings with present problems raised by the new biotechnologies. And this is exactly what we find. Empirical studies on public perception, policy debates and the political regulations of modern biotechnology show great differences between the European states. On the basis of a vast amount of empirical data, the authors of a comparative review on "biology in the public sphere" come to the conclusion:

> That there is no unified public discourse about biotechnology in Europe. In terms of public policy, we have found different European countries dealing with modern biotechnology over very different timescales and in very different ways. In terms of media coverage, we have found that a commonly held discourse of progress and benefit is paralleled by rather different patterns of media reportage in the European countries. Last but not least, we have seen from the results of Eurobarometer 46.1 that the different European countries tend to have widely differing levels of engagement with, knowledge about and attitudes towards biotechnology. In light of these results, it is a brave person indeed who would hazard a general conclusion about 'the European view of biotechnology' (Bauer, Durant & Gaskell, 1998, p. 226).

What is stated here with regard to the public perception of biotechnology in general can also be confirmed with regard to the *ethical* aspects of biotechnology and biomedicine. There is impressive evidence from the available data that ethical appraisal by the public of important questions like the moral status of the human embryo encompasses enormous diversity (a) *within* the different European countries; and (b) *between* the different European countries; consequently, the opinions concerning biomedical options like stem cell research, embryo experimentation, IVF and PGD are very controversial (Solter et. al., 2003, pp. 157-203). The controversy concerning "therapeutic cloning", reported in the introduction to this paper, may be seen as an illustration of the actual lack of consensus in important bioethical questions and as a warning against too much hope (or anxiety) regarding the possibility of a consensus. Official documents like the "Bioethics Convention" are always programmatic and prospective in character, and therefore never offer a true picture of the given situation, stressing the reached agreements and leaving unmentioned all those questions on which agreement proved to be impossible. It becomes obvious that the realm of disagreement remains considerable if we focus on what is not regulated in the text of the Convention. Two especially important areas may be mentioned here.

The *moral status of the human embryo* is one of the key questions on which Europe remains far from any consensus. The "Bioethics Convention" states in Article 1 that the parties to this shall protect the dignity and integrity "of all human beings and guarantee everyone, without discrimination, respect for their integrity". Since the decisive terms "human being" and "everyone" are not defined, it remains an open question as to whether the human embryo is included.[9] This is not by accident, as the "Explanatory Report" says explicitly:

> In the absence of a unanimous agreement on the definitions of these terms among member states of the Council of Europe, it was decided to allow domestic law to define them for the purposes of the application of the present Convention (Council of Europe, 1997b, § 18).[10]

This makes it possible for very different regulations concerning several important medical options to continue to exist in different European states. (a) The first and most important of these options is abortion. There are states with strict prohibition of any kind of *abortion,* like Ireland, and others with very liberal regulations. (b) The same holds true for the question of *embryo experimentation,* where one finds three groups of countries. One group with very liberal regulation, explicitly allowing embryo research (UK); a second group with restrictive regulation, allowing research only if it directly benefits the embryo itself (Germany); and a third group which allows embryo research under certain specifically defined circumstances (Spain), (Solter et. al., 2003, pp. 111-155). (c) The third option to mention here is *preimplantation genetic diagnosis,* which is forbidden in Austria, Switzerland and (de facto) Germany, but allowed in Great Britain, France, Sweden and Belgium.

A second important question to which there is no common European answer is that of *euthanasia.* The "Bioethics Convention" remains silent here, too. The deep divergences at the level of national regulations became obvious when on 14th April 2001 the first chamber of the Netherlands parliament decided to legalise (under carefully defined circumstances) assisted suicide and the killing of terminally ill persons; in Belgium a similar bill is currently in preparation. Reactions in other European countries were very similar to those some weeks earlier with regard to the British decision to extend the grounds for research using early embryos. The Prime Minister of the German State of Bavaria declared euthanasia to be "a break with our Christian and humanistic tradition"[11] (Frankfurter Allgemeine Zeitung, 2001, p. 8). A group of (mainly Christian and Green) members of the European Parliament announced their intention to bring an action against legalized euthanasia to the European Court because of violation of Art. 2 of the *European Convention on Human Rights* (1950), which forbids the intentional killing of persons. These reactions appeal to "European values", but they show at the same time how controversially these values are being interpreted. Many people think that these values have never been static and must be adapted to the contemporary conditions. Current intensive discussions in several European countries are intended to develop European values further in the direction of giving more weight to autonomous personal decisions. In some of these countries, including France and Switzerland[12], a future liberalization of the still existing restrictive regulations seems to be likely.

Moreover, it should not be overlooked that the "Bioethics Convention" is a product of political construction, drawn up by a small group of experts at the level of governmental agencies. It is the result of political bargaining and therefore formulates a compromise rather than a consensus. For two reasons it cannot and does not precisely express "the European bioethical point of view". (a) There is, as we have seen, no consensus *between* the different states in important questions, and even in general attitudes, manifested in the fact that the Convention has yet to be signed by several countries, including Belgium because it is too restrictive, and Germany because it is not restrictive enough. (b) There is no consensus *within* the different states. "Europe" does not consist only of states, but also (or mainly) of many individual people. Among them we find a lot of partly converging, partly diverging opinions and convictions. "Consensus" in the sense of 100% agreement by an entire population is a rare thing in all modern societies; and biomedical problems are no exception to this rule (cf. the contributions in Bayertz, 1994). There are many and even fierce debates on bioethical problems in many European countries and it would be simply false to say that *the* British favour stem cell research and "therapeutic cloning" while *the* Germans or French reject it. There are ongoing controversies in all these countries; and what we find at the end of the British parliamentary decision process is not consensus, but a majority decision: the House of Commons voted 366 to 174 and the House of Lords 212 to 92. Similarly, in the Netherlands the law concerning euthanasia was accepted by the first chamber of parliament by 46 to 28 votes.

What are the reasons for and causes of these disagreements? At the most fundamental level it is the fact that, as explained above, the common cultural and moral identity of Europe has *never* been a homogenous and uniform system, but always more of a unity-in-diversity. If one looks more closely at the field of bioethics and concentrates on the differences *between* the countries, one will find some especially important factors of divergence:

A. Religious Differences

The general importance of religious differences should be clear; it is visible in the divergent opinions of Churches or confessions to specific biomedical options. The religious situations in the different European countries being very different, this can be expected to have a considerable effect on opinions and regulations. There are at least four groups of countries: (a) some predominantly Catholic: France, Italy, Ireland, Poland, (b) others predominantly Protestant: Great Britain, Scandinavia, (c) others mixed: Germany, Switzerland, Netherlands, (d) some predominantly Orthodox: Greece, Cyprus. Moreover, the influence of religious communities differs in degree from country to country: it can be very direct and strong (Poland, Italy, Germany), but there can be less involvement elsewhere (France, Great Britain). As a matter of fact, the bioethical positions held by the various religious denominations differ gravely. One illustration of this is the opinions issued in the debate on the abovementioned revised edition of the British *Human Fertilisation and Embryology Act* by the Catholic Church, by the Church of England and by a Jewish Chief Rabbi: the first strictly negative, the second and the third cautiously positive regarding therapeutic cloning (House of Commons 2000, p. 50-54). Empirical findings show clearly that the divergence of religious orientation is one of the most important factors explaining the divergence of opinions *within* and *between* the states on bioethical questions (Solter et. al., 2003, pp. 183-186, 194-196).

B. Different Legal Systems

In Europe the legal systems and legal cultures also differ from country to country. The contrast between the British and continental legal cultures immediately comes to mind. The following quotation pinpoints the British and French attitudes to biomedical legislation and regulation:

> There is in human nature a scale of different possible reactions to the slogan: from ethics to law. At one extreme is the temperament which feels: if it's wrong, we must legislate at once. Let us forbid it in the Penal Code, or at least write it into the Civil Code, and if we can't do either of those, then let us outlaw it in some other code or body of law, such as the Public Health Code. The British think that is the French way. At the other extreme is the temperament which feels: if it's wrong, let us educate everybody to know that it is wrong, and that will surely solve the problem. At the very most, let us hope the professionals will regulate it in their own codes of practice; medical nursing and so on. Above all, no new law. The French think that is the British way[13] (Fluss, 1998, p. 13).

This may be ironic exaggeration; but in fact we find very different legal situations in Europe. There is detailed legislation concerning biotechnology and medicine in countries such as Austria, Germany, the Netherlands and Switzerland, whereas Italy has become noteworthy for its lack of regulation. Such differences can have far-reaching consequences for the public discussion:

> The fact that Italy still has no law governing organ transplants or artificial insemination has meant that the philosophical, juridical, sociological and medical debate on these issues has become progressively harsher, with positions that are becoming increasingly radical and polarized. At the same time the arguments put forth by the different parties have become shallower and poorer. The result is that today the positions of the opposing factions are even further apart than they were a few years ago (Mazzoni, 1998, p. 5).

C. Different Mentalities

The common European tradition and culture has not prevented the development of different mentalities in different peoples and countries. The British, for example, are said to be "pragmatic", while Germans tend to be "principled". Of course, such differences and oppositions tend to be commonplaces or national(istic) stereotypes; and the analytic power of the concept of "mentality" is doubtful. Nevertheless, at least some national differences in opinions about and regulation of bioethical matters can be explained by such diverging mentalities. Especially illuminating is the situation in multi-ethnic countries like Switzerland. In fact, we find here that the voting behaviour of the German population in referenda on bioethical questions differs gravely from that of the Roman (French and Italian) population, in being more restrictive.

D. Historical Differences

History plays an important role in current bioethical debates. This is especially true for Germany, where the burden of the past still casts a dark shadow on all contemporary discussions. Without knowledge of the crimes committed during the Nazi period it would be impossible to understand the often very restrictive legal regulation in Germany, as well as certain tendencies in the German discussion, which oppose any kind of pragmatism in bioethical questions and may therefore seem to be somewhat "fundamentalist". Many objections to the "Bioethics Convention" in Germany have their roots in an intention to avoid the barbarities of the past. This is especially the case with respect to such questions as euthanasia, eugenics, or experiments with non-competent humans. Other countries which have a different history can deal with the bioethical problems of the present time more easily and more pragmatically.[14]

E. Ethical Differences

European countries differ in their philosophical traditions. Even if it would be an oversimplification to say that Great Britain is uniformly Utilitarian, Germany uniformly Kantian, and France uniformly Cartesian, it cannot be denied that these traditions have a strong influence and shape the philosophical and public debates in those countries. It has been pointed out that these differences in "ethical culture" lead to different prevailing styles of ethical argumentation. One can roughly distinguish a consequentialist and need-oriented type of moral reasoning in countries like Great Britain, the Netherlands and Scandinavia from a deontological and value-oriented type of reasoning prevailing in France or Germany. The difference can easily be identified in recent statements concerning the cloning of human beings. Although all these statements agree in the rejection of this technology and in their plea for a prohibition of cloning, at least momentarily, they have significantly different justifications for this. The British opinions refer mainly to the risk of harm for human beings inherent to this method; the French and German opinions primarily argue the danger to values, especially to human dignity (Birnbacher, 2000, p. 158). Another example of strong disagreement is the question of medical research on persons unable to consent. The "Bioethics Convention" allows for such research under certain conditions; in Germany this has caused strong protests from several groups, with the result that Germany has not signed the Convention.

> The discussion of this issue in different European countries exhibits the difference between ethical cultures. In countries like Great Britain and the

> Netherlands without a collectivist past and perhaps with a stronger utilitarian tradition, the principle of 'group benefit' has met with much less opposition than in Germany. Part of this opposition stems from the Kantian tradition: in the case of experiments without consent and benefit for the person involved, the categorical imperative never to use a human being merely as a means does seem to be violated [...] What the example shows is, in my view, the very relevance of diversity between cultures, both regarding their philosophical traditions and their moral-political experiences, for important questions of science-ethics (Siep, 1997, p. 129).

III. Morality as a Political Construction

Modern societies are essentially and increasingly self-observing and self-reflecting societies. They have developed special organs and institutionalised procedures for this self-observation and self-reflection; publicity and the media being the most important of these. It is trivial, but nevertheless important that this self-observation and self-reflection is not only descriptive, but always with a *normative* dimension: whatever becomes a topic of public concern will not only be reported but evaluated, too. It is obvious that matters of medicine and health care *are* a topic of public concern and it can be presumed that bioethics has assumed the role of a social institution of normative self-observation and self-reflection regarding the field of medicine and health care; and moreover, it has become a tool in the social problem-solving process and has thereby unavoidably been "politicized". Bioethicists are being appointed to committees and councils; they are expected to produce useful recommendations, directives or guidelines; their reasoning gains a practical impact not only occasionally or accidentally, but rather regularly and systematically (Bayertz, 2002). Possibly the most important instrument of problem solving and, therefore, the goal of bioethical activity is the construction of *consensus.* It seems to be self-evident today that consensus on moral questions and answers is a good thing. But this self-evidence is an illusion which decays rapidly if we look back at former times, where consensual agreements played only a minor role in politics. The attractiveness and necessity of moral consensus is a typical feature of modern societies which lack any authoritative and binding ideology, philosophy or religion. Under these circumstances it becomes difficult to legitimize political decisions (e.g., on biomedical problems) by appealing to unquestionable values and norms. Such decisions may then seem to be arbitrary and lacking in moral foundation. A consensus suggests itself as a substitute for a moral foundation on such values and norms and is eagerly sought by political decision-makers whenever they have to provide answers to morally relevant questions. Modern societies seem to face a problem here, which may be called the *paradox of consensus*: the fewer unquestionable values and norms providing a legitimation basis for political decisions there are, the greater the need for consensus as a substitute for safe legitimation becomes; but at the same time the smaller the normative basis for such a consensus will be. What—instead of genuine consensus—will be feasible under these conditions, will be only more or less substantially contingent political compromises.

The increasing social institutionalisation and political involvement of bioethics, and its increasing attempts to achieve consensus, are not restricted to the national level, but extend to the supranational level, too. The *Universal Declaration on the Human Genome and Human Rights,* which was adopted unanimously by the General Conference of UNESCO in 1997, is one example of this tendency; the efforts of the European Council and the European Union to develop a common bioethical framework are another. There are a number of reasons given for this need for supranational agreements and regulations:

(a) Most important is a widespread perception in major parts of the public and the political class that the progress of modern biotechnology and the biomedical sciences on the one hand, and globalization on the other, imply serious ethical risks; and that these risks not only touch peripheral problems but the very core of what morality is all about. It has become a widespread assumption that at least some bioethical problems (e.g., germ-line intervention and reproductive cloning) are *human rights* problems,[15] the solution of which cannot be left to individual nation states. As far as Europe is concerned, the European Council then seems to be the appropriate institution for developing and implementing such regulations because it was founded during the Cold War to defend human rights.

(b) Some major health care problems (AIDS, SARS) are supranational in their dimensions and, therefore, have to be met at a supranational level. Moreover, the progress of modern biomedical sciences and technology is essentially a supranational development; the ethical problems arising from this development cannot be sufficiently solved at a national level alone. This is especially true for Europe, where geographical distances are very short and where the borders between different states—especially within the EU—have lost their former importance dramatically during the last decades; traffic and tourism are increasing. This implies that medical services which do not exist or are forbidden in one country can easily be obtained by going to a neighbouring country. During the 1960s many German women went to the Netherlands to have an abortion; today they go to Belgium for preimplantation diagnosis. Many, especially politicians, see this as a problem which has to be solved; and the solution can consist only in a harmonization of national legal regulation, which presupposes common ethical standards.

(c) The member states of the European Union are cooperating more and more closely in certain political fields, including science and technology. In fact, the European Union has increasingly established its own supranational policy in this field. An important example is provided by biomedical research and development, which has become a major beneficiary of funding by the central institutions of the European Union. This presupposes a certain amount of agreement on the ethical permissibility of this research. In most cases this will not be difficult to obtain; in other cases, however, strong disagreements exist: embryo research is certainly one of the most important research options for which no ethical agreement exists. There are many inter-European consultations and negotiations to develop a common ethical framework, within which the EU may continue to extend its biomedical policy. In addition the European Commission, as the executive organ of the EU, decided in 1991 to set up a "European Group on Ethics in Science and Technology" with the following terms of reference: (i) identification and definition of ethical issues raised by biotechnology; (ii) appraisal of the ethical aspects of Community activities in the field of biotechnology and their potential impact on society and the individual; (iii) advising the Commission in the exercise of its powers as regards the ethical aspects of biotechnology.[16]

The reasons given for the need for a common European bioethical framework range from practical-political reasons, resulting from a closer cooperation within the European Community, to very fundamental considerations concerning the character of challenge posed by modern biomedicine. Especially these latter considerations make it impossible—for the political class as well as for major parts of the public—to treat the challenges of biomedical progress in a merely pragmatic way. These challenges are perceived as genuine and deep *ethical* problems; and they are perceived as ethical problems whose solution cannot be left to a spontaneous moral discourse, which may have a contingent or arbitrary outcome. Instead, the solution must be pushed ahead institutionally and controlled by legitimised political organs. The "Bioethics Convention" is by no means the only, but maybe the most significant attempt to *construct* a common European morality for dealing with matters of medicine and health care policy. This at least is the bioethical agenda of the political authorities and of major parts of the general public[17]. And this agenda fits very neatly into what we have already seen above: the identity of Europe in general, and its moral identity in particular exist mainly in the form of an idea or a postulate. This can easily be detected from the fact that talk about "European bioethics" is in most cases counterfactual: it does not refer to a given reality but to something which we either have lost or forgotten (and, therefore, should recall); or which would be good to have or which may even be necessary in order to solve threatening problems.

But what about the prospects of all these attempts to construct a common European bioethics? Will they be successful? Will Europe within the foreseeable future be dominated by one comprehensive bioethical outlook? It is obvious that there is a process of Europeanization in biopolitics, a tendency towards the "harmonization" of regulations. And this process is accompanied and legitimated by a broad range of bioethical activities and arguments, which will certainly not remain without its effects on public opinion. Biopolitics thereby seems to fit a general pattern of cultural development within Europe: a development towards less diversity and more homogeneity[18]. Recent empirical studies in different, but similar fields show that specific attitudes and policies in different European countries (such as the liberal Dutch drug policy, the restrictive Nordic alcohol control policy, and the conservative Irish policy towards sexual morality) are under pressure originating from the expansion of European governance; they come to the conclusion "that national peculiarities are shrinking and that a modest rate of cultural convergence has occurred" (Kurzer, 2001, p. 2). The increasing amount of activities in the field of bioethics at a European level seems to point in the same direction and intentionally aims at this direction.

Nevertheless, it would be hasty to expect this process to be overwhelmingly successful within a short time-span. There are several reasons not to be either too optimistic (or, if one prefers, too pessimistic) with respect to the Europeanization of bioethics, biolaw and biopolitics. I wish to mention three of them. The *first* emerges from what has been said about the counterfactual character of the idea of a European identity and about the diversity of European culture during most of its history. It seems very unlikely that the efforts of one (or even a few) generation of politicians, bureaucrats and bioethicists to harmonize opinions and regulations will be able to sweep away what has grown over centuries. To be sure, laws and regulations can be made easily and changed easily; but mentalities and traditions certainly cannot. We have to expect, therefore, that there will be a considerable amount of obstinacy with respect to deeply rooted mentalities and traditions, preventing a straightforward bioethical homogenisation of Europe. There will be agreement and consensus; but there will be disagreement and dissensus, too. *Second:* This is exactly what we find if we look carefully at what has actually been achieved in matters of a common "European bioethics". Especially instructive is the most important of these achievements: the "Bioethics Convention". It has already been mentioned that this document does not provide any complete and consistent regulation of bioethical matters, but leaves important questions open (especially, but not only the questions of the moral status of the human embryo and of euthanasia). In practice, this means that these questions are being answered in very different ways by national law. Moreover, even where the Convention provides regulations, considerable scope for national differences remains. The Convention provides only minimal standards of protection and allows explicitly for national regulations going beyond what is prescribed by the Convention. *Third:* We must bear in mind the simple fact that regulation does not guarantee homogeneity. We know from many contexts that the same rule can be interpreted and implemented very differently and that the *setting* of standards is one thing, the *enacting* of standards quite another.[19] Empirical findings show that regulations may not be as universalizable as one might expect:

> Rothstein et. al. have recently reviewed the issues of regulatory convergence and Europeanisation, taking the agrochemicals sector as their case study. They concluded that Europeanisation goes along with difference and that moves towards standardisation can serve to re-emphasise the significance of local mechanisms for interpretation and implementation. Their empirical finding was that a distinction of considerable importance exists between standard setting and standard enactment. In the context of agrochemicals regulation, they found that a subtle and diverse series of negotiations goes on within the process of regulation concerning 'what regulatory requirements really mean' (Wilkie, 2000, p. 120; the author summarizes the findings of Rothstein et. al., 1999).

There is no reason to expect that the gap between regulation and implementation will suddenly disappear when it comes to bioethics and biolaw. Even if European supranational regulations will be comprehensive and pervasive one day (which is not likely), this would not necessarily mean the end of all national or regional diversities.

All this seems to indicate that we do not have to expect a thorough process of ethical homogenisation of European bioethical thinking and regulation. The supposition that bioethical diversities will continue to exist is supported by other empirical studies which deal with similar problems. In her above mentioned book on the evolution of national attitudes and policies in several European countries, Kurzer comes to the conclusion that her findings:

> Do not point to an end to Europe's famous mélange of cultural diversity and lend support to the contention that not much will fundamentally change in the foreseeable future. Changes are taking place and the direction of adaptation is towards mainstream EU thinking, but the pace is slow and change is piecemeal. Whether this is good or bad depends on one's vision for Europe and one's hope for the future. One thing is sure, however. Genuine political union will take a long time to emerge. For the reasons sketched out in this study, on morality norms and national culture member governments face a loss of national sovereignty and are required to make adjustments that they do not necessarily desire. But national institutions package reforms in such a fashion that adjustments are ultimately modest and perhaps inconsistent with what prevails in the rest of Europe. Furthermore, the main pressure for change comes from the abolition of borders and the desire of consumers to enjoy goods and services not easily available at home (Kurzer, 2001, pp. 184f).

Moving from the empirical to the normative level, we finally have to come to an overall assessment of the present European situation, of its (likely) development in the future and, especially, of the struggle for a common European bioethics. The starting point for such a normative assessment should be the insight that ethics basically has to do with the freedom and well-being of human individuals. This means, with regard to the problems we are dealing with in this paper, that the central question we have to ask is not whether bioethical regulations come from national political authorities or from supranational institutions; instead, the central questions are:

(a) Are these regulations simply politically imposed, or do people agree with them, do they accept them?
(b) What is the content, the aim and the effect of the regulations; especially, do they restrict the freedom of individuals and infringe their well-being or do they enlarge their freedom and foster their well-being?

The first question pertains to political legitimation, not only in a narrow or formal sense. It is realistic to say that there is a certain suspicion among the public in all European countries concerning EU regulations *in general.* The EU institutions seem to exist and to decide far removed from the citizens who are subject to their regulation. Moreover, these citizens are accustomed to national parliaments passing laws and national governments enforcing them. However, this aversion against supranational institutions and law should not be overestimated; it equally exists with regard to national governments. It is often forgotten that national law is a recent achievement and its "naturalness" an illusion stemming from a deficient historical memory.[20] What seems to be "natural" may change within a few decades and people may soon become accustomed to EU-law just as they have become accustomed to national law. Whether this will happen depends on several factors which can hardly be anticipated, one of them certainly being the content of EU-law and its appreciation by the citizens. Remarkably, some (very few) available data show that just with respect to *bioethical* questions there is a widespread opinion that regulation at a EU level is necessary; at least with respect to embryo experimentation in eight of nine European countries, a majority among the population prefers common regulations for the whole EU to national regulation (Solter et. al., 2003, pp. 198-200). It is hard to judge if this finding can be generalized; it indicates, however, that common EU regulations of bioethical matters have at least a good chance of being accepted by a majority of the population.

Ethically more important is the second question. If we take seriously the insight that the central ethical question pertains to the freedom and well-being of individuals, we shall immediately see that there is nothing inherently moral in any kind of national diversity and/or supranational homogeneity. Diversity and homogeneity *become* morally relevant if they satisfy human needs and individual preferences, if they provide opportunities for human beings to decide their own destiny and live their own life. If we look at European bioethics and biolaw from this perspective, we have to establish that there certainly has been no general tendency to narrow individual freedom. Quite the contrary: any sober recapitulation of the history of the last three or four decades shows clearly that the overall tendency during this period has been a continuous extension of room for autonomous decisions concerning individual bodies, sexuality and health. The proliferation of biotechnological options on the one hand, and a step-by-step retreat of the state[21] on the other have created an increase in individual liberty which would have been inconceivable half a century ago.

If this is the case, which role has the EU played in this process and which will it presumably play in the future? It would be a grave exaggeration to pretend that European unification has played a dominant role in this process; this is elucidated by the fact that EU regulations of bioethical matters began when this process had not only already begun, but had also already reached a considerable momentum. The main factors have been the technological development and a general and pervasive cultural change not only in Europe but in other developed countries of the world, too. But the European institutions and their activities have promoted this tendency (a) by weakening the importance of national boundaries between the European states, intensifying traffic and commerce, and by guaranteeing free movement for patients and professionals. It is hard so see how the prohibition of PID in some countries (e.g., Germany) will continue to exist in the long run, while it is available in surrounding countries; and (b) by a constant pressure on the individual nation states to make possible and facilitate access to biotechnological options and health care services. The admission and availability of abortion in almost all European states is probably the most striking, but not the only example. With regard to the few European countries in which abortion is still forbidden or severely restricted, in 2002 the European Parliament accepted a Report which recommended "that, in order to safeguard women's reproductive health and rights, abortion should be made legal, safe and accessible to all" and called upon governments of the Member States and the Accession Countries "to refrain in any case from prosecuting women who have undergone illegal abortions" (European Parliament, 2002, p. 9, 17). If this (very controversial, of course) Report is successful one day, there will be less national diversity in Europe, and there will be more individual freedom for pregnant women in Ireland, Poland or Portugal.

There is one final objection to this analysis. We have seen in this paper that the common European bioethics and biolaw which has been constructed and implemented during the recent past includes at least some substantive moral values, "human dignity" being the most prominent among them. These values build a (rough scaffold of a) particular moral vision, a vision of what human beings essentially are and how they have to behave in the biomedical world. As a corollary of this vision and of its legal implementation, the freedom of choice in some fields is confined. The prohibition of a commercialization of the human body and its parts, of surrogate motherhood, and of predictive genetic testing outside the established health-care system show that "human dignity" not only guarantees the protection of individuals from unwanted third-party interventions, but restricts their freedom even where no infringement upon the interests of others occurs. From a liberal or libertarian point of view it seem obvious that a common European bioethics of this kind will impose a particular substantive morality on autonomous persons and thereby not widen, but narrow the range of individual liberty. It is undeniable that there is a tendency in this direction and that there are influential groups (mentioned above) who favour and push for a common European bioethics exactly because they take this to be morally necessary.

If we look at the entire struggle for a common European bioethics from a distant perspective and try to put it in its proper place we will have to come to the conclusion that its effects are not only limited, but—more importantly—are essentially ambivalent. Many of the possibilities and opportunities offered by technologically advanced biomedicine amount to a provocation for the historically grown moral convictions of major parts of the population. The substantive moral values of a common European bioethics are robust remnants of these convictions and form a barrier to certain forms of use of these possibilities and opportunities. But it would be hasty to conclude that this barrier is impermeable or insurmountable. German constitutional lawyers, trained in dealing with the value or principle of human dignity, like to say that while the *violation* of human dignity is *not* allowed, its *interpretation* is. And via interpretation the strong substantive content of "human dignity" can be gradually changed into flexible procedural norms. Values can be preserved by thinning them out; and this is what happens to many of them. The prohibition of predictive genetic testing unrelated to any health-purposes certainly restricts the free choice of individuals by preventing them from using this technology. The term "health purposes", however, can be interpreted in a way which will minimize the number of occasions on which people will be refused the availability of this kind of diagnostics. The requirement of therapeutic legitimation for all kinds of biomedical interventions restricts only marginally the free choice of individuals; it can be argued that its factual effect is to make available (almost) everything, provided that some kind of justification in medical terms can be given.[22] Apart from some exceptions, such as the sale of organs or surrogate motherhood, the European way of regulating biomedical action may in the long run prove to be an effective device for paving the way for a widespread use of modern biotechnology by autonomous individuals.

IV. Summary and Conclusion

During the recent past there have been many intensive efforts to construct and implement a common European bioethics. Among the reasons why this has been judged necessary are immediate political and pragmatic ones, which have to do with the fact that a growing part of research and development in biotechnology and medicine has been shifted from the individual states to the European Union. More importantly from an ethical point of view, however, is a certain assessment by many opinion leaders, ideological groups and politicians that there are two pervasive developments which form a deep threat to human rights and dignity on the field of bioethics: (a) the revolutionary progress of bioscience and biotechnology and (b) the economic, social and cultural changes epitomized as "globalization". The "Bioethics Convention" of the European Council is the most important document reflecting this struggle for a common European bioethics which is intended to form a bulwark against this threat.

When we look at the agents of these efforts, we find a variety of groups and their (partly harmonizing, partly diverging) ethical world-views. This is what should have been expected in a part of the world which consists of modern pluralist societies. And it should come as no surprise when we find that these groups are trying to take advantage of these efforts to construct and implement a common European bioethics, to bring their respective ethical world-views into play, and to take this opportunity to enforce their world-view through the authority of the state(s). What is going on, therefore, may well be described as a battle about the should-be European bioethical identity. An especially strong and influential party in this battle consists of a big coalition of otherwise competing groups which are unified (negatively) by a certain sceptical appraisal of modern science and technology as well as of globalisation; and (positively) by a certain substantial image of the human essence and a content-rich conception of the good. They tend to identify "Europe" with one of its ideological and moral traditions (preferably with the Christian one) and to marginalize the other traditions and moral world-views.

One of the main theses of the present paper has been that it is crucial to make a clear distinction between what the moral aspirations of people or groups are on the one hand, and the European reality on the other. If we look at the latter we will find that attempts to homogenize European bioethics have not been very successful so far. The plurality of standpoints, judgements and traditions has proved to be rather resistant to efforts to construct and implement one common bioethical identity. Although there is considerable pressure in the direction of homogenization, there are also robust factors which have guaranteed European bioethical diversity so far. And there is no evidence that there ever will be such a thing as a common European bioethics.

This does not preclude that a certain harmonization of the different European legal systems will take place; and that in this context a (more or less) common biolaw will originate. It is still an open question how far this process of mutual assimilation of the national legal systems will go. Even if it will go—in the long run—very far, we have every reason to remain sober in this respect. The diversity of the national legal systems is a historically very recent fact and should not be furnished with any intrinsic moral worth. National differences have no value of their own. Morally valuable are not differences between states, but the possibility of *individuals* to decide their own destiny and thereby become different from each other.

While unlikely, it is certainly conceivable that there will some day be one common European or even global bioethics without forming any threat to moral diversity and ethical pluralism. The condition is that this common European bioethics reduces to some essential but thin procedural norms which leave it to the individual moral subjects to make their own medical decisions and to use (or not to use) modern biotechnology according to their own values as long as others are not affected. The beginnings of a European bioethics of today are far from this. But if one considers the developments during the last decades one can hardly overlook the fact that some important steps in this direction have been taken.

Notes

1. "Les perspectives très sérieuses qu'ouvrent aujourd'hui les thérapies cellulaires en matière notamment de lutte contre les maladies dégénératives méritent un débat approfondi. Il faut l'aborder avec une grande prudence. Ce débat ne doit pas faire prévaloir une conception utilitariste de l'être humaiu, qui mettrait en cause les fondements mêmes de notre civilisation et porterait atteinte à la dignité de l'homme. Mais il ne peut pas non plus priver l'humanité de la possibilité de faire reculer ses souffrances." And concerning therapeutic cloning: "Par ailleurs, je ne suis pas pour ma part favorable à l'autorisation du clonage thérapeutique. Il conduit à créer des embryons à des fins de recherche et de production des cellules, et, malgré l'interdit, il rend matériellement posssible le clonage reproductif et il risque de conduire à des trafics d'ovocytes."
2. For a more general analysis of this change in ethical thinking cf. Bayertz (2002). Within the present volume the contribution by David Solomon (2006, pp. 235-261) gives an analysis of the origin and the prospects of applied ethics, while the paper by Kevin Wildes (2006, pp. 362-379) deals more specifically with bioethics.
3. Cf. the papers under this heading in Mazzoni (1998).
4. As a substitute for many other references I only mention the essays collected by Anthony Pagden, 2002.
5. The *Council of Europe* must not be identified with the European Union. The *Council of Europe* was founded during the Cold War in 1949 to foster the idea and the implementation of human rights in Europe, and in 1950 it issued the *European Convention on Human Rights.* Today, it has more than 40 member states, among them all members of the EU, as well as most East-European countries including Russia, and Turkey and Cyprus. For a short history of the activities of the Council of Europe see (Council of Europe, 1995); the appendix of this report lists many documents related to bioethics adopted by the Council of Europe.
6. Valuable information concerning the background and history of this convention is offered by de Wachter (1997}. The process of globalization as an important background of the "Bioethics Convention" is stressed by Honnefelder (1999).
7. It should be emphasized that this impression is not restricted to intellectuals like

Habermas. The (former) French Prime Minister Lionel Jospin formulated a concept of Europe as a specific way of living, based on a common history and on common values, which is clearly invoked as a counter-model to the effects of globalization: "Il existe un *‚art de vivre'* à l'européenne, une facon propre d'agir, de défendre les libertés, de lutter contre les inégalitées et les discriminations, de penser et d'organiser les relations de travail, d'accéder à l'instruction et aux soins, d'aménager le temps. Chacun des nos pays a ses traditions et ses règles mais celles-ci composent un univers commun" (Jospin, 2001).

8. "Il ne peut être porté atteinte à l'intégrité du corps humain qu'en cas de nécessité thérapeutique pour la personne." The next sentence requires the consent of the person (Loi No. 94-653, Art. 16-3). The German penal code in its § 228 regards interventions in bodily intactness as punishable bodily harm if they "offend public decency", even if the person affected freely agrees.
9. A detailed analysis of the notion of the human being as depicted in the "Bioethics Convention" is provided by Reuter (2000)—The European Court of Human Rights judged in 2004 "that the issue of when the right to life begins comes within the margin of appreciation which the Court generally considers that States should enjoy in this sphere" and "that there is no consensus on the nature and status of the embryo and/or fetus" (European Court of Human Rights, 2004, §§ 82 and 84).
10. Even more explicit is the "Report giving an Opinion on the Draft Bioethics Convention": "The interpretation which the European Commission of Human Rights places on the terms—such as 'human life', 'person', 'everyone', etc.—should facilitate the acceptance of the text of the bioethics convention which does not include a definition of these terms. Otherwise, given the philosophical, scientific, ethical and religious implications, we might become involved in an interminable debate, which would reveal our inability to address rationally and respond adequately to a dynamic situation in which science and technology increasingly enter into the activities of everyday life" (European Council, 1995, p. 9f).
11. Frankfurter Allgemeine Zeitung, March 8, 2001. p. 8.
12. In Switzerland active euthanasia is forbidden; assistance to suicide is legal only when it is not egoistically motivated. There have been two initiatives in the Parliament in 1994 and in 2000 for a liberalization of the law but a consensus has not yet been reached.
13. Lord Kennet in an unpublished paper, quoted from Fluss (1998, p.13).
14. An impressive analysis of the historical roots of differences in the debate on euthanasia in the Netherlands and in Germany is provided by Gordijn (2000).
15. This assumption has been disputed. In his critical analysis of the "Bioethics-Convention" Gilbert Hottois comes to the conclusion that some of the underlying assumptions of the Convention are not in accordance with, but conflict with the human rights tradition: "...the presence in the convention of some items—for example, technoscientophobia focused on research and development in genetics; the 'right not to know'; the subtle influence of the 'slippery slope' argument raising doubts about the value of knowledge, information, education, ethics of responsibility and the individual capability of judging freely; the poor explanation of a progressivist and ethical policy—all run counter to the human rights philosophical tradition" (Hottois, 2000, p. 145).
16. Cf. the detailed overview by Hottois (1998).
17. It is worth noting that the vast majority of the general public in EU member states

prefers regulation on embryo experimentation by EU authorities to regulation on the level of nation states (Solter et. al, 2003, pp. 198-200).

18. It is an open question whether this general process of a decline in specific regional or national cultures is restricted to Europe and caused by the process of European unification. There are arguments and theories which state similar processes in many areas of the world and predict an end to national cultures. The Europeanization of culture and morality described in this paper would then be nothing but an element of a worldwide comprehensive tendency of cultural development in general.
19. The reader will find a possible philosophical interpretation of this often overlooked fact in the paper of Joseph Boyle (2006, pp. 300-334). According to him, Thomas Aquinas makes a distinction between self-evident moral principles on the one hand, and judgments based on reasoning that must take into account a variety of moral circumstances on the other. "It certainly seems that bioethical judgments generally fall along a continuum between the immediate implications of moral principles and the detailed casuistical judgments that require the analytical expertise of trained casuists... Consequently, recognising general moral standards should not be expected to remove controversy. When the full details of the circumstances of troubling decisions come to light, controversy must be expected as a matter of the structure of moral reasoning, and any bioethics, global or other, will not remove that" (p. 14f).
20. "Present-day Europeans live under their national systems of law, which are almost invariably codified... European courts of justice, the European Commission, the European Parliament and European laws have not yet altered the basic fact that people live under national laws which were produced by the sovereign national states. And most people, no doubt, find this a natural state of affairs, as natural as their various languages. What they do not realize and would be surprised to find out, is that this 'natural state of affairs' is, on the time scale of European history, quite recent (going back only one or two centuries) and that the rise of the European Union may turn into a brief and transient phase" (van Caenegem, 2002, p.1).
21. My assessment differs from Angelo Petroni's diagnosis on this point, who writes: "In all European countries health care is monopolised or heavily regulated by the state. While in past years the state has rolled back from the control of the economy, there is no sign that the same is happening as far as health care is concerned. One could be tempted to say that the contrary holds. The more the states are losing control over the economy as a result of the common European market and globalisation, *the more they have the tendency to extend their control over other aspects of human life*" (p. 26f). A possible explanation for this disagreement may be that my analysis focuses mainly on the question of how strongly individual choice concerning the use of biomedical options is infringed upon by state regulations. My thesis here is that in many cases state regulation is a *form* through which autonomous individuals gain more freedom in biomedical matters: Voluntary euthanasia has become a real option for people in the Netherlands by *state regulation*.
22. My analysis converges neatly with the findings of Dominique Memmi, who in her analysis of "statal administration of the human body" comes to the—seemingly paradoxical—conclusion that individual autonomy concerning the human body has been *encouraged* and *made possible* by activities and regulations of the modern

state. "Ce qu'on voit apparaître ici au total, c'est la coexistence de trois phénomènes qui sont qu'apparemment contradictoires entre eux: la montée des l'autocontrôle comme idéal, son encouragement mais aussi son encadrement par les instances représentatives de l'État, enfin l'avènement d'un *sujet triomphant,* curieusement encouragé *par les dispositifs de contrôle eux-mêmes...* L'étape contemporaine du processus d'individuation apparaît alors comme un produit de l'État moderne: c'est un processus par lequel les agents sociaux intériorisent les discours de l'État plutôt que de les subir sous forme de sanctions juridiques imposées à des pratiques déviantes. Ils peuvent d'ailleurs se contenter d'une adhésion minimale, purement discursive, leur permettant d'être capables de les produire au moment voulu (il suffit d'assister à une demande d'avortement ou d'une procédure de conciliation de divorce, pour s'en convaincre). Le seul contrôle qui importe alors, c'est celui par lequel sont encadrés les discours que le ‚je' produisent sur eux-mêmes" (Memmi, 2000, p. 14f).

References

Bauer, M. W., Durant, J., & Gaskell, G. (1998). 'Biology in the public sphere: a comparative review,' in J. Durant, Bauer, M.W., & Gaskell, G. (Eds), *Biotechnology in the Public Sphere.* A European Sourcebook (pp. 217-227). London: Science Museum.

Bayertz, K. (Ed.) (1994). *The Concept of Moral Consensus. The Case of Technological Interventions into Human Reproduction.* Dordrecht: Kluwer.

Bayertz, K. (1996). 'Human dignity: problems and paradoxes,' in K. Bayertz (Ed.), *Sanctity of Life and Human Dignity.* Dordrecht: Kluwer.

Bayertz, K. 2002. 'Self-enlightenment of Applied Ethics,' in R. Chadwick & Schroeder, D. (Eds.), *Applied Ethics* (pp. 36-51). Vol. I. London: Routledge.

Birnbacher, D. (2000). 'Bioethische Konsensbildung durch Recht? Das Dilemma des Menschenrechtsübereinkommens zur Biomedizin,' in Dietmar Mieth (Ed.), *Ethik und Wissenschaft in Europa. Die gesellschaftliche, rechtliche und philosophische Debatte* (pp. 156-163). Freiburg/ Münchern: Alber.

Boyle, J. (2006). 'Natural law and global bioethics,' in this volume.

Center for Ethics and Law. (1999). *Dignity. Ethics and Law. Bibliography.* Copenhagen.

Chirac, J. (2001). *Allocution de Monsieur Jacques Chirac, Président de la République, à l'occasion de l'ouverture du forum mondial des biotechnologies.* [Online]. Available : (http://www. elysee.fr./cgibin/auracom/aurw.../fil?aur_file=discours2001/BIO0102. html)

Council of Europe. (1982). Parliamentary Assembly, *Recommendation,* 934(1982),1.

Council of Europe. (1995). Parliamentary Assembly. *Report giving Opinion on the Draft Bioethics Convention* (Rapporteur: Mr. Palacios). Document 7210.

Council of Europe. (1997a). *Convention for the Protection of Human Rights and Dignity of the Human Being with regard to the Application of Biology and Medicine: Convention on Human Rights and Biomedicine.* Printed in: *The Journal of Medicine and Philosophy.* (2000). 25(2), 259-266.

Council of Europe. (1997b). *Explanatory Report to the Convention for the Protection of Human Rights and Dignity of the Human Being with Regard to the Application of Biology and Medicine: Convention on Human Rights and Biomedicine.* Strasbourg.

de Wachter, M. A. M. (1997). 'The European Convention on Bioethics.' *Hastings Center Report,* 27 (1), 13-23.

Engelhardt, H. T., Jr. (1996). 'Unavoidable pluralism: rethinking secular morality and community at the end the 20th century.' *Dialektik*, 3, 105-118.

Engelhardt, H. T., Jr. 'The search for a global morality: bioethics, the culture wars, and moral diversity,' in this volume.

European Court of Human Rights. (2004). Case of Vo v. France (Application no. 53924/00). Judgment.

European Parliament (2002). Report on Sexual and Reproductive Health and Rights (2001/2128 (INI)).

Fluss, S. S. (1998). 'An International Overview of Developments in Certain Areas, 1984-1994,' in C.M. Mazzoni (Ed.) *A Legal Framework for Bioethics* (pp. 11-37). The Hague: Kluwer.

Gordijn, B. (2000). Die Debatte um Euthanasie in den Niederlanden und Deutschland. Ein Vergleich aus historischer Sicht. In: B. Gordijn and H. ten Have (Eds.), *Medizinethik und Kultur. Grenzen medizinischen Handelns in Deutschland und den Niederlanden* (pp. 303-343). Stuttgart- Bad Cannstadt.

Habermas, J. (2001). ,Warum braucht Europa eine Verfassung?' *Die Zeit*, 27, 7

Haferkamp, B. (1996). 'The concept of human dignity: an annotated bibliography,' in K. Bayertz (Ed.), *Sanctity of Life and Human Dignity* (pp. 275-291). Dordrecht: Kluwer.

Hegel, G. W. F. (1845). *Hegel's Philosophy of Mind: Being Part Three of the Encyclopaedia of the Philosophical Sciences* (A. V. Miller, Trans.). Oxford: Clarendon Press.

Herodotus: *History*.

Honnefelder, L. (1999). 'Biomedizinische ethik und globalisierung: zur problematik völkerrechtlicher grenzziehung am beispiel der menschenrechtskonvention zur biomedizin des Eurparates,' in A. Eser (Ed.), *Biomedizin und Menschenrechte. Die Menschenrechtskonvention des Europarates zur Biomedizin. Dokumentation und Kommentare* (pp. 38-58). Frankfurt am Main: Josef Knecht.

Hottois, G. (1998). 'Bioéthique européenne: l'apport du GCEB,' in C. M. Mazzoni (Ed.), *Un Quadro Europeo per la Bioethica?* (pp. 17-40). Florence: Leo S. Olschki.

Hottois, G. (2000). 'A philosophical and critical analysis of The European Convention of Bioethics.' *The Journal of Medicine and Philosophy*, 25(2), 133-146.

House of Commons. (2000, December 3). *Stem Cell Research and Regulations under the Human Fertilisation and Embryology Act 1990.* House of Commons Research Paper 00/93. [On-line]. Available: http://www. parliament.uk

Jospin, L. (2001, May 28). *Intervention sur ,L'avenir de l'Europe élargie'*. [Online]. Available: http:/www.premier-ministre.gouv.fr

Kurzer, P. (2001). *Markets and Moral Regulation. Cultural Change in the European Union.* Cambridge: Cambridge University Press.

Locke, J. (1667). 'A letter concerning toleration,' in *The Works of John Locke in Ten Volumes*, Vol. VI. London.

Loi No. 94-653 du 29 Juillet 1994. Relative au respect du corps humain. in Gazette du Palais (pp. 576-579).

Mazzoni, C. M. (1998). 'Bioethics needs legal regulation,' in C. M. Mazzoni (Ed.), A *Legal Framework of Bioethics.* Dordrecht: Kluwer.

Memmi, D. (2000). 'Vers une confession laique? La nouvelle administration étatique des corps.' *Revue Française de Science Politique*, 50, 3-19.

Pagden, Anthony (Ed.). (2002). *The Idea of Europe: From Antiquity to the Europen Union.* Cambridge: Cambridge University Press.

Petroni, A. M. 'Perspectives for freedom of choice in bioethics and health care in Europe,' In this volume.

Reuter, L. (2000). 'Human is what is born of a human: personhood, rationality, and the European Convention.' *Journal of Medicine and Philosophy,* 25(2), 181-194.

Rothstein, H., Irwin, A., Yearly, SA., & McCarthy, E. (1999). 'Regulatory science, Europeanisation, and the control of agrochemicals.' *Science, Technology, and Human Values,* 24(2), 241-264.

Siep, L. (1997). 'Ethics and culture,' in P. J. D. Drenth, Fenstad, J.E. & Schiereck, J.D. (Eds.), *European Science and Scientists Between Freedom and Responsibility* (pp. 123-130). Amsterdam.

Solomon, D. (2006). 'Domestic disarray and imperial ambition: contemporary applied ethics and the prospects for global bioethics,' in this volume.

Solter, D., Beyleveld, D., Friele, M.B., Holowka, J., Lilie, H., Lovell-Badge, R., Mandla, C., Martin, U., & Pardo Avellaneda, R. (2003). *Embryo Research in Pluralistic Europe.* Berlin: Springer

Ten Have, H. A., & Welie, J. V. (Eds.). (1998). *Ownership of the Human Body. Philosophical Considerations on the Use of the Human Body and its Parts in Healthcare.* Dordrecht: Kluwer.

van Caenegem, R. C. (2002). *European Law in the Present and the Future. Unity and Diversity over Two Millenia.* Cambridge: Cambridge University Press.

Weber, M. (1920). ‚Vorbemerkung,' in *Gesammelte Aufsätze zur Religionssoziologie (9th ed.) Vol. III* (pp. 1-16). Tübingen: J. C. B. Mohr.

Wildes, K. W. (2006). 'The limits of moral reason in a multi-cultural world,' in this volume.

Wilkie, T. (2000). 'The need for ethical subsidiarity,' in D. Mieth (Ed.), *Ethik und Wissenschaft in Europa. Die gesellschaftliche, rechtliche und philosophische Debatte* (pp. 111-125). Freiburg/ München: Alber.

Perspectives for Freedom of Choice in Bioethics and Health Care in Europe

Angelo Maria Petroni

Europe is traditionally the land of diversities. Its very long history in civilisation, the variety of races and religions, the existence of strong borders, made the Old Continent a mosaic of different institutions, languages, morals, and laws. On these grounds, the difference with countries like the United States or Japan used to be striking.

The situation is changing at an unexpected speed. As a matter of fact, Europe is experiencing a homogenising process that is likely to radically affect its spiritual as well as its material aspects. This process is partly due to the effects of cultural and economic globalisation. From this point of view there is no special difference between Europe and others parts of the developed world. But the main reasons of the rapid changes are due to the building of the institutions of the European Union, and to the spreading of its policies through the fifteen member states.

This process equally affects bioethics and health care. This paper will explore how biomedical diversity in Europe is in the course of being put under stress by the European Union. It will therefore propose an alternative model of how a higher degree of interaction and exchange in Europe could be made compatible with the preservation and the enhancing of national diversities and individual freedom in matter of bioethics and health care.

H.T. Engelhardt, Jr. (ed), *Global Bioethics* (pp. 238–270).

I. What Kind of Institution Is the European Union?

As is well known, from the historical and legal point of view, there is no such thing as an EC, but three Communities established with the Treaties of Paris of 1951 (the European Coal and Steel Community) and of Rome of 1957 (the European Economic Community and the European Atomic Community). The three Communities were unified with the Treaty of Amsterdam (1997). In 1992 the Treaty of Union has established the single European currency and—even more important for the purposes of our paper—the principle of a European citizenship.[1]

In order to evaluate the positive as well as the normative aspects of the intervention of the EU in the fields of bioethics, biomedical research, and health care, one has to address first the question of whether the founding treaties of the EC (or EU) have to be considered as purely international agreements amongst sovereign states.

The origin and the structure are, of course, that of multilateral treaties signed by representatives of the states and they have been ratified and empowered according to the principles of international law. However, both the content of the treaties, and in particular the treaty establishing the EEC, and the jurisprudence which has arisen from their implementation qualify them as something essentially different from the classical treaties between states retaining their national sovereignties. Let me recall here the two basic elements, which justify this statement.

In the first place, contrary to the basic principles of international law, the Treaty of Rome endows the Community with powers, which *apply directly* to the citizens of the states concerned. This is established, for example, by Article 189 (now Article 249 in the Consolidated Version) of the Treaty. In this way the citizens of the member states are subjects both to their national law and to Community law. By the same token, as Michel Massenet writes, "contrairement aux traités internationaux de type classique, les traités communautaires confèrent aux particuliers des droits que les juridictions nationales ont le devoir de sauvegarder" (Massenet, 1990, p.11). Individuals can protect the rights guaranteed by the Treaty by appealing to the Court of Justice. According to Article 187 (now 244) of the EEC Treaty the sentences of the Court of Justice are valid *directly in the territory* of the member states. National authorities are obliged to enforce the sentences of the Court against their nationals without an *exequatur* (Art. 192, now 256). This also constitutes a strong element of difference between the Treaty of Rome and classical international treaties.

Second, the jurisprudence elaborated by the Court of Justice in interpreting the Treaties has constantly ruled in favour of the pre-eminence of the Treaties over national law—including constitutional law. In turn, EC regulations prevail over national (non-constitutional) law. In the famous Costa sentence (1964) the Court ruled that:

> by contrast with ordinary international treaties, the EEC Treaty has created its own legal system. (...) By creating a Community of unlimited duration, having its own personality, its own legal capacity (...) and, more particularly, real powers stemming from a limitation of sovereignty or transfer of powers from the States to the community, the Member States have limited their sovereign rights (Court of Justice of the European Communities, 1964, p. 593).

This limitation is *definitive.*

In another famous sentence the Court ruled that, "It is not for the Court (...) to ensure that the rules of internal laws, even constitutional rules, enforced in one or other of the Member States are respected" (Court of Justice of the European Communities, 1960, p. 438). A *monistic* point of view (in the sense used by Hans Kelsen) is followed in the relationship between the Treaties and derived jurisprudence, on the one hand, and national laws, on the other. In particular, the national judge is obliged to apply Community law and to consider, on this own authority, as invalid any national law (be it past or future) which might conflict with it.

Are these characteristics of Community sufficient for us to affirm that the Treaties (and their interpretation) represent a *constitution*? As you would expect in such cases, much (too much) depends on the content you attribute to the concept of constitution. If "constitution" means an explicit agreement made by individuals upon the basic rules of their society, then obviously Treaties are not a constitution, and Community/Union law is not a constitutional law. However, it is even truer that following this criterion there would be no "true" constitutions around at all.

On the other hand, if—from the viewpoint of legal positivism—the constitution is taken to mean the highest law valid in a given territory, then the situation becomes more complex. Provided that member states have agreed to accept both the content of the Treaties *and* the interpretations of the Court of Justice, the Community/Union law is the highest law. Albeit in very different ways, all the highest legal authorities of the EC/EU states have accepted the supremacy of Community/Union law over their national law.[2]

At the same time, Community/Union law is not the source of the validity of all the other laws enforced in the European states. If this logical dependence is considered an essential feature of a constitution, as it is in a contractarian view, or even in some legal positivism perspective, then obviously Community law is not constitutional law. However, by this same token, would the American Constitution be a constitution? And would there exist at all any constitutional law in England? Note that, even if you consider nation-states with civil law systems such as Italy or France, it is very difficult to affirm that there is a strict logical dependence of the bulk of the law on the constitution. Normally laws remain relatively unchanged when a new constitution is adopted, and the pre-eminence of constitutional law means those previous laws that conflict with it are abolished.

II. Does the Constitutional Framework of the European Union Represent a Liberal Order?

Some years ago Norman Barry stressed the difference between the traditional liberal meaning of "constitution" as "a set of substantive rules protecting a fully-fledged individualistic political morality, or as a set of neutral but rigorously strict procedural rules" and the "mistaken idea of constitution (...) prevalent in much of contemporary welfare economics". The liberal constitution is not designed to implement the people's choice "but to impose significant constraints on government, whatever form it takes (majority rule or otherwise)"(Barry, 1990, pp. 270-271).

In terms of this distinction, *Community law is very close to the concept of a liberal constitution.* It imposes constraints on national governments and majorities on the basis of individual freedoms (the "four freedoms" stated in the Treaty of Rome of 1957: free movement of goods, persons, services and capital).

As a matter of fact, Community law has represented a remarkable instrument for taming the all-pervasive power of the European nation-states over their citizens. The establishment of the EC/EU was tremendously instrumental for opening the European markets, deregulating national markets, and downsizing the huge state-owned industry.

However this is just a part of the story. Starting from the end of the Eighties, *the EC has increasingly turned into machinery aimed at centrally re-regulating markets, abolishing national and regional diversity, and finally reducing individuals' choices.* This situation is often expressed with the statement that the European Union is turning into a "super-state", whose powers are more distant from the citizens than the powers of the nation-states, and whose democratic legitimacy is therefore weak.

The fear that the European institutions are destined to turn into a superstate is as old as the Community itself. Perhaps nobody expressed it better than Wilhelm Roepke; writing in 1958, he saw in the Community institutions the way towards generalised economic and political planning—a European Saint-Simonism—which would have been even more dangerous than planning at the national level. According to Roepke, the traditional divide between socialists and liberals did no longer represent the fundamental cleavage of our societies. The real divide was between "centrists" and "decentrists". In his own words:

> The problem if the ideal world is the decentralisation or the centralisation; if the fundamental factor should be the individual (and the small group) or the large collective bodies, namely the state, the nation, or even a single state encompassing the entire world has become the real watershed of the opposite opinions.

For the "de-centrist":

> The political and economic strengthening of Europe must be realised by saving what is really essential: unity in variety, freedom in solidarity, and the respect of the human person in its individuality. Decentrism is an essential factor of the European spirit. The willingness of organising Europe from a centre, to make it the object of a planning bureaucracy, to fuse it in a compact block, is tantamount to betray Europe and its spiritual heritage. A continental nationalism and economic *dirigisme* do not represent a progress in comparison to the nationalism and the *dirigisme* of the single nation states (Roepke, 1958, pp.120-121).

Undoubtedly the Community, and now the Union, has always had two "souls": one liberal, the other *dirigiste*. This reflects in the EC Treaty, which contains several Articles which leave plenty of room for heavy state intervention in the economy. If one considers that the Treaty was written at the high point of intellectual and political support for planning, this is hardly surprising. As is well known, the Treaty of Union was written from a point of view much more favourable to the free market. However, it is easy to see that the two "souls" are very well present even in this Treaty, as is shown by the "Social Charter", which corresponds to a *dirigiste* and socialist ideology.

III. The Treaty Establishing a Constitution for Europe

In December 2001 the European Council decided to set up a special body, named "European Convention on the Future of Europe", which was given the following aim:

> [...] draw up proposals on three subjects: how to bring citizens closer to the European design and European Institutions; how to organise politics and the European political area in an enlarged Union; and how to develop the Union into a stabilising factor and a model in the new world order (European Convention, 2003, p.1).

The European Convention produced a final report in July 2003. The report is a fully-fledged text that systematises all previous European Treatises. The Inter-Governmental Conference that opened in October 2003 was aimed ad adopting the text (with some changes) as the new "Constitution" of the European Union.

The Inter-Governmental Conference failed to adopt the text in the meeting of December 2003 in Brussels. The failure was largely due to a contrast concerning the number of votes to be attributed to large, medium and small member States. The most likely scenario is that an agreement will be eventually found in 2004, and that the text issued from the European Convention will still be the basis of the "constitution" of the Union.

As far as the purposes of this paper are concerned, the main changes introduced by the Treaty establishing a Constitution for Europe can be summarised as follows:

a. The European Union is given legal personality. This means that it will act as an sovereign state *vis-à-vis* of other states;
b. The range of action of the European Union is much widened, especially in the fields of foreign policy, defence, fiscal policy, economic policy, criminal justice, social policy;
c. The notion of "shared competence" between the Union and the member states is introduced, as well as a so-called *Kompetenzkatalog*. As a matter of fact, shared competence applies to the following principal areas: internal market; area of freedom, security and justice; agriculture and fisheries, excluding the conservation of marine biological resources; transport and trans-European networks; energy; social policy; economic, social and territorial cohesion; environment; consumer protection; common safety concerns in public health. The notion of shared competence—which is directly derived from the German Constitution—is defined as follows: "[...] the Union and the Member States shall have the power to legislate and adopt legally binding acts in that area. The Member States shall exercise their competence to the extent that the Union has not exercised, or has decided to cease exercising, its competence" (European Convention, 2003, p.11);
d. The notion of "supporting, coordinating or complementary action" by the Union is introduced. The areas concerned by this kind of Union's action are the following: industry; protection and improvement of human health; education, vocational training, youth and sport; culture; civil protection. In these areas the legally binding acts adopted by the Union "[...] may not entail harmonisation of Member States' laws or regulations" (European Convention, 2003, p.14). This means that member states should not be superseded in their competence in these areas;
e. The general principle of majority voting within the EU institutions is affirmed, leaving unanimity ruling as an exception;
f. It is affirmed as a constitutional principle that "The Constitution, and law adopted by the Union's Institutions in exercising competences conferred on it, shall have primacy over the law of the Member States" (European Convention, 2003, p. 10).
g. It is a matter of debate if the text produced by the European Convention—differently from the previous Treaties—does represent a fully-fledged constitution. As a matter of fact, the juridical form is still a treaty amongst sovereign states, as it is proved by the fact that any future revision of the text will need to be decided by the unanimous agreement of the member states.

However, from a substantive point of view there is no doubt that much more power is conferred to the European Union, and that the potential for centralisation has enormously increased.

IV. The Competence of the EU in the Fields of Bioethics and Health Care

The founding Treatises of the Fifties provided no competence for the EC in the field of health care. The competence was established only in 1992 with the Treaty of Union. As a matter of fact, there was the insertion of a "Public Health" Title, which opened the way to formal co-operation between member states in this area. In parallel, Article 3 raised health protection to the rank of a Community objective.

The Treaty of Amsterdam has better defined the role of the European Union in public health. As a matter of fact, Article 152 affirms that:

> A high level of human health protection shall be ensured in the definition and implementation of all Community policies and activities. Community action, which shall complement national policies, shall be directed towards improving public health, preventing human illness and diseases, and obviating sources of danger to human health. Such action shall cover the fight against the major health scourges, by promoting research into their causes, their transmission and their prevention, as well as health information and education.... Community action in the field of public health shall fully respect the responsibilities of the member states for the organisation and delivery of health services and medical care.

No reference to any bioethical issue exists in the previous Treaties, as well as in the text produced by the European Convention. As a consequence, the competence of the EU in this field derives from other legal sources that will be described later on.

V. EU Policies in Health Care

At the present the European Union is not a federation in the classical meaning of this term. As a matter of fact, until the drafting of the Treaty establishing a Constitution for Europe, the limitation of powers of the member states that was implied by the Treaties and by the jurisprudence of the Court of Justice did not extend itself as to include such essential powers as criminal law and defence. At the same time the EU is something more than a confederation, since the member states accepted that the limitation of their powers is definitive (the so-called "*acquis communautaire*"). This point can be made more clear by reminding that the member states accepted that in some policy matters of the Union collective decisions can be taken not by unanimity but by (qualified) majority. As a consequence, sovereignty is not just *limited,* but is *surrendered* by nation states.

Differently from classical federations, there is no clear-cut vertical division of powers within the EU. The system of governance of the Union is (or should be) based on the so-called "subsidiarity principle". Subsidiarity does not belong to the classical political concepts. As a matter of fact, it originates in the social doctrine of the Catholic Church in the late XIX century. Originally, the concept was instrumental in tracing the boundaries between the proper functions of the state on the one side, and the functions of individuals, families and organised social bodies on the other. It was intended as a *limit* to the power of the state—e.g., in education and health care.

The concept of subsidiarity entered into the constitutional framework of the EC with the EC Treaty and the Treaty of European Union, as a result of Conservative British concerns about national sovereignty and the loss of state control, Christian Democratic/Catholic social philosophy concerning the importance of allowing lower units of authority to achieve their own ends, and German regional politics based on the constitutionally protected competencies of the Laender.

Article 5 of the EC Treaty established that:

> The Community shall act within the limits of the powers conferred upon by this Treaty and of the objectives assigned to it therein. In areas which do not fall within its exclusive competence, the Community shall take action, in accordance with the principle of subsidiarity, only if and in so far as the objectives of the proposed action cannot be sufficiently achieved by the Member States and can therefore, by reason of the scale or effects of the proposed action, be better achieved by the Community. Any action of the Community shall not go beyond what is necessary to achieve the objectives of this Treaty (European Commission, 1993, Art. 5).

The same concept is now expressed by Article 9 of the text of the European Convention (European Convention, 2003, p. 9).[3]

Despite the fact that its use has rapidly spread within the Community law and legislation, the meaning of subsidiarity is far from being clear. Roughly, the principle is meant to achieve two main functions: (1) to draw a boundary between the sphere of competence of the Community and the sphere of competence of the member states; (2) to avoid excessive centralisation and an inexorable increase in Community action and influence at the expense of other and "lesser" political units.

As applied to health care, the concern for subsidiarity was stressed in section 4.b of Article 152 of the EC Treaty, stating that the Council will act "excluding any harmonisation of the laws and regulations of the member states". "Harmonisation", of course, is the typical EU jargon for the more crude but clearer term "unification". As a matter of fact, any "harmonisation" simply means that laws and regulations laid top-down by EU institutions replace different national laws and regulations.

In the text produced by the European Convention, the concern for subsidiarity as far as health care is concerned is expressed by the fact that—as we saw before—"protection and improvement of human health" is considered as an area of "supporting, coordinating or complementary action" (European Convention, 2003, p. 14) where no power should be removed from member states. The matter makes now the object of Article III-179 of the Treaty establishing a Constitution for Europe.

However, a major change was introduced by the Treaty establishing a Constitution for Europe, whose consequences are likely to be far-reaching. As we saw before, "common safety concerns in public health matters" is now classified an area of shared competence between the Union and the member states. According to the very definition of "shared competence", this means that the Union will be able to replace national legislation with its own legislative acts in all health issues that may be defined as "common" to all member states, or to a significant number of member states. Since no clear-cut distinction may be drawn between "public health" and "health", the foreseeable conclusion is that the Union will be given increasing powers at the expenses of national policies and regulations.

Following the content of Article 152 of the EC Treaty, and now of Article III-179 of the text laid down by the European Convention, as well as the subsidiarity principle, the competence of the EU in health care should be focused and limited to the following aspects. In the first place, the EU should have competence in all aspects of health care that have "spill-over effects", or "negative externalities" that go beyond the boundaries of the single member states. In the second place, the EU should have competence in all aspects of health care where there are aims that are considered by all member states as desirable to be attained, but no single member state is individually able to do so.

Both areas of competence correspond to the spirit of a federal framework. *Per se,* they do not imply any kind of unification of the laws and regulations of the several member states. *However, it is clear from the programmes in health care laid down by the EU that reality is different from the letter and the spirit of the Treaties.*

In one of the first documents produced by the EU Commission after the Treaty of Union it was stated that:

> The member states in partnership with their health professionals and individuals involved, are concerned with the financing and delivery of care and treatment. However, the Commission may assist the member states in improving their collaboration on health care matters, as for example on fundamental health choices, and may provide assistance to them in actions desired to improve the quality of health care and treatment (European Commission, 1993, p. 4).

None of these tasks assigned to the Commission corresponds to the proper functions of a federal power, since they do not concern neither spill-over effects nor aims that are considered by all member states as desirable to be attained, but no single member state is individually able to do so. As a matter of fact, they are aimed at directly influencing the proper characteristics of the several health policies of the member states.

Significantly, this centralising bias was much reinforced in the document of May 2000 by the Commission presenting the "Action in the field of public health 2001-2006" of the Community. The document starts by paying lip service to the subsidiarity principle: "The Community's situation is not the same as that of member states. It does not itself manage health services or medical care, which under the Treaty is the clear responsibility of the member states. The Community' role in public health is to complement their efforts, to add value to their actions and in particular to deal with issues that member states cannot handle on their own"(Commission of the European Communities, 2000b, p. 6). Then a classical argument for super-national collective action is proposed: "Infectious diseases, for example, do not respect national borders; neither does air and water pollution. This is why the Treaty has given the Community an important responsibility to tackle health concerns in the widest sense" (Commission of the European Communities, 2000b, p. 6).

One might wonder about the general argument that *any* spill-over effect, or any "negative externality", is a *sufficient* ground for justifying the imposition of centralised rules and legislation. This may be proved to be false as far as pollution is concerned.[4] But the case is even more untenable as far as the case of infectious diseases is concerned. As a matter of fact, the argument relies on the (tacit) assumption that a single political domain (e.g., a state) would have an interest in doing nothing—or doing less than it is necessary—for eliminating or adequately reducing the effects of an infectious disease on its own citizens in the presence of negative externalities produced by the disease over the citizens of other political domains. This is patently absurd. The negative consequences for the citizens of a given political domain of an infectious disease are not reduced by the fact that the disease spreads over other political domains. There is noting in common between this situation and the classical examples of negative externalities—e.g., the interest in doing little for avoiding to pollute a river that flows into a land owned by somebody else.

Starting from these false premises, one should not wonder that the Commission rapidly expanded the scope for Community action:

> People rightly want to be protected against illness and disease. They demand that their food is safe and wholesome, and that the products and services on the market meet high safety standards. They want to bring up their children in a healthy environment and they expect their workplace to be safe and hygienic. (...) In all these areas the Community has a vital role to play (Commission of the European Communities, 2000b, p.6).

The subsidiarity principle is made ineffective, and any proper exclusive sphere of competence for the member states is vanishing.

The ideology of centralisation is followed by the facts. The "Specific objectives and actions" of "Action in the field of public health 2001-2006" include the following:

> *Strengthening the capacity to tackle other health threats.* 1st Objective: To develop strategies and mechanisms for responding to non-communicable disease threats. Review and develop strategies on responses to non-communicable disease threats, including, if appropriate, developing a Community network with links to existing surveillance, notification and alert mechanisms; 2nd Objective: To promote the formulation of guidelines and measures on electromagnetic fields and other physical agents. Review and further develop guidelines and advice on protective and preventive measures on exposure to: 1) electromagnetic fields; 2) other physical agents, such as optical and ultra-violet radiation, laser radiation, pressure, noise and vibration (Commission of the European Communities, 2000b, p. 35).

It easy to see that non-communicable diseases *by definition* do not cross national borders, and that the consequences of ultra-violet radiation over Sicilian people do not have any spill-over effects over Scottish people.

Many other objectives for Community actions follow. Fellow readers on the other side of the Atlantic are likely to be surprised to apprehend that this wide range of objectives will cost to the EU no more than 300 millions of euros (roughly, 260 millions of dollars) for the whole period 2001-2006! Considering the budgets for health policies allowed to central governments in unitary states as well as in federal states one might be tempted to say that the danger of reducing diversity and freedom of choice in health care in Europe as a consequence of EU policies is just irrelevant.

This conclusion would be wrong. For understanding why, it suffices to refer to another objective listed in the above-quoted document:

> Developing strategies and measures on socio-economic health determinants. Objective: To contribute to the formulation and implementation of strategies and measures on socio-economic determinants. (1) Develop a methodology for benchmarking and linking strategies to identify health inequalities using data from the Community health information system, and, if appropriate, develop Community instruments relating to health services and insurance arrangements and to the impact on them of Community policies and activities. Actions will also cover questions related to consumption, cost-effectiveness and expenditure on medicinal products (Commission of the European Communities, 2000b, p. 36).

The obvious aim of these "strategies and measures" *is to create a levelled ideological field for unifying health policies of the several member states of the EU.* The underlying ideology is, of course, the standard social-democratic view, which consider that inequalities are bad in themselves, irrespectively of the absolute income level of a given local or national community.

Here we lie at the core of the problem of choice in health care in Western Europe. The EU has a very small budget, amounting to 1.27 per cent of GDP of the member states. As a consequence, in the present situation it would be impossible to imagine that the EU could play the role of centralising Europe in the same way as in the United States the federal government progressively did after the New Deal, namely, by shifting the bulk of the resources collected by taxation from the states to Washington.

Centralisation in the area of the EU is a post-modern centralisation. EU is in the way to centralise Europe neither by military force nor by shifting the main power to tax from the periphery to the centre, but by unifying laws, regulations, and national policies. Since in Europe more than the half of GDP of most countries is taken and re-distributed by the state, this unification is tantamount to be tremendously effective in homogenise values, lifestyles, and social institutions.

It is worthwhile to remark that centralisation in the field of health care was often justified by EU institution under the cover of the creation of an European single market.

As it is well known, in economic theory there are various approaches to the very idea of market, about its principles and how it works. According to the standard neo-classical view, efficiency is reached when markets are in equilibrium, or near to the equilibrium. In turn, higher levels of economic equilibria are reached when transaction costs are lowered. In order to lower transaction costs, all the different areas included in a given market should have the same regulations. In real world, this means that economic efficiency requires a central legislative authority that lays down rules replacing—if necessary—the several rules previously holding in the different areas.

A very different approach follows from the so-called "Austrian economics", represented by such scholars as Ludwig von Mises and Friedrich von Hayek. According to this view, the state of equilibrium as defined by neoclassical economics does not properly describe the real advantages of market economy over other modes of production. The advantages of markets derive from the fact that they foster innovation of products and services. Markets are never in equilibrium, and happily so. Market is a *discovery* process, where different alternatives are tried and selected by consumers' choices. As long as the production of goods and services requires a legal and regulatory framework, different legal and regulatory system are also put in competition and tried out. Consequently, *competition between legal and regulatory systems is as good as competition for final goods and services.*

The EU approach follows the first view. As a matter of fact, Article 94 of the EC Treaty states that "The Council shall, acting unanimously on a proposal from the Commission and after consulting the European Parliament and the Economic and Social Committee, issue directives for the approximation of such laws, regulations or administrative provisions of the member states as directly affect the establishment or functioning of the common market". The same concept is reaffirmed in Article III-64 of the Treaty establishing a Constitution for Europe. "Approximation" is, of course, a diplomatic wording for "unification". Since the above-reminded Article 152 of the EC Treaty and Articles 16 and III-179 of Treaty establishing a Constitution for Europe forbid "any harmonisation of the laws and regulations of the member states" in the field of health policies, an obvious source of conflict arises here between the competence of the member states and the establishment of uniform rules for a common market of health services.

Empirical evidence everywhere in the world shows that central levels of government seldom restrain themselves from the temptation of invading the competence of lower levels of government. This rule is confirmed in the case of health market in the EU. As a matter of fact, the Council and the European Parliament interpreted Article 94 (and Article 95) as extending their competence as to violate the prohibition stated by Article 152. This fact was made evident when the European Court of Justice was called to decide about the issue of a Directive banning advertising for tobacco. The Court ruled that:

> The Directive is concerned with the approximation of laws, regulations and administrative provisions of the member states relating to the advertising and sponsorship of tobacco products. The national measures affected are to a large extent inspired by public health policy objectives. The first intent of Article 129 (5) [corresponding now to Article 152] of the Treaty excludes any harmonisation of laws and regulations of the member states designed to protect and improve human health. But that provision does not mean that harmonising measures adopted on the basis of other provisions of the Treaty cannot have any impact on the protection of human health. Indeed, the third paragraph of Article 129(1) provides that health requirements are to form a constituent part of the Community's other policies. *Other articles of the Treaty may not, however, be used as a legal basis in order to circumvent the express exclusion of harmonisation laid down in Article 129(4) of the Treaty* (Court of Justice of the European Communities, 2000, p.I-8419. Italics are added).

As it frequently happened in its history, the European Court of Justice has represented an effective countervailing against the centralising tendency within the Community.[5] However one should not expect that the Court would have a sufficient power as to curb the logic of centralisation. A very significant example of this fact is that the European Parliament in 1999 established a "Temporary commission on human genetics and other new technologies of modern medicine". This commission lasted until the end of the legislature (2004) and had a very broad mandate. The commission, as a main juridical basis for its action, explicitly invoked articles 94 and 95. The claim is that progresses in genetic therapies and drugs should be monitored and evaluated by the European Parliament, and that EU legislation is justified in order to avoid obstacles to the internal market and "distortion of competition."[6]

VI. The New European Ideology: The "Precautionary Principle"

The European Union is not just centralising rules about health policies and services in Europe. *It is creating a new ideology about health care* and the protection of the environment. The basis of this ideology is the so-called "precautionary principle", which is now affirmed in the Treaty establishing a Constitution for Europe by Article III-129, concerning Union policy on the environment (European Convention, 2003, p.118).

In 1997, the Treaty of Amsterdam stated that:

> The Commission, in its proposals (...) concerning health, safety, environmental protection and consumer protection, will take as a base a high level of protection, taking account in particular of any new development based on scientific facts. Within their respective powers, the European Parliament and the Council will also seek to achieve this objective (Article 95).

As any relational concept, the expression "a high level of protection" does mean little if one does not specify what he does mean for a "low" level of protection. However, the connotation of the concept is clear: *The European institution was committed to policies privileging the reduction of risks.* This is confirmed by Article 174, stating that "Community policy on the environment shall aim at a high level of protection taking into account the diversity of situations in the various regions of the Community. It shall be based on the precautionary principle (...)". The text is now contained in Article III-129 of the Treaty establishing a Constitution for Europe.

The precautionary principle does not originate from the creativity of European bureaucrats. One of the first instances was in the Ministerial Declaration of the Second International Conference on the Protection of the North Sea (1987):

> In order to protect the North Sea from possibly damaging effects of the most dangerous substances, a precautionary approach is necessary which may require action to control inputs of such substances even before a causal link has been established by absolutely clear scientific evidence.

A new Ministerial Declaration was delivered at the Third International Conference on the Protection of the North Sea (1990). It fleshes out the earlier declaration, stating that "the participants (...) will continue to apply the precautionary principle, that is to take action to avoid potentially damaging impacts of substances that are persistent, toxic and liable to bioaccumulate even where there is no scientific evidence to prove a causal link between emissions and effects."

The precautionary principle is also listed as Principle 15 of the "Rio Declaration" of 1992 among the principles of general rights and obligations of national authorities:

> In order to protect the environment, the precautionary approach should be widely applied by states according to their capabilities. Where there are threats of serious or irreversible damage, lack of full scientific certainty shall not be used as a reason for postponing cost-effective measures to prevent environmental degradation.

Clearly, there is a sharp difference between the two formulations. In the first case the principle is tantamount to adopt a "zero-risk strategy". A given class of actions should be forbidden even when there is no scientific evidence that they are conducive to an undesired result. In the second case the principle is tantamount to assume a "low-risk strategy". A given class of actions should be forbidden when scientific evidence exists that they are harmful, even if no scientific certainty may be attained.

The second formulation is compatible with standard rational behaviour theory. In the presence of prospective catastrophic losses, a relatively low degree of evidence suffices for refraining from taking a given course of actions. But the first formulation is incompatible with standard rational behaviour theory. If evidence for a causal link between a given action and a given consequence is zero, then no basis exists for refraining from taking that action. *There is no difference between this version of the precautionary principle and plain superstition.*

It is far from being clear that the institutions of the EU are realising what is at stake here. A few examples will make the issue clear. In the Communication of 30 April 1997 on consumer health and food safety, the Commission stated "the Commission will be guided in its risk analysis by the precautionary principle, in cases where the scientific basis is insufficient or some uncertainty exists" (Commission of European Communities, 1997). Since *some* uncertainty *always* exists, risk analysis is tantamount to mean nothing at all. The Commission therefore stated that:

> The Treaty requires the Community to contribute to the maintenance of a high level of protection of public health, the environment and consumers. In order to ensure a high level of protection and coherence, protective measures should be based on risk assessment, taking into account all relevant risk factors, including technological aspects, the best available scientific evidence and the availability of inspection sampling and testing methods. Where a full risk assessment is not possible, measures should be based on the precautionary principle (Commission of the European Communities, 1997).

If "full risk assessment" requires that "*all* relevant factors" are taken into account the inescapable conclusion is that no risk assessment is possible at all, since one may never be sure about what are all relevant factors of any phenomenon—even of the simplest one.

The issue of the precautionary principle has become so important in EU policies that the Commission, in February 2000, has felt necessary to summarise its guidelines. The conclusion of the paper is illuminating:

> When the available data are inadequate or non-conclusive, a prudent and cautious approach to environmental protection, health or safety could be to opt for the worst-case hypothesis. When such hypotheses are accumulated, this will lead to an exaggeration of the real risk but gives a certain assurance that it will not be underestimated (Commission of the European Communities, 2000, p.28).

The consequences of this conclusion are far-reaching. As standard rational decision-making theory teaches, in any course of action to act on the basis of the *worst* possible consequence is completely irrational. On these grounds, one should never take a flight or cross a street. Even more relevant for the issue of health care *one should never engage himself (and patients) in clinical trials of new drugs or new medical treatment.*

Supporters of the precautionary principle systematically ignore the fact that any human action involves the so-called "opportunity costs", i.e., the costs that people must bear as a consequence of the fact that new situations, such as new products or new technologies, are not produced because the decision was taken of not engaging in alternative course of actions. Therefore, there are opportunity costs of the decision of doing nothing, or little. The decision of delaying the pace of scientific, technological and economic change as a consequence of the willingness to avoid any kind of risk implies the costs of renouncing to all benefits that would have followed from change—better procedures, better products, better technologies. Included in these costs is the fact that humans will have fewer instruments for facing future changes in the environment where they live. They will have fewer chances facing the appearance of a new threat, such a new virus. *On the long run the systematic application of the precautionary principle will lead to a less safe and a more unpredictable world.*

The high relevance given by the EU to the precautionary principle corresponds to the technocratic view of the EU institutions and policies. Bureaucrats and politicians are seeking for the widest control over scientific research, technology, and agricultural and industrial production. Complete or almost complete harmonisation within Europe becomes the inescapable conclusion. As a matter of fact, if policies—including health policies—must be based on zero (or near to zero) risk strategy, then there can be no variety of policies, since every difference in rules and resource allocation will result in a different level of risk for the individuals. Therefore the precautionary principle is likely to act *as a strong centralising drive within the EU.* As we saw before, in the field of health policy EU institutions are far from respecting the subsidiarity principle. The precautionary principle is conferring them further powers. For example, it allows EU institutions to intervene directly in biomedical scientific and technological research carried out in the several member states on the ground that the resulting products must be "safe" for all consumers of the European common market.

But the precautionary principle also has an anthropological aspect that should not be underestimated. As a matter of fact, it corresponds to a view of society that wants to deprive individuals from their freedom of choice. It is a part of this freedom that individuals should be allowed to choose the level of risk—and corresponding costs—they prefer about food, health care, personal lifestyles. Policies based on the precautionary principles strongly reduce this freedom. Individuals are not seen as free and responsible beings, but as minors needing to be guided by bureaucrats and politicians.

VI. Enter Bioethics

The issue of bioethics is coming at the hearth of the process of creating an "European identity" superseding the several national and regional identities.

In 1991 the Parliamentary Assembly of the Council of Europe began drafting a Bioethics Convention. The Council of Europe was established in 1949 to promote political, legal and cultural relations among member states. It is juridical distinct from the European Union, but in the issues of bioethics the areas of overlapping are enormous. In fact it would be difficult to draw a sharp line of distinction between EU legislation and the legal documents of the Council of Europe. In 1991 the Committee of Ministers of the Council of Europe issued a directive to the Committee on Bioethics to "study the set of problems posed for law, ethics and human rights by progress in the biomedical sciences (...) *with a view to harmonising the policies of the member states as far as possible*" (European Parliament, 2001c, p. 52). The European Convention on Human Rights and Biomedicine was finally agreed to by the Committee of Ministers of the Council of Europe in November 1996. The decision of the Council of Europe resulted in the "Convention for the Protection of Human Rights and Dignity of the Human Being with regard to the Application of Biology and Medicine: Convention on Human Rights and Biomedicine", signed in Oviedo in 1997.

For the purposes of this paper, the main interest of the Oviedo Charter lies in the *limitations* it states, and in the relationships between the "rights" guaranteed by the Charter and the national laws.

Limitations are manifold. Article 13 ("Interventions on the human genome") states that "An intervention seeking to modify the human genome may only be undertaken for preventive, diagnostic or therapeutic purposes and only if its aim is not to introduce any modification in the genome of any descendants". Article 14 ("Non-selection of sex") states that "the use of techniques of medically assisted procreation shall not be allowed for the purpose of choosing a future child's sex, except where serious hereditary sex-related disease is to be avoided." Article 21 ("Prohibition of financial gain") states that "the human body and its parts shall not, as such, give rise to financial gain". *All these statements pose limits to individual freedom, not to the power of the states over their citizens.*

It is interesting to consider the general view underlying the Charter. As a matter of fact, the reasons adduced for such a Convention were twofold. In the first place, it was argued that advances in biomedicine were moving at such a pace that the laws in the various member states were not able to keep pace with the developments. In the second place, concerns were emerging that given the rapid pace of developments, and the fragmentation of approach among member states, "havens" could emerge for research where scientists could exploit lack of regulation in order to evade the legal restrictions in force in their own countries.

Both reasons correspond to a *dirigiste* view, wholly unacceptable from a liberal standpoint. The *dirigiste* view assumes that variety and diversity is bad, and that homogeneity is good. The point at stake here is not just a value standpoint. It is also a factual point. Why a centralised legislation extending to many states should be better suited than national laws to keep pace with scientific or technological developments? The contrary holds. Centralised legislation is necessarily the result of a long process of negotiation between states, interest groups, bureaucrats and politicians. Is a compromise between ideologies, parties, and religious belief. There is no reason to assume that this process will be faster than legislation by the single states. Furthermore, the fact that different states have different laws allows for different "experiments" to be tried. In this diversity it is likely that new solutions will emerge that will prove to be more effective than others are, and that will spread by imitation in other legal systems.

But the most striking ideological element underlying the Convention is the idea that "lack of regulation" in some states is bad because it allows scientists to carry out research forbidden in their own country. *This means that more value is given to prohibitions than to freedom of research.*

The "Convention for the Protection of Human Rights and Dignity of the Human Being with regard to the Application of Biology and Medicine" has been the forerunner of the main document about rights produced by the European Union[7], namely, the "Charter of Fundamental Rights of the European Union", ratified in December 2000. With the Treaty establishing a Constitution for Europe the Charter was included in the legal framework of the European Union, as Part II of the Treaty (European Convention, 2003, pp. 47-60).

The reasons in favour of drafting a specific charter of rights for the European Union were essentially political. As a matter of fact, the Charter was intended to help to establish an "ever closer union" among the European peoples by calling for a specific juridical identity as a basis for fully-fledged European citizenship.

The idea that drafting a charter of rights might be crucial in building a new citizenship seems to stem from the German debates of the last decade or so around the concept of "constitutional patriotism". Indeed, in the history of European nations cultural, ethnic or political identities stand before the establishment of constitutional rights. To a lesser degree, the idea reflects a long-lasting trend in French political culture, as summarised in the famous dictum "C'est l'Etat qui fait la Nation". In providing the basis for a European citizenship, the Charter rests on the assumption that, beyond national diversities, there is a wide area of "common values" shared by all European people (*Preamble,* 3). These values provide the basis for the statement of the rights that the Charter guarantees to "each person" (*Preamble,* 7). In this way, rights are made dependent on values. This dependence is likely to have a far-reaching effect on the relationships between the Charter and the rights guaranteed by the constitutions of the Member States.

It is crucial to stress that the Charter establishes no hierarchy of rights. As a matter of fact, the Charter is articulated in six broad areas (Dignity, Freedom, Equality, Solidarity, Citizenship, Justice). In the *Preamble,* dignity, freedom, equality and solidarity are qualified as "indivisible, universal principles", while—quite surprisingly—"the principle of democracy and the rule of law" is set apart. This means that none of the statements of the Charter is made dependent upon the fulfilment of any other. In this way the right guaranteed by Article 28 ("Everyone has the right of access to a free placement service") is given the same constitutional relevance as the right guaranteed by Article 2.1 ("Everyone has the right to life"). One may easily appreciate which kind of view of men and morality underlies the Charter. The willingness to give "positive" rights, proper of the socialist tradition, the same ranking of the "negative" values, proper of the liberal tradition, produced wholly absurd consequences.

Biomedical rights are stated in Article 3 ("Right to the integrity of the person") of Chapter I, "Dignity", and in Article 35 ("Health care") of Chapter IV, "Solidarity".

Article 3 states that:

1. Everyone has the right to respect for his or her physical and mental integrity.
2. In the fields of medicine and biology, the following must be respected in particular:
   - the free and informed consent of the person concerned, according to the procedures laid down by law,
   - the prohibition of eugenic practices, in particular those aiming at the selection of persons,
   - the prohibition on making the human body and its parts as such a source of financial gain,
   - the prohibition of the reproductive cloning of human beings.

Article 35 states that:

> Everyone has the right of access to preventive health care and the right to benefit from medical treatment under the conditions established by national laws and practices. A high level of human health protection shall be ensured in the definition and implementation of all Union policies and activities.

The ideology of the Charter of Fundamental Rights of the European Union is therefore the same of the ideology of the Oviedo Charter. Technically, the Oviedo Charter is not submitted to the subsidiarity principle. The Charter is intended to grant a kind of "basic" level of rights protection. This protection can be strengthened by the states if they want so. This possibility is stated in Article 27 ("Wider protection"):"None of the provisions of this Convention shall be interpreted as limiting or otherwise affecting the possibility for a Party to grant a wider measure of protection with regard to the application of biology and medicine than is stipulated in this Convention." The same logic was adopted by the Charter of Fundamental Rights of the European Union, that states that human rights and fundamental freedoms granted by the member states' constitutions should not be restricted or adversely affected by the Charter. In this way the autonomy of the several states should be fully respected.

It is not so. Having to establish a *minimum commune,* certain specific features of national constitutions are necessarily not fully reflected in the Charter, and innumerable potential conflicts arise. Let me show this point with a comparison between the Charter and the Italian constitution as far as economic and social rights are concerned.

The Italian constitution provides for a strongly egalitarian view. This is especially reflected in Article 3.2 ("It is the duty of the Republic to remove all economic and social obstacles which, by limiting the freedom and equality of citizens, prevent the full development of the individual and the participation of all workers in the political, economic and social organisation of the country") as well as in Article 42.2 ("Private ownership shall be recognised and guaranteed by laws which shall determine the manner by which it may be acquired and enjoyed, and its limits, in order to ensure its social function and to make it open to all").

There is no article in the Charter that can be considered as the equivalent of Article 3.2. In turn, Article 42.2 of the Italian constitution is only partially reflected in Article 17 of the Charter:

> No one may be deprived of his possession, except in the public interest and in the cases and under the conditions provided for by the law, subject to fair compensation being paid within a reasonable period for their loss. The use of property may be regulated insofar as is necessary for the general interest.

No claim is made about a "social function" of private property or about its availability to all citizens. The point at stake here is that the *additional* level of social rights guaranteed by the Italian constitution conflicts with the stronger protection of private property rights guaranteed by the Charter.

Of course, reverse examples could be found, namely, that the Oviedo Charter and the Charter of Fundamental Rights of the European Union adversely affect rights guaranteed by national laws. Let us consider Article 14 of the Oviedo Charter ("Non-selection of sex"):"The use of techniques of medically assisted procreation shall not be allowed for the purpose of choosing a future child's sex, except where serious hereditary sex-related disease is to be avoided". Clearly, this prohibition conflicts with constitutionally guaranteed rights to the non-invasion by the state in the field of sexuality. One might also wonder about the moral basis of such a restrictive legislation, given that almost all European countries make abortion legal. Finally, one cannot help but to agree with Corinna Delkeskamp that "contradictions within the (Oviedo Charter) arise with regard to respect for autonomy, the unlimited extension of rights bearers, and the granting of a right to health care itself" (Delkeskamp, 2006, p. 56).

VIII. The Case of Legislation About Research on Human Embryos and Medically Assisted Reproduction

Research on human embryos has become the most important bioethical issue in Europe. *It has also become one of the driving forces of "harmonisation" of biomedical legislation in Europe.*

The issue is dealt in Article 18 of the Oviedo Charter ("Research on embryos *in vitro*": "1. Where the law allows research on embryos *in vitro,* it shall ensure adequate protection of the embryo. 2. The creation of human embryos for research purposes is prohibited"). One might wonder if any serious meaning can be given to a "law" that allows experiments on embryos and at the same time claims that embryos should be "protected"! This is really a good example of how attempts to unify several laws are often leading to unworkable rules.

Laws and regulations concerning research on human embryos, as well as medically assisted procreation, are considerably different in the several member states of the EU. This difference reflects the existence of large differences in perception and judgement by the citizens of different countries.[8] In Britain, for example, the current law prohibits only the substitution of the nucleus of an embryonic cell by a nucleus removed from a cell of a person or an embryo. It thus permits cloning by nuclear transfer provided this takes place prior to fertilisation and also cloning by means of splitting. Furthermore, no prohibition exists about creating embryos for research purposes.[9] Since United Kingdom has not ratified the Oviedo Charter, and since the Charter of Fundamental Rights of the European Union does not prohibit this creation, there is no legal base for any of the bodies of the EC to interfere with the British law or with any other similar national law.

The situation is different. In the "Resolution on the Protection of Human Rights and Dignity with regard to the Application of Biology and Medicine" adopted in October 1996, the European Parliament declared that:

> 1. Consumptive research on and the production of human embryos for research purposes must be prohibited; 2. In artificial human insemination no more than three embryos must be in a women during one cycle; the preservation of frozen embryos is admissible only in exceptional circumstances if implantation is not possible during one cycle on medical grounds; 3. Cryoconservation after the fertilisation treatment is completed must be forbidden (European Parliament, 1996, p.1268).

The resolution of the European Parliament was void of legal consequences. But is not void of political consequences, and it does not represent at all an isolated case. As a matter of fact, the tendency by the EU organs to centralise legislation about human embryos, stem cells, medically assisted procreation, is strong.

The issue of research on human embryos and stem cells has gained considerable momentum in connection with the Sixth Framework Programme issued for the years 2003-2006. According to the Commission, the Programme had to fund embryonic stem cells research, leaving to national legislation the right to allow or to forbid such kind of research. The proposal of the Commission followed a decision taken in 2002 by the Parliament and by the Council.

However, facing the opposition of several member States, in order to find an agreement a moratorium was declared on the funding of research on embryonic stem cells, expiring on the 31st of December, 2003.

The proposal of the Commission did not pass the legislative procedure of the Union by the end of the deadline. Short of a final decision concerning the inclusion of funding of embryonic stem cells, research in the general guidelines of the Sixth Framework Programme, the Commission has declared that the European Commission and EU governments will have to scrutinise each proposal to use EU funds on a "case by case basis". Since huge differences exist between national legislation, and since embryonic stem cells research is forbidden – or severely restricted - in several countries, such as Germany, Italy, France, Austria, and Ireland, the approval of the proposal of the Commission would be tantamount to shift resources from some member States to others.

However, money is not the main point at stake here. As a matter of fact, of the EU's 17 billion Euro research budget for 2002-2006, stem cell scientists are likely to receive an amount of the order of 50 million Euro. The point at stake is the extension of the legislative and regulatory power of the EU over matters that do not fall into any of its own competences. The Research Commissioner Philippe Busquin affirmed that the proposal was not an attempt to set guidelines for member State policies towards embryonic stem cell research, and neither did it aim to provide universal ethical principles. However, it is quite obvious that the funding by the EU of embryonic stem cells research will put considerable pressure over member States that do not allow such kind of research to change their own legislation.[10]

The several committees of bioethics that were created by the Council, the Commission, and the Parliament play a crucial role in the process of creating a centralised legislation. "Experts" compose them that *invariably*—but not surprisingly—*suggest that more power should be given to the EU.*

The most important and influential committee is probably the "European Group on Ethics in Science and New Technologies", established by the EC Commission in 1991. The EGE is composed by twelve scholars, and provides opinions to the Commission and to the Parliament. One of the most relevant of them deals with "Ethical aspects of human stem cell research and use"

(November 2000). The recommendations for political action by the EU that the document provides are revealing. The document pays the usual lip service to pluralism within the EU: "Pluralism is characteristic of the European Union, mirroring the richness of its tradition and adding a need for mutual respect and tolerance. Respect for different philosophical, moral or legal approaches and for diverse cultures is implicit in the ethical dimension of building a democratic European society" (EGE, 2000, p.15). But then proposed policy recommendations are just the opposite of these claims. For example the EGE considers that "(...) it is crucial to place embryonic stem cell research, in the countries were it is permitted, under strict public control by a centralised authority" (EGE, 2000, p.16). In this way, the EGE allows itself to interfere in the national laws, fostering a strong *dirigiste* and anti-federalist view. The EGE then recommends to the Commission and to the Parliament that "(...) cell banks should be regulated at European level in order to facilitate the implementation of a precautionary approach" (EGE, 2000, p.19). This proposal is fully in contrast with the fact that legislation about stem cell research is a matter reserved to the member states, which may adopt different policy approaches, founded on different ethical views.

One further point about the relationships between the EU and bioethics is worth to be stressed. In the period 1994-1998 (Fourth Framework Programme) the European Union had financed bioethical research for an amount of 30 millions of euros, involving 700 research centres in Europe. Given the orientations of the Commission and of the other organs of the EU, one may reasonably assume that the main reason for spending such a large amount of money was not fostering progress in bioethical knowledge, but "*building a consensus*" about the very idea that the European Union should have a key role in the biomedical field.

One may easily realise this point by looking at the ideological activities done by the EU institutions. For example, an important conference was recently organised by the Commission on "Genetics and the Future of Europe". Here is one of the statements from the official synthesis of the debate: "Pluralism can enrich any debate, but could there be a risk that our diversity of sensitivities, of national and regional cultures, might preclude even minimal European agreement on a basic set of ethical principles? Geographic boundaries are not necessarily the determining factor: *"The diversity of ethical values and beliefs is often greater within each member state than between states of the Union"*. This means we must build on a consensus based on *"a foundation of common European values"* such as democracy, human rights, solidarity, and sharing. *"Finally, all of us are equally affected by the genetic risk"*[11]. The first statement is by Professor Octavi Quintana-Trias, the second by Professor Axel Kahn, and the third by Professor David McConnell—three distinguished scholars. The statement by Quintana-Trias is particularly interesting, at least for two reasons.

The first reason is that it is an example of a classical cognitive and statistical error. Statements about "within each member state" refer to individuals' properties, while statements about "between states" refer to statistical averages. The two data cannot be compared, or can be compared only in a trivial and scientifically uninteresting sense. For example, one can say that there are people within the USA that differ about preferences for wine vs. beer, and that those who prefer wine have something in common with French people rather than with their fellow citizens who prefer beer. You may extend the "argument" by saying that the percentage of population that prefers wine to beer in California is similar to the percentage in France, while is different from the percentage in Oregon. You may also find other statistical "results". For example, that New York people earning more than 10 million dollars a year drink as much champagne as wealthy Paris people, and not as little as New York homeless people.

The second reason is that, should one take seriously the statement by Quintana-Trias, the logical consequence would be exactly the contrary of the thesis that we should have a unified European bioethics. If we seek to maximise utility, we should rather be *downsizing regulations as to abolish even national legislation,* and consequently be allowing individuals to adhere to ethical "clubs" in the meaning given to this word in economic theory by James Buchanan.

IX. Is This Situation the Result of a Democratic Processs?

Supporters of the current policies of the EU claim that they are the result of a democratic process. Citizens directly elect the European Parliament, the ministers of member states compose the Council, and members designated by the governments of member states compose the Commission. The result of the political process made by the interplay of these institutions—including harmonisation/centralisation—may be considered as efficient or non-efficient, but cannot be judged as undemocratic. Therefore, EU policies reflect the preferences of the majority of citizens, and must be consequently respected.

As straightforward as it may seem, the argument is basically flawed. The essential point at stake here is that the fact that the players of the EU game have democratic legitimacy does not means that their decisions reflect the preferences of the majority of European citizens. One might suspect so from the fact that in half a century of story of the European institutions only a handful of times the peoples of Europe were called to express themselves by referenda on the major steps. For example, never were the Germans called to vote if they agreed upon abandoning the German mark for the euro. Most likely, European people will not be called to vote about the enlargement of the EU towards central and East European countries. When referenda were held in some member states, the result was often a rejection.

We have abundant theoretical and empirical evidence that shows how centralisation of unitary states as well as of federations was the result of several factors, none of which can be considered as the expression of the plain will of the electorate. Vested interests, lobbies, the so-called "fiscal illusion" (in Wicksell's sense), the rent-seeking behaviour of politicians, are the most likely factors that account for the shifting of the vertical balance of powers from the local to the central level. There is also abundant empirical evidence that this is happening in Europe today, and that the citizens' preferences do account nothing, or little, for the fact that the EU has harmonised the size of condoms and apples[12]. For the purposes of this paper, one might wonder if harmonisation in bioethical rules or in health care carried out by the EU is derived from the attempt to reflect the preferences of its citizens, or is rather the result of a largely self-feeding political process.

X. Is This Situation the Result of a Process Towards a Global Ethic?

There are good reasons to assume that the process toward a European unified ideology in matter of bioethics and health care has much to do with the movement toward a Global Ethic. As a matter of fact, the reasons that are brought in favour of a European unified ideology bring many elements in common with the ideology of the Global Ethic.

In the *Declaration toward a Global Ethic* of the Parliament of the World's Religions the statement is made that "We are interdependent. Each of us depends on the well-being of the whole, and so we have respect for the community of living beings, for people, animals, and plants, and for the preservation of Earth, the air, water and soil" (The Parliament of the World's Religions, 1993, p.11). The statement is a curious mix of Renaissance-style pantheism and New Age views. But it is also the expression of the idea that the world is so strictly interconnected as to impose to all humans to follow common ethical rules for the purpose of their material well being. The same idea is expressed in more political terms in the 1995 report *Our Global Neighbourhood* by the Commission on Global Governance. The report states that:

> It is now more difficult to separate actions that solely affect a nation's internal affairs from those that have an impact on the internal affairs of other states, and hence to define the legitimate boundaries of sovereign authority. [...] Increasingly, countries are having to accept that in certain fields sovereignty has to be exercised collectively, particularly in respect of the global commons. [...] States continue to perform important functions, and must have the powers to fulfil these functions effectively. But [...] they are also limited by the fundamental interests of the humanity, which in certain severe circumstances must prevail over the ordinary rights of particular states (Commission on Global Governance, 1995).

It is easy to recognise in these statements the age-old arguments in favour of reducing the sphere of self-government, and centralising power toward more comprehensive levels, the last being the whole world. Clearly, the ideology of a unified European bioethics and health care policy removing the ultimate responsibility from local communities and member states of the EU is based on the very same views.

However, this is just a part of the story. The building of a unified European bioethics and health care policy is driven by the view that Europe presents a peculiarity in respect to the rest of the world. This peculiarity is represented by the European model of the welfare state. As it was put:

> The extension of the notion of responsibility in the modern welfare state implies that the welfare state must in legislation and legal practice continue the protection and care for the individual human body, something which was earlier a question of private activity or just handed over to social institutions like the church and the medical profession. The implementation of the basic principles in modern legal practice, is not only present in civil and criminal law but also in social, health and labour law. The actual legal development shows an extended protection of the human person as the driving force in bioethics and biolaw (Rentdorf, 1998).

The EU bioethical and health care policy should be, therefore, based on the principles of the welfare state. *E converso,* implementing a unified European bioethical and health care policy is presented as the only chance to preserve the welfare state. As a matter of fact, a centralised EU policy would make sure that no competition would exist between the member states in order to lower the costs imposed upon individuals and firms for the purpose of finding the resources for financing the health care systems.

XI. Perspectives for Change

People that praise individual liberty and responsibility in biomedicine and health care cannot help but look pessimistically at the European situation. In most European countries, the largest parts of biomedical research are carried out in public institutions, or are publicly funded. In all European countries, health care is monopolised or heavily regulated by the state. While in past years the state has rolled back from the control of the economy, there is no sign that the same is happening as far as health care is concerned. One could be tempted to say that the contrary holds. The more the states are loosing control over the economy as a result of the common European market and globalisation, *the more they have the tendency to extend their control over other aspects of human life.*

The peculiarity of the European situation is that this phenomenon is coupled with another phenomenon, namely, the creation of a super-national state that has the tendency to assume on itself most of the new regulatory functions. Systematically, the European Union acts for de-regulating the internal markets and legal framework of the states in order to re-regulate them according to its own rules. The result of this situation is that "(...) if one compares the degree of harmonisation in Europe with that in Canada, the United States, and other federations, one is impressed by the extent to which it is greater in Europe than in the federations" (Breton, 1996, p. 276).[13]

Bioethics is an example of this fact. In the case of bioethics, since national legislation is generally incomplete or does not cover all aspects, *the attempt of the EU is to directly lay down new rules valid for all member states.*

Of course, one cannot but agree with the remark by Kurt Bayertz that the so-called "European moral identity" is not "(...) a homogeneous system of values or ideals, which would (or at least could) function as the basis of a comprehensive moral consensus" (Bayertz, 2006, p. 209). Bayertz is right in stressing the religious, legal, psychological, historical and ethical differences that exist in Europe, and that are reflected in the differences between the national regulations in matter of bioethics. However, one should not forget the very making of the history of the European nation-state. As a matter of fact, the centralistic states emerged from ethnic, cultural, and linguistic differences which were extremely strong (see Weber, 1976, in particular, chapter 7). And differences have a strong tendency to be reduced as economic and cultural exchanges increase.

The fact that all-pervasive harmonisation in Europe is conducive to a situation were individual freedom, cultural differences and economic efficiency are put in danger is not going unrecognised, even at political level. A very significant example was the position taken by the European People's Party (the largest political formation in the EU) in the last congress held in Berlin in January 2001. The document affirms that:

> Europe will not be a federation in the conventional sense, but a new form of federal system, of which economic and monetary union is the precursor. European federalism is competition-based federalism. Economic and monetary union has centralised just one element—monetary policy—of one key area of public policy, the economy. The others, in contrast to a federation, remain the responsibility of participating states. Competition between member states, the essence of the competition-based federalism, is essential to find best practices, and to give member states enough room for manoeuvre to adapt themselves to new challenges in respect of their specific problems, needs, and experiences. (...) Within this new federal system of economic and monetary union, the objectives of federalism – welfare, equality, and justice— *are therefore not primarily the outcome of transfers and harmonisation as in classical federal states, but the result of a fair and rule-based competition between the member states* (European People's Party, 2001, italics are added).

Unfortunately, the position taken in this document was completely overturn by the choices made within the European Convention by the representatives of the European People's Party, as they were at the forefront of the extension of the Union's competence and regulatory powers. This was particularly true of the German members. This may be seen as a further evidence of the powerful drive in favour of centralisation that supersedes ideology.

While harmonisation reduces the opportunities for individual choice, competitive federalism increases them. *As a matter of fact, individuals become free to choose among as many sets of rules as the states that are members of the federation.* Moral diversity *is not sacrificed to the need of extending the area of cultural and economic exchange.*

The view of "competitive federalism" is largely alternative to the ideology followed today by the European Union. But competitive federalism was and is not completely absent from EU history and policy, as is proved by the relevance of the so-called "principle of mutual recognition".

The principle entered the legal framework of the EU in an irreversible way after a decision by the European Court of Justice known as the *Cassis de Dijon* ruling.[14] Up to then, the sale of Cassis was forbidden in Germany, as the German law envisages a mandatory minimum alcohol content for alcoholic beverages to be marketed. The provision relating to the minimum wine-spirit content for potable spirits laid down in the German *Branntweinmonopolgesetz* was an obstacle to the import of a consignment of Cassis de Dijon originating in France, as its alcohol content was between 15 and 20%. In the absence of common rules, the Court of Justice, though recognising that the member states had the right to legislate the sale of products within their own territories, affirmed that this national right could not counter Art. 28 of the EC Treaty (formerly Art. 30), which would be violated whenever the import of a good lawfully produced and marketed in another member state was impeded.

According to the principle of mutual recognition, no European country should be compelled to modify its own laws and, while maintaining them, it cannot impede the import of goods, services and capitals from other member states with different laws. *In this way, harmonisation of national laws is not necessary, and their substitution with EU laws is not necessary either.*

Critics of the principle of mutual recognition point out the fact that it would lead at an increase of transaction costs, while harmonisation would lower them. There is some truth in this argument, but transaction costs should not be overestimated, and economic advantages of harmonisation—independently from the losses of freedom it involves—should be compared with its cost[15]. *As far as health care is concerned, the argument is even less decisive.* As a matter of fact, there might be good reasons in favour of the fact that such things as labelling of drugs or information about sanitary products were "harmonised" in such a way as to make easier their use in all European countries. But this has nothing to do with the idea that one should harmonise such things as therapeutic protocols, the authorisation procedures for the commercialisation of new drugs, or the procedures for clinical trial. *In all these matters the logic of competition among different rules is almost isomorphic with the very concept of scientific research.* The plurality of approaches does not represent at all a "cost", a limit to overcome, but an essential factor of progress.

Strictly speaking, mutual recognition and competitive federalism do not coincide. As a matter of fact, competitive federalism is based on the simultaneous application of two principles.

The first principle is the coincidence between territorial domain and collective decisions. This, in turn, implies the "principle of exclusivity", namely, that competence about collective action are distributed—vertically and horizontally—in such a way as to avoid that different institutions are responsible of the same functions. There must be no superposition of the power of the federal government and the power of the federate states. The repartition of powers should be made considering what is the "optimal area" of collective action that is most likely to satisfy the preferences of citizens. The second principle is the opening of territories and markets of the federate states to the people, goods and services of any other federate state.

The first principle without the second is conducive to the pre-modern and pre-state, when there was a plurality of separate sovereign territorial powers. The second principle without the first is conducive to the centralised national state, which is the opposite of the federalist model.

Mutual recognition is perfectly compatible with these two principles. However, this compatibility comes under stress if mutual recognition is extended as to include the possibility that sets of rules of a member state of the federation might be *applied directly* on the territory of other member states. French people could go work in Germany being paid according to French and not German standards. Medical treatment could be given in Spain by British (or Dutch) doctors according to British professional and bioethical rules. Hospitals could be built in France respecting Danish regulations, and vice-versa. Hospital could be built in Italy respecting German regulations (but hopefully *not* vice-versa...). In this way, mutual recognition would be leading to a substantial de-coupling of rules from geographical location of people. This is tantamount to deprive the principle of exclusivity of most of its content. As a matter of fact, there would be no more coincidence between territorial domain and collective action.

The extension of the principle of mutual recognition leads to a more libertarian institutional framework, which would mirror Buchanan's theory of clubs. In recent years, Bruno Frey prospected this possible world with his theory of FOCJ, an acronym for *Functional, Overlapping, Competing Jurisdictions.*[16] FOCJ are jurisdictions because they have coercive powers over their members. But adhesion to a FOCUS is a voluntary one. In some cases, federal or state governments might decide to compel their citizens to adhere to a given class of FOCJ, as in the case of those which provide education for children or basic medical treatment. However, governments would not have the right to impose on their citizens to what specific FOCUS to adhere. From the economic point of view, FOCJ are conducive to a high degree of respect of the principle of "fiscal equivalence"—which is the cornerstone of fiscal federalism—and to lower negative externalities.

In comparison with the extended version of the mutual recognition principle, FOCJ further enlarge individual liberty as they are not necessarily limited to state and public jurisdiction, but may include privately created and enforced jurisdictions. *Health care is a most natural field where several FOCJ could develop and flourish,* bringing together people that in different states and regions share the same moral values, the same risk propensity, and the same ranking of preferences concerning medical treatment and its cost.

From the point of view of individual freedom, the theory of FOCJ is the highest approximation to a purely libertarian world, where there would be no coercive collective action. As desirable as this might be seen, it seems most unlikely that it might represent a realistic alternative for the future of the Old Continent.

XII. Conclusion

Facing the many unpalatable consequences of the harmonisation policies in Europe, several traditionalist and nationalist forces are calling for a return to the *status quo ante* the birth of the European Community. They favour a return to the all-encompassing, self-contained national states that could guarantee the survival of the different traditions and morals.

There are many reasons to believe that this return is impossible and undesirable, since it would be tantamount to dramatically reduce the enormous advantages that derive from the extension of the European market and from freedom of movement of people within Europe. At the same time, it should not be forgotten that all-encompassing, self-contained national states were for two centuries the main cause of wars, restriction of individual rights, and reduction of cultural diversity as represented by regional and sub-regional cultures.

Differently from a romantic appeal to the virtues of the national states, the systematic application of the principle of mutual recognition could bring many benefits. Replacing the logic of harmonisation with the logic of mutual recognition represents the necessary condition for turning the process of building the European institutions in a great opportunity for fostering individual liberty and economic prosperity, while preserving the variety of morals and customs that constitutes the true spirit of Europe.

Unfortunately, after the approval of the Treaty establishing a Constitution for Europe, there is little chance that the future of Europe will significantly deflect from the pattern of explicit as well as of creeping centralisation that history has proved to be the reality of most large-scale political institutions, be they democratic or un-democratic.

Notes

1. See Article 2: "The Union shall set itself the following objectives: (...) to strengthen the protection of the rights and interests of the nationals of its Member States through the introduction of a citizenship of the Union".
2. See Isaac (1990, pp. 172-182).
3. Since the there is widespread concern about the effectiveness of the principle of subsidiarity as a way to keep the proper balance between the Union and the member states, the Treaty establishing a Constitution for Europe contains a specific Protocol on the Application of the Principle of Subsidiarity and Proportionality (see European Convention, 2003, pp. 229-231). The Protocol states that, if one-third (or one-fourth, for some specific matters) of the parliaments of the member states consider that Union's action has violated the twin principles of subsidiarity and proportionality, then the Commission is obliged to reconsider the legislation laid down. However, there is no obligation for the Commission or the other bodies of the Union to revert their decision.
4. As it was shown by the so-called "market ecology", externalities can be appropriately dealt with by the introduction of an efficient system of property rights.
5. On this issue see Petroni (1997). These outcomes were not the result of chance, of course. They were basically the result of the traditional judicial practice followed by the Court, which considers opposed parties as being equal before the law. This allowed individual rights and free-market principles to prevail over wide *and* strong interests. One could scarcely expect a majoritarian democratic process to produce better or equivalent outcomes.
6. See European Parliament (2001b).
7. There is no reference to the "Convention for the Protection of Human Rights and Dignity of the Human Being with regard to the Application of Biology and Medicine: Convention on Human Rights and Biomedicine" in the *Preamble* of the Charter of Fundamental Rights of the European Union. The reason is that at that time the Convention was not ratified by all member states of the EU. The Charter is still under the process of ratification by national parliament. Till now only a handful of states completed the process.
8. A very interesting statistical survey is given by the report of Eurobarometer (2000). The survey includes attitudes toward bioethical issues such as human cloning and genetic therapy.
9. See European Parliament (2001). In September 2000 the European Parliament has called on the UK Government "(...) to review its positions on human embryo cloning" and called on the United Kingdom's Parliament "to reject the proposal to permit research using embryos created by cell nuclear transfer." The European Parliament also repeated its call "to each member state to enact binding legislation prohibiting all research into any kind of human cloning within its territory and providing for criminal penalties for any break" (Document n. A5-0168/2000).
10. See http://communities.msn.se/CellNews, as well as http://europa.eu.int/commm/research

11. The conference was hold in Brussels on 6 and 7 November 2000. Available: http://www.europa.eu.int/research/quality-of-life/genetics.
12. On this topic see Petroni and Caporale (2000).
13. The interesting explanation given by Breton is that there is so much harmonisation in Europe because the institutional framework of the EU is not federal enough, namely, that the EU institutions do not have the power to effectively enforce the rules of a "fair" competition for the common market. States do not want to give to the EU this power fearing that it would infringe their sovereignty: "But to be able to enjoy a stable Union structure, they impose upon themselves a series of harmonising measures that transform them into the simile of a unitary state—thereby metamorphosing their individual sovereignty into symbol!" (*ibidem*, p. 276).
14. Contrary to widespread opinion, the "Cassis de Dijon" sentence—unfortunately!—did not establish mutual recognition as a principle replacing harmonisation. It was, instead, a device for preventing the *"acquis communautaire"* from being made ineffective, in view of the fact that harmonisation—explicitly contained in the EEC Treaty—will take a long time to be accomplished.
15. As a matter of fact, new technologies—e.g., computers and Internet—drastically reduce information costs, which are the main part of transaction costs.
16. See for example Frey (2000).

References

Barry, N. (1990). 'The liberal constitution: rational design or evolution?' *Critical Review*, 3(2), 267-82.

Bayertz, K. (2006). 'Consensus and dissensus in matters of health care policy and bioethics in Europe,' In H.T. Engelhardt, Jr. (ed.), *Global Bioethics: The Collapse of Consensus*, pp. 207-237.

Breton, A. (1996). *Competitive Governments. An Economic Theory of Politics and Public Finance.* Cambridge: Cambridge University Press.

Commission of the European Communities. (1997). *Green Paper on the General Principles of Food Law in the European Union.*

Commission of the European Communities. (2000, February 2). *Communication from the Commission on the Precautionary Principle.* Brussels: COM (2000), 1 final.

Commission of the European Communities. (2000b, May 16). *Communication from the Commission to the Council, the European Parliament, the Economic and Social Committee of the Regions on the health strategy of the European Community.* Brussels: COM (2000), 285 final.

Commission on Global Governance (1995). *Report: Our Global Neighbourhood.* [Online]. Available: http://www.cgg.ch.

Court of Justice of the European Communities. (1960, 15 July). *Reports,* Geitling vs. High Authority.

Court of Justice of the European Communities. (1964, 15 July). *Reports,* Flaminio Costa vs. ENEL.

Court of Justice of the European Communities. (1979, 20 February). *Reports,* Rewe-Zentral AG vs. Bundesmonopolverwaltung fuer Branntwein.

Court of Justice of the European Communities. (2000, 5 October). *Reports,* Federal Republic of Germany vs. European Parliament and Council of the European Union.

Delkeskamp-Hayes, C. (2006). 'Implementing health care rights versus imposing health care cultures: the limits of tolerance, Kant's rationality, and the moral pitfalls of international bioethics standardization,' In H.T. Engelhardt, Jr. (ed.), *Global Bioethics: The Collapse of Consensus*, pp. 50-94.

European Convention. (2003). *Draft Treaty Establishing a Constitution for Europe.*

Eurobarometer. (2000). 52.1 *The Europeans and Biotechnologies.* Brussels: Commission of the European Communities.

European Commission (1993, 24 November). *Commission Communication on the Framework for Action in the Field of Public Health.* Brussels: COM (1993), 559 final.

EGE-European Group on Ethics in Science and New Technologies to the European Commission. (2000). *Ethical Aspects of Human Cells Research and Use.* Opinion n.15.

European Parliament .(1996, October 28). Resolution on the Protection of Human Rights and Dignity with Regard to the Application of Biology and Medicine. *Official Journal C 320.*

European Parliament. (2001). Directorate General for Research, STOA-Scientific and Technological Options Assessment, *Embryos, Scientific Research and European Legislation,* Briefing Note n.14/2001 (PE303.112). Luxembourg.

European Parliament. (2001b). Temporary Commission on Human Genetics and Other New Technologies of Modern Medicine, *Report* PE 300.121.

European Parliament. (2001c). Directorate General for Research, STOA-Scientific and Technological Options Assessment, *The Ethical Implications of Research Involving Human Embryos* (PE289.665/Fin.St.). Luxembourg.

European People's Party. (2001, January 11-13). *A Union of Values.* [Online]. Available: http://www.eppe.org/archive/congress2001.

Frey, B.S. (2002). *A Utopia? Government without Territorial Monopoly.* Zuerich: University of Zuerich.

Isaac, G. (1990) *Droit communautaire général.* Paris: Masson.

Massenet, J. (1990). *Le droit de l'Europe.* Paris: Institut Euro 92.

Petroni, A.M. (1997). 'A liberal view on a European constitution,' in A. Weale & Lehning, P. (Eds.), *Citizenship, Justice and Rights in the New Europe.* London: Routledge.

Petroni, A.M, & Caporale, R. (2000). *Il federalismo possibile. Un progetto liberale per l'Europa.* Soveria Mannelli: Rubbettino.

Rentdorf, J.C. (1998, April). *Basic Principles of Bioethics and Biolaw* [Online]. Available: http://www.bu.edu/wcp.

Roepke, W. (1958). *Jenseits von Angebot und Nachfrage.* Erlenbach-Zuerich: Eugen Rentsch Verlag.

The Parliament of the World's Religions. (1996). 'Declaration toward a global ethic,' in H. Kung (Ed.), *Yes to a Global Ethic.* New York: Continuum.

Weber, E. (1976). *Peasants into Frenchmen: The Modernisation of Rural France, 1870-1914.* Stanford, CA.: Stanford University Press.

Bioethics: Globalization, Communitization, or Localization?

Ruiping Fan

I. Introduction: How Should We Deal with Moral Dissensus?

Kurt Bayertz and Angelo Maria Petroni portray the recent experience of European approaches to bioethics and health care policy. As they show, the European Union, a supernational institution of Europe, is playing a more and more powerful role in providing "standard" bioethical norms to direct the biomedical research and health care policy of its member states. This constitutes a unique phenomenon in today's overwhelmingly state-centered and state-dominant world. No continent other than Europe has had such a formal supernational power in addressing moral issues. Thus, the European Union could set an example for other continents. Since bioethical issues cross borders and affect people in different states, continentalizing bioethics might facilitate the approach of states to such issues. If Europeans can unify their bioethics this way, why not people in other continents, such as the Americas and Asia?

Is it because Europeans hold sufficient bioethical consensus so that they can form a unified bioethics? Both Bayertz and Petroni inform us this is not the case. There is no generally agreed European identity or "European

H.T. Engelhardt, Jr. (ed), *Global Bioethics* (pp. 271–299).

bioethics" in Europe. Instead, the unity of Europe has always been a unity-in-diversity. As Petroni points out, "Europe is traditionally the land of diversity. Its very long history in civilization, the variety of races and religions, the existence of strong borders, made the Old Continent a mosaic of different institutions, languages, morals, and laws" (p. 1). Bayertz identifies numerous points in which European countries differ from one another: religions (some countries are predominantly Roman Catholic, others predominantly Protestant, and still others mixed), legal systems (British vs. Continental), mentality ("pragmatic" vs. "principled"), ethics (Utilitarian vs. Kantian vs. Cartesian), and history (pp. 13-15). Given these differences, it is no surprise that there have been dramatic disagreements and dissensus regarding bioethical issues and health care policies among European countries (e.g., Bayertz identifies two issues of particular dissensus: the moral status of the human embryo and euthanasia, see pp. 11-12). Accordingly, the "European Bioethics" affirmed by the European Union may only reflect the ethical view of some European people, but not all of them. It may represent the temporary hegemony of one group and its ideology over others.

Indeed, as Bayertz observes, there is hardly any consensus regarding any important ethical issue in contemporary societies, if by "consensus" one means 100 percent agreement by the people involved (p. 12). This is a difficulty not only for the European Union. There is no consensus at any international level. There is also no consensus at any national level, either. One should add that there is often no consensus even at a local level—simply imagine the situation of a small city, town, or village in any country today. Since people from different moral and cultural backgrounds move everywhere (let alone the diffusion of information by media) in today's world, there are often dissenters about important ethical and bioethical issues in any place. There is also dissensus regarding when there is moral authority for the political imposition of a particular morality. If unjustified bioethical coercion is wrong, it is wrong at any level, international, national, or local. How should we, then, deal with moral dissensus in order to solve bioethical issues and formulate health care policy?

Bayertz and Petroni provide a number of views and arguments around this important issue. This essay recognizes that, generally speaking, liberalism and libertarianism—the two most influential modern Western social and political philosophies—have been widely used to deal with moral dissensus in contemporary societies. Liberalism argues for global ethics and bioethics based on a doctrine of human rights and individual liberties. Libertarianism argues for the limited moral authority of the state based on its view of individual rights as side constraints and for allowing a non-geographically-located communitarian ethics and bioethics. More specifically, liberals attempt to resolve moral dissensus by promoting individual self-determination as a fundamental value, whereas libertarians by taking individual self-determination as a fall-back limitation. This essay argues that neither liberalism nor libertarianism can adequately address bioethical dissensus or the issue of proper bioethical deportment. It offers a critical response to the very ways in which Bayertz and Petroni characterize the issues, problems and disputes. By drawing on the Confucian insight into the nature of human civilization, the essay argues that the strategy of localization based on a thin principle of the Confucian virtue is the only appropriate strategy for handling moral and bioethical dissensus among different moral communities and areas.

II. Bioethical Globalism: The Liberal View

In spite of obvious cross-religion, cross-culture and cross-community moral diversity and dissensus, various liberal strategies for a global ethics and bioethics have been proposed. The most popular of them is the minimalist strategy: to establish a minimal ethic to bind all communities and individuals in the world (e.g., Kung, 1996, p. 2). Generally speaking, liberals see a set of basic human rights and individual liberties composing the minimal ethic for all human beings. For instance, a well-known American liberal bioethicist, Tom Beauchamp, has incessantly argued for "the common morality" for all the people. For him, this common morality is not merely one morality differing from other moralities embraced by communities or traditions of practice. Rather, it is the universal core of all moralities and is represented by universal human rights as its favored category of claims in recent years (see, e.g., Beauchamp, 2001, p. 613).

More specifically, the contemporary liberal strategy of handling moral diversity constructs an overarching theory of justice to guide people in dealing with moral disagreements and making public policy. For instance, John Rawls' political liberalism proposes a theory of justice[1] which, he believes, makes possible "a stable and just society of free and equal citizens profoundly divided by reasonable though incompatible religious, philosophical, and moral doctrines" (1993, p. xviii). This theory is meant to allow for "a diversity of doctrines and the plurality of conflicting, and indeed incommensurable, conceptions of the good affirmed by the members of existing democratic societies" (1985, p. 225). The political liberal ideal is that, with the principles of justice established, individual rights, liberties and other primary social goods will be fairly distributed to individuals so that each of them will be able to live up to whatever (reasonable) religion, morality, or a way of life as he/she sees fit to him/her in contemporary pluralist society.

According to the liberal understanding of persons, personhood lies in the capacity to autonomously and critically choose ends for oneself, including religions, moralities, and ways of life. The emphasis is not on the substance or content of any particular religions, moralities, or ways of life. Rather, these function as value contexts (e.g., areas of "spiritual" and moral concern) within which various particular concerns (e.g., with nature, sex and the ultimate) can be arranged in particular compositions. The various concerns like pieces of a mosaic are at the disposal of individuals to choose, determine and arrange. It is up to each of them, at any particular time, to "autonomously" decide which composition is more appropriate, satisfactory, or interesting to him/her.[2] Accordingly, liberalism focuses on the individual as the source and determinant of value. It emphasizes a particular notion of individual liberty, namely, the value of promoting individual sovereignty over oneself, self-fulfillment, and self-satisfaction. Consequently, the cardinal values underlining contemporary liberal views are individual independence, autonomous choice, and self-determination. Individuals are thus liberated from any structures claiming special communal authority, either religious or familial. In the liberal culture, one would be ridiculed as immature if one submits to one's parents for a marriage arrangement or to one's teachers for a career plan. In the health care context, liberals insist on the principle of informed consent not only for precluding medical interventions opposed by the patient. The principle is also voiced as a requirement for the patient to choose among alternative therapies, thereby directly making health care decisions by him/herself. Moreover, patients are strongly encouraged to select another individual in advance as one's exclusive surrogate decision maker to make decisions according to one's wishes and values when one becomes incompetent. In this way one is believed to extend one's sovereignty over oneself to the stage when one is incompetent. In short, liberalism takes individual self-determination as a fundamental value and gives it the first priority in moral decision-making.

However, not all people are sympathetic to this liberal understanding of individual liberty or autonomy as a cardinal value with priority. As Bayertz observes, although the value of autonomy is by no means alien to European ethical thinking, it has played no central role in the European tradition of medical ethics. While individual autonomy is currently emphasized by the European Bioethics Convention, it is also recognized that autonomy should be restricted by considerations of human dignity as well as concerns for solidarity (pp. 7-8). For the Chinese people in the Confucian tradition, individual autonomy is normally understood in the context of family autonomy. For instance, the authority to give consent to or refuse medical treatment belongs to the patient's whole family, not the patient individually. Chinese take the family as an ultimate autonomous unit from the rest of society. When ill, the patient is supposed to relax and rest. The family, having a responsibility, must shoulder the fiduciary obligation of care for the patient, including taking care of the burdens of communicating with the physician and making medical decisions and signing a consent form for the patient. Moreover, when a fatal diagnosis or prognosis is involved, the patient is often prevented from the truth. It is understood as unsympathetic and uncaring if such harsh information is directly disclosed to the patient. If we attempt to understand this Confucian familist pattern of medical decision making in terms of a liberal contractarian model (namely, the patients have voluntarily chosen or agreed to such a familist pattern), we would distort the Confucian way of life. Confucianism understands humans as beings living in natural (appropriate) human relations, such as husband-wife, parent-child, and brother-sister. Such relations are existential, rather than contractarian, forming the living condition of humans. They generate certain natural moral obligations binding everyone, whether or not they agree. For instance, it is the natural obligation of the family to take care of its members in illness. And in illness what one should want is the interdependence of the family rather than one's own independence. Moreover, it is too individualistic to be appropriate for the Chinese to pick out one single family member (much less an extra-familial person) as one's exclusive surrogate decision maker, because this breaks the unity of the family as a whole. When the whole family makes medical decisions for the patient even when the patient is competent, it is only appropriate that the whole family continues to shoulder the obligation when the patient becomes incompetent. It would be woefully embarrassing for the Chinese to designate one family member, ignoring the others, to be one's single decision maker. To do this is to destroy the unity and harmony of the entire family.[3]

In short, Confucian Chinese cannot accept the liberal cardinal value of liberty or autonomy as self-determination. Instead, their cardinal value is family-determination. This constitutes the first fundamental disagreement between liberals and Confucians in ethics and bioethics.

Moreover, the liberal understanding of individual liberty and its priority easily leads to unacceptable egalitarian requirements of equality of opportunity. As autonomous choosers of their ends and life plans, individuals need opportunity to realize them. If everyone, as liberals see it, is *equally* an autonomous chooser of their ends, everyone should have equal opportunity to realize their ends. That is the liberal logic of justice. For instance, Rawls argues that the state should not only ensure formal equality of opportunity, it should also affirmatively act to maintain fair equality of opportunity. The formal equality of opportunity that simply requires eliminating *formal or legal barriers* (such as race, class, gender, etc.) to persons seeking jobs and positions will not suffice. In addition, fair equality of opportunity requires taking positive steps (e.g., through the public educational system) to enhance the opportunity of those disadvantaged by social factors, such as family backgrounds. Such social factors, for Rawls, are arbitrary from a moral point of view, because none of us deserves the advantages conferred by accidents of birth. Therefore, Rawlsian liberal justice requires the state to step in to maintain equality of opportunity unless inequality is beneficial to the least advantaged individuals (Rawls, 1971, pp. 72-74). This means that the state should offer various types of welfare programs, ranging from state-subsidized education and redistributed taxation to affirmative action, in order to maintain fair equality of opportunity. In health care, since disease and disability affect individuals' opportunity, justice requires establishing a comprehensive health care system to satisfy everyone's basic health care needs. Only those medical services that do not essentially affect individual opportunity may be left to the private health care sector (Daniels, 1985).

When European bioethicists emphasize equal access to health care in Europe, they are in congruence with this liberal view of equality. However, Confucians cannot support this view because it contradicts the Confucian view of the autonomy of the family. Confucianism requires family-based opportunities autonomously provided by families, rather than the so-called "fair" equality of opportunity imposed by the state. The autonomy of the family is the requirement that decisions and activities within a given family governing the development of its children should not be coercively interfered with by the state (Fishkin, 1983, pp. 35-36). Evidently, families can give their children significant advantages by promoting their opportunities in society: a secure home environment, congenial home culture, successful role models, private schools, private lessons, an advantaged peer group, trips abroad, and nutritious meals and advanced health care. All of these can substantially enhance the children's opportunities for seeking offices and positions in society. Given that such advantageous family opportunities may not benefit the least favored children in society, and given that Rawls' account of justice requires equality of opportunity unless unequal opportunities are to the benefit of the least fortunate people, Rawlsian liberal justice would require the state intervene in this regard. Since mere leveling-up strategies of assisting poor families cannot fully meet the requirement of fair equality of opportunity when the institution of the family exists, Rawls' liberalism will have to support leveling-down strategies in restricting advantageous family opportunities so as to equalize life prospects of all children with similar natural endowments.[4] This leads to the conflict with the Confucian autonomy of the family.

Unequal opportunities provided by parents to their children have always been taken for granted by the Confucian understanding of an appropriate society. Parents, guided by the Confucian view of the parental virtues, are always encouraged to enhance their children's opportunities by, e.g., providing them the best educational programs. It is true that the fundamental Confucian moral principle of *ren* requires loving all humans. But it also requires loving humans with differentiation, distinction, and relativity of importance. One should always "love with distinction" and "care by gradation" in terms of different human relations. In particular, one must start one's love from the family and give preferential treatment to one's family members. The parents are obliged to work hard for achieving better life chances for their children, and the children are obliged to exercise filial piety in taking care of their elderly parents. Since the Rawlsian requirement of fair equality of opportunity has to use state-controlled measures to restrict parents from pursuing better educational opportunities or health care services for their children, it contradicts the fundamental Confucian moral conscience of *ren* with preferential love given to one's own family. For Confucians, even if the existence of better educational programs or better basic tiers of health care for families' voluntary purchases does lead to unequal opportunity for young people, that is just right and legitimate. A state-imposed egalitarian health care system prohibiting unequal private basic health care is in contradiction with the fundamental Confucian moral sentiment in favor of the family.

Evidently, even if liberalism only requires the government to achieve as much equal *basic* health care as possible without absolutely prohibiting private basic health care, liberalism may still require restricting the family autonomy in order to rule out the threat by market-based private health care services undercutting the basic egalitarian health care system by luring away resources and the best physicians. Without some such restrictions, affluent families would invest significantly in the private sector, good physicians would move to the private sector, the quality of the public sector would not be maintained. That is, the liberal ideal of equality cannot be reconciled with the Confucian value of the family autonomy. The more equality is pursued, the less family autonomy can be respected. Finally, an egalitarian health care system is inevitably expensive and requires heavy taxation. Confucianism has always required that a government of *ren* make the taxes and levies light and leave resources to families for pursuing welfare for their family members (see, e.g., *Mencius*, 1970, 1A: 5). The position of Confucianism is that the provision of welfare is primarily the responsibility of the family. It is morally misleading for the state to coercively imposed an egalitarian welfare system.

Liberalism holds that the principles of justice specifying individual liberties and rights do not depend for their justification on any particular conception of the good life. In other words, liberalism appeals to the method of separating the right from the good to defend its account of justice. This method fails. It is illusory that the contemporary liberal theories of justice are justified independently of any particular conception of the good life.[5] Any account requires a particular ranking of primary goods. Further, even if we assume that this method works, a liberal theory of justice and a set of liberties and rights will fail to provide any coherent moral approach to a series of bioethical issues. This is the case because, first, these liberal rights and liberties are always normal-adults-oriented. They cannot give sufficiently specified guiding regarding the status of non-adult humans. For instance, it is unclear what grounds have been offered by the liberal view of rights for coping with the issue of research using early human embryos. Secondly, the meanings of individual rights and liberties in the liberal account are often vague and ambiguous in specific bioethical contexts. For instance, what does "human dignity" mean for the issue of organ sale? Is it that the individual is promoting his dignity when he is able to sell part of his body as he wills? Or is it that his dignity is maintained when he is prohibited by the state from commercializing his body and its parts?

Particular answers to these questions require a particular ranking of goods and a particular view of human flourishing. As a result, if contemporary liberals have offered a full-fledged moral approach to bioethical issues, it cannot be the case that the approach has been established independently of any particular moral tradition. A full-fledged moral approach is inevitably a conceptual reconstruction of a moral perspective nested in a particular moral tradition. A moral perspective includes rich moral resources and content, such as moral narratives, exemplars, examples, commitments, and rules. When liberals argue that they are defending their views independently of any particular moral perspective, what is actually happening is that they are reconstructing various moral perspectives according to their general moral theory or some abstract moral principles that they hold. This is why their views often sound incomplete or even fragmented—they are not deeply committed to any coherent moral tradition, but at the same time they touch on the views of several different moral traditions. Hence, liberalism can only obtain "half-way" or fragmented moral content from different moral perspectives.

For instance, when the European Parliament demanded the British Government to withdraw all plans for allowing human embryos to be cloned for research by arguing that such research poses a profound ethical dilemma and crosses a boundary in research norms (Bayertz, 2006), it is hard for a Chinese reader to make sense of the argument except by placing it in the context of the traditional Christian view of life. But the Parliament fails to draw a full implication from the traditional view because it aspires to rely on liberal "universal" reason to reach its conclusions. Since it does not draw on any complete moral tradition, Christian or other, the result is only fragmented, even incoherent, moral views being claimed. On the one hand, the European Parliament prohibits the creation of human embryos for research. On the other hand, however, it allows research on already created embryos *in vitro* and believes that such research will ensure adequate protection of the embryo. How can anyone, as Petroni comments, give any serious meaning to such a "law" that allows experiments on embryos and at the same time claims that embryos are "protected" (Petroni, 2006, pp. 258-259).

Evidently, liberal bioethical views are ultimately from somewhere. They are inheritors of particular Western religions, moral traditions, and ways of life, although not full-fledged inheritors of any of them. These are not self-evident. They are self-evident only to those who already share those views. In this sense, liberalism is philosophically disingenuous in claiming that its views can be justified independently of any particular religion, morality, or the conception of the good. To the contrary, since its views, though fragmented, are still reconstructions of particular moral or religious perspectives implicit in particular moral traditions, the liberal claims advanced are not nested in a universal moral perspective or "reason." Claiming that the commitments of liberalism are a universal foundation able to ground a global bioethics is morally misleading and politically arrogant. Since many people do not accept these particular liberal views and commitments, imposing them everywhere in the name of global bioethics can be the source of social unease and even disturbance.

To summarize, contemporary liberalism cannot deal with moral dissensus. First, its particular idea of liberty or self-determination as a cardinal value is not accepted by many non-liberal people in the world. Second, its requirement of equality of fair opportunity is in contradiction with the Confucian autonomy of the family. Finally, its particular view of liberty, as well as its lexical priority, is the result of a particular moral tradition without a justified claim to universality. Its protest to the contrary notwithstanding, liberalism draws on particular moral and religious traditions for its resources which are not universal. Accordingly, as a series of European examples offered by Bayertz and Petroni in their papers shows, attempts to establish a liberal ethics and bioethics as a state bioethics, a continental bioethics, or a global bioethics, fail to be rooted in a foundation that all must affirm. The foundation in the end turns out to be particular and contingent. The aspiration of liberalism to a global bioethics fails.

III. Bioethical Communitization: The Libertarian View

As liberals, libertarians also take individual rights and liberties seriously. Their theories are also theories of entitlement. However, their view of rights and liberties sharply differs from the liberal view. Essentially, libertarian rights and liberties are not values to be promoted. Rather, they are constraints by individuals against others – when individuals have rights, there are things no person or group may do to them (Nozick, 1974, p. ix). This is why libertarians style fundamental rights and liberties as "side constraints." For them, no one should be coerced to do anything that is taken to be valuable by others (for instance, no one should be forced to make decision about his own health care, even if some people, like liberals, take self-determination to be a cardinal value). Similarly, no one should be coerced not to do anything that is taken to be wrong by others (for instance, no one should be forced not to commit suicide, even if many people believe suicide is morally wrong). Compared to liberals, libertarians are proud of themselves being coherent in not taking liberty as a value, thus leaving enough room for individuals to choose what to do or not to do according to their own views, as long as their action does not involve coercing innocent, non-consenting others. Consequently, under the libertarian view the function of the state must be minimal—only maintaining the order of the free market in which consenting individuals contract and collaborate with each other for their preferred ventures.

Why do individuals have such rights as side constraints? Tristram Engelhardt has offered an impressive argument for this libertarian view in consideration of the possible solutions to moral controversies[6]:

> On the one hand, many of the controversies depend on different foundational metaphysical commitments, as with respect to the significance of abortion and the production of embryos for research, and infanticide (i.e., whether entities involved should be considered as persons on a par with competent adult humans). As with most metaphysical controversies, resolution is possible only through the granting of particular initial premises and rules of evidence. On the other hand, even when foundational metaphysical issues do not appear to be at stake, the debates turn on different rankings of the good. Again, resolution does not appear to be feasible without begging the question, arguing in a circle, or engaging in infinite regress. One cannot appeal to consequences without knowing how to rank the impact of different approaches with regard to different interests (e.g., with respect to liberty, equality, prosperity, and security interests). Nor can one uncontroversially appeal to preference satisfaction unless one already grants how one will correct preferences and compare rational versus impassioned preferences, as well as calculate the discount rate for preferences over time. Appeals to disinterested observers, hypothetical choosers, or hypothetical contractors will not avail either. If such decision-makers are truly disinterested, they will choose nothing. To choose in a particular way, they must be fitted out with a particular moral sense or thin theory of the good. Intuitions can be met with contrary intuitions. Any particular balancing of claims can be countered with a different approach to achieving a balance. In order to appeal for guidance to any account of moral rationality, one must already have secured content for that moral rationality (2006, pp. 35-36; also see his 1996, Ch.2).

This is to argue, facing various incompatible and incommensurable moral traditions, views and theories in contemporary pluralist society, we are not able through sound philosophical argument to establish a standard morality to bind all communities and individuals. As a result:

> the only source of general secular authority for moral content and moral direction is agreement. To rephrase the point, because there are no decisive secular arguments to establish that one concrete view of the moral life is better than its rivals, and since all have not converted to a single moral viewpoint, secular moral authority is the authority of consent. Authority is not that of coercive power, or of God's will, or of reason, but simply the authority of the agreement of those who decide to collaborate (Engelhardt, 1996, p. 68).

Engelhardt's basic idea is that since no one is able to prove or justify a particular moral view to be the right view without begging the question, by default, every individual obtains a right not to be treated by unconsented-to force from others. Thus, through a type of moral epistemological (not metaphysical) skepticism, Engelhardt offers a by-default philosophical argument for the libertarian understanding of rights as side constraints. Again, Engelhardtian libertarian rights are not rights as values. They are only by-default entitlements. With this view, it is incorrect to say that every individual has a right to self-determination because self-determination is taken to be a value. Rather, every individual has a right to give up self-determination if they so prefer. What is crucial for libertarians is that no one be treated by unconsented-to force. As to what one should consent to, the libertarian argument cannot offer a concrete answer. For Engelhardt, you have to join a particular moral community to find an answer.

Not many libertarians emphasize the role of specific moral communities for moral substance. But Engelhardt, for one, strongly argues that one cannot find content-full meaningful morality except through joining a moral community (such as a religious group) that carries a specific moral tradition. For him, a true libertarian is at the same time a true communitarian. If you are lucky enough, you could even join the right community and find the right morality. Accordingly, instead of seeking the liberal ideal of ethical and bioethical globalization, the Engelhardtian libertarian ideal is to pursue ethical and bioethical communitization:

> With the advent of a general, worldwide, peacekeeping authority limited by the morality of mutual respect (which is to say, with the coming of the secular millennium), one could be assured of the possibility of individuals freely joining in various associations, which need not be limited to any particular geographical area. One might think here of the ways in which individuals of different faiths may proceed to gain a divorce in Israel, on the basis of the rules of their particular religious groups. In such associations, individuals could pursue their views of the good life. Each association could in its own way provide a level and kind of health care in accord with its guiding view of the good life. Such associations would tax their members. Some associations (e.g., religious) would establish a thick set of regulations and canons. The result would likely be a world in which individuals would belong in different ways to different associations. As a consequence, individuals could have complex entitlements to health care and other support (Engelhardt, 1996, p. 175).

This ideal is true communitarianism in the sense that each moral community is shaped by its own fundamental moral views of rights, goods, and virtues which are shared by its members. Such communities can easily move beyond the borders of the state and become cross-state organizations. True Christians, for example, should not be distinguished by being Americans or Chinese. They would be the members of the same community, a community that is not in its essence geographically fixed. No doubt, such non-geographical communities can play a significant function in weakening the unjustified power of the state, which power remains one of the main sources of people's suffering and disaster in today's world. Finally, when such communities recognize that they cannot, through rational argument, prove their moral view to be more true than their rivals', they should tolerate (in the sense of forgoing force against) the practice of other morals and do not attempt coercively to use control over other people. Hence, members of different moral communities may peaceably collaborate with each other domestically and internationally.

Engelhardt's account of moral epistemological skepticism is clear-cut and persuasive. Facing today's moral diversity and disagreement, an honest scholar has to concede that he has no general rational argument for establishing a particular moral view as canonical without ultimately begging the question, arguing in a circle, or engaging in infinite regress. Now the question is where we can go from this moral epistemological skepticism? Is Engelhardt's by-default argument for the libertarian view of rights as side constraints a sound argument? I will turn to this issue in the next section. Here I have a major practical concern: is Engelhardt able to combine his libertarian requirement of rights as side constraints and his ideal of ethical and bioethical communitization into a feasible comprehensive moral system for practice? I think he is not. This is not feasible because in practice his communitarian ideal cannot be pursued given his requirement of individual rights as side constraints. The reason is as follows.

In the first place, many people today do not live a communitarian moral life. That is, they do not belong to any particular, coherent moral community. As Engelhard himself recognizes:

> What if the chaos of the moral life is such that many people possess no coherent understanding of the right, the good, and the virtuous? Thoroughly post-modern persons that not only have no moral narrative to share with others but also no coherent moral account of their own lives are exactly such individuals. Life happens to them, including their passions. They are persons without a moral plot for their own biographies. They have desires, impulses, urges, needs, wants, and concerns, but no moral projects that shape and unite their lives as a whole (2000, p. 137).

Can emphasizing libertarian rights as side constraints help those people stop being post-modern cosmopolitans and join particular moral communities? I think the answer is "no"—at least for most individuals. This is because enjoying the moral commitments of a moral community requires active moral cultivation that is not available within a general libertarian ethos regulated by the libertarian rights as side constraints. To the contrary, emphasizing libertarian rights will most probably induce individuals to seek liberation from the constraints of traditional moral communities and become liberal cosmopolitans. For most individuals, libertarian rights as side constraints can be used more easily for gratifying their immanent physiological impulses or whims than fulfilling their moral hungers. Again, as Engelhardt himself observes:

> [b]ecause sex sells and self-indulgence is appealing, a market ethos can thus favor a liberal cosmopolitan critique of asceticism, Christian tradition, and

> heterosexist ideals. The general affirmation of consensual sexual gratification becomes the norm. By appealing to immediate and simple gratification, or refined self-satisfaction (admittedly a smaller market niche), the focus becomes robustly thisworldly and openly post-metaphysical (2000, p. 142).

It is simply natural for most individuals to find self-indulgence easy and appealing, moral commitments hard and demanding. This is why traditional religions and moralities, such as Confucianism, have always emphasized the significance of overcoming self-indulgence through gradual moral discipline and cultivation so as to form a good moral habit. This is to say, a commitment-required communitarian moral life requires training, nurturing, and disciplining, which is thereby hard to live, while a life of self-indulgence is easy going. Given that the very tone of individual rights as side constraints makes self-indulgence sound proper and confident ("I have a right to do it, even if it is wrong"), it is no surprise that many individuals holding such rights will naturally go for it. Moreover, from such "rights" many individuals can easily make an additional step to reach the position of supporting the liberal ideal of welfare state: the state ought to ensure basic welfare to every individual so that they are ensured to live up to whatever kind of life they prefer. Accordingly, pace Engelhardt, stressing libertarian rights induces many individuals to become liberal cosmopolitans rather than moral communitarians. It would, in fact, accelerate the emerging dominance of liberal cosmopolitan culture in every region of the world. As a result, ever fewer will still take particular moral communities seriously.

To summarize, the libertarian strategy of dealing with ethical and bioethical dissensus is to establish individual rights as side constraints by which individuals can join non-geographical moral communities so as to pursue their substantive ethical and bioethical goals. However, many individuals today no longer belong to any coherent moral community, and emphasizing libertarian rights as side constraints does not help them in joining or maintaining particular moral communities. Rather, it helps with the process of ensuring a worldwide dominance for liberal cosmopolitanism. In this sense, the entire Engelhardtian libertarian system (consisting of both the requirement of individual rights as side constraints and the ideal of bioethical communitization) has become self-defeating in practice, even if it is not self-contradicting in theory.

IV. Bioethical Localization: The Confucian Insight

If liberal globalization is unjustified and libertarian communitization is infeasible, do we have any other suitable strategy to deal with ethical and bioethical dissensus? For this difficult issue, I would like to invite us to draw on the insight of a great Chinese master, Confucius (551-479, B.C.), for useful instruction. Confucius lived in a time of immense social conflict and turmoil in Chinese history. By his time, China already had thousands of years of civilization, including the great system of rites (*li*) established in the Former Zhou Dynasty (about 1066-771 B.C.). *Li* originally identified holy rituals or sacrificial ceremonies performed by the family in memory of the ancestors (Ho, 1992). Given the sacredness, seriousness, and sublimity of such rituals or ceremonies, the Chinese found them a significant metaphor for understanding human life as distinguishable from animal existence. Accordingly, the Zhou Chinese used a system of *li* metaphorically to mean more broadly human behavior patterns that had been established and accepted as appropriate, including what we call rites, rituals, ceremonies, manners, etiquettes, customs, and social and political systems. This system organized human lives, regulated human relations, directed individual actions, and shaped social institutions.[7] However, the glory of *li* was declining at Confucius' time. Some rich and ambitious feudal lords wanted to grasp more political power. The states began to wage wars against each other, subjects murdered their princes, and children killed their parents. They no longer followed the rites that they used to venerate seriously. As the rites were undergoing disintegration, the Chinese society was experiencing moral corruption, degeneration, and chaos. A dozen of the greatest minds China had ever produced began to reflect on the nature of human civilization and seek solutions to its contemporary difficulties. Confucius was among them and proved to be the most profound, although he did not offer an elaborate philosophical argument. To make the long story short, I take that Confucius' reflections can be summarized into the following points.

First, distinctively human civilization is embodied in human rites (*li*). Confucius recognizes that civilized humans are ceremonial beings – they are acting on reasons and following rules in cooperation, rather than simply reacting by instinct. The image of the original memorial ceremony of the family's ancestors becomes a metaphor of authentic human existence because it brings out forcefully not only the harmony and beauty of human intercourse, but it also discloses the historical root and moral perfection of human development manifested in achieving one's ends by dealing with others in the ceremonial way. Hence, the very feature of acting on reasons and following rules in rite-performance distinguishes human behavior from mere animal reaction. For Confucius, no human civilization can exist in any geographical region without such symbol-rich and somewhat mystic rites, rituals, or ceremonies. They constitute the essential character of human civilization. Metaphysically, rites relate humans to the transcendent—which is incomparably higher than humans—so as to give human life an eternal meaning. Humans have no way of getting access to the transcendent (whether it is God, Dao, or their deceased ancestors and parents) except through performing such rites. Aesthetically, rite-performance offers opportunities for humans to enjoy the beauty and sublimity of their lives. Morally, rule-following rite-performance assigns sanctity to human actions that other animals can never obtain in their instinct-driven behaviors. Finally, virtue is cultivated in rite-performance, and virtue in turn strengthens human civilization (see the subsequent argument in this section). Accordingly, for Confucius, human civilization is impossible without rite-performance.[8]

Moreover, more specifically, distinctively human civilization is rooted in the following of the constitutive rules of human rites (*li*). Rites are possible because they are rule-governed activities, with constitutive rules to define them. These rules are rules of propriety about how to perform rites. You cannot perform a rite without following rules. For instance, the rules of a sacrificial ceremony tell you about when you begin to join, where you stand, how you move, and what you say... This does not mean that every act in a rite is predetermined by rules—an act in ritual performance is not determined by ritual rules any more than each move in transportation is settled by traffic laws. Instead, a rule stands like a sign-post: it does restrict one's behavior—at a no-left-turn sign one should not turn left, but it also opens the possibilities of one's action—one can go straight or turn right without being caught in chaos. With this insight, Confucius was not far from the later Wittgenstein in recognizing that humans are rule-following animals. However, it is very important to understand that, for Confucius, such rules of propriety are constitutive of concrete rites or rituals and thereby are highly context-sensitive. They are rite-bearing rules for real practice, not philosophical abstracts for general theorizing. As a result, particular rules characterize particular rites. For instance, the rules of truthfulness in human rites are never so abstract as philosophically articulated claims of an absolute obligation for "truth-telling." In one culture, the rules of truthfulness cover the requirement of not telling the truth to elderly great-aunts who invite their young relatives to admire their new hats. In another culture, they cover the requirement of not telling the truth to the terminally ill parents who still hold hope for survival. The rules of truthfulness vary from culture to culture because people are performing different rites with specific constitutive rules.

Third, rules exist only when people (especially children) are appropriately educated to follow them. Human civilization cannot be maintained and developed if the established rites and rules are not duly respected. Again, rites are possible because there are constitutive rules to define them. Rules are possible because a certain convention or consensus on their meanings dominates. Consensus is possible only when people are educated and trained in ways in which their passions and impulses are regulated and reshaped by rules so that their capricious impulses to violate the rules cannot prevail in the disguise of a legitimate or moral reason. Accordingly, for Confucius, in order to maintain human civilization, individuals must be trained to control their impulses and follow rules of propriety. This is why he insistently emphasized the importance of subduing impulses and complying with established rules (*Analects* 12:1). Indeed, humans are not self-sufficient individuals who just happen to consent to a social contract. They become truly human as their raw impulses are recast by the rules of propriety, which make them authentic persons in the process of performing appropriate rituals. A man is born as "raw material" who must be civilized by education through rites, and thus becomes truly human. He must be taught and trained to follow the established rites and rules of propriety so as to direct his attention to the traditional social pattern of conduct and relationships (Fingarette, 1972, p. 34). This is why education is crucially significant for Confucians.

Finally, rites are morally meaningful because they are indispensable to the fulfillment of a fundamental human virtue. The Confucian theory of virtue is grounded in the Confucian understanding of human nature. Confucius reflected on human nature and recognized that humans are never atomistic, discrete, self-serving individuals coming to construct a society through contract. They are first and foremost characterized by the familial roles that they take on: husband, wife, father, mother, son, daughter... A human cannot come into being without the combination of a man and a woman. Children cannot grow up without being looked after by their parents. And elderly parents cannot survive without being taken care of by their adult children. For every human individual, this familist way of existence is not chosen, but given. Accordingly, Confucius held that humans are by nature familist animals, possessing the potential to form the family. More importantly, Confucius found in familial relations a most significant and noble aspect of human nature: a propensity to sympathize with each other.[9] This natural sympathy constitutes the human disposition of love. For Confucius, the natural love between parents and children and between siblings sets down the root of a fundamental human virtue, *ren* (*Analects* 1: 2). This Confucian virtue of *ren* as love is not only a feeling, but is more foundationally a potential, a power, and a character, from which the feeling of love is cultivated and regulated. However, a root is not a trunk yet, much less a fruit. The fundamental virtue of *ren* as the best aspect of human nature is only a potential, which must be cultivated, nurtured and developed in order to fully realize itself. For Confucius, the only way of cultivating and exercising this virtue is to follow rites. He clearly taught that the method of realizing *ren* is: "do not look at what is contrary to rites; do not listen to what is contrary to rites; do not speak what is contrary to rites; and do not make a movement which is contrary to rites" (*Analects* 7:1). In this way rites become morally significant because they are indispensable to the fulfillment of the fundamental human virtue (*Analects* 3: 3).

The Confucian concept of love implicit in the fundamental human virtue of *ren* illustrates a particular type of human love. This love is not *erosic.* Neither is it *agapic.*[10] If we must coin a name for it, it is *relational* love. The love between the parent and the child is the primordial case of this Confucian vision of love. On the one hand, a father loves his son not because his son has certain valuable properties so that he is attracted to love the son. Even if he knows that his son has much less merits compared to his neighbor's son, he still loves his son more than his neighbor's son. The same goes for the son's love for his father. Thus this type of love is not *erosic.*[11] On the other hand, the father's love of the son or the son's love of the father does have a reason: "he is *my* son" or "he is *my* father." Thus it differs from God's love of humans or Christian neighbor-love. God's love of humans goes beyond any human reason. God loves humans not because humans are the creatures of God. Rather, God loves humans because God is God—His nature is to love. Hence, *agapic* love is exclusively subject-centric, while Confucian relational love is relation-centric. As a result, Confucius set up a view of love—relational love—differing from either erosic or agapic love. A significant Western question is: should we promote erosic love (like the love a person has for God) or agapic love (like the love that God has for persons) in order to shape a good society? A typical Confucian question is: how should we promote relational love to shape a good society?

The Confucian answer is ritualization—one should perform different rites with different people in order appropriately to practice relational love. Relational love is by nature not egalitarian—it is not loving everyone without distinction. If a requirement of loving all humans equally means that one should exercise the same rituals with everyone, it would basically conflict with the Confucian view of relational love manifested in ritualized human relationships. Again, for Confucius, relational love is rooted in the familial-tie between parent and child and between siblings (*Analects* 1: 2). This love illustrates the best part of human nature, ren, disclosing that the moral nature of human relationships is love (*Analects* 12: 12).[12] Although this love is naturally granted inside of the family, it can be nurtured, promoted and extended to other people outside of the family. Confucians require relational love to be universally-applied to all the people, although it should begin from the family and be gradually-extended to other people and be differentiated in terms of human relationships. When some fault Confucianism for no clear way to extend familist love (e.g., taking care of the family) into love for all (e.g., aiding strangers) (Wong, 1989), they fail to recognize the Confucian strategy of ritualization. As is well-known, the five basic relations emphasized by Confucianism have formed general pattern of traditional Chinese society. "Between father and son, there should be affection (*qin*); between sovereign and minister, righteousness (*yi*); between husband and wife, attention to their separate functions (*bie*); between old and young, a proper order (*xu*); and between friends, fidelity (*xin*)" (*Mencius* 3A: 4).13 These different virtues, *qin, yi, bie, xu,* and *xin,* manifest specific relational love in different rituals. A filial son is one who exercises the rituals of greeting his parents every morning, speaking to them in a gentle tone, solving their problems actively... Faithful friends are those who exercise the rituals of visiting each other from time to time, drinking together joyfully, helping each other in need… In short, relational love is ritualized love. It is in the exercise of relevant rites that the love is manifested, nurtured, and promoted.

What do these Confucian reflections have to offer us for dealing with ethical and bioethical dissensus we face today? A couple of heuristic points are following from the above discussion. First, in order adequately to deal with moral dissensus, we need to understand the nature of moral dissensus in terms of human rituals. If the differences of civilizations, cultures, and moralities can better be understood in terms of different rituals being performed, then moral and bioethical dissensus must imply the possibility of different rituals. Consider people's painful disagreements about abortion, infanticide, female circumcision, polygamy, homosexuality, or euthanasia. The adherents of euthanasia, for instance, intend to perform a type of medical rituals sharply different from that performed by the opponents. Second, what is crucially important for the maintenance of human civilization is virtue, shared rituals, not individual rights. What is most destructive to human civilization is vice, de-rituralization, not disagreements. Indeed, moral dissensus is always there in human society. It occurs not only across moral communities carrying different moral traditions. It also occurs inside a moral community carrying the same moral tradition. It is not rare that individuals disagree about the moral standing of some ritual-constitutive rules, and there may not always be a sound rational argument to settle the status of a controversial rule or the meaning of a controversial rite even within a moral community (e.g., *Analects* 17: 21). Decision-making procedures are always necessary for the unity of a moral community. In fact, such procedures constitute part of the accepted rites of each sustaining moral community. They are rites about rites, "metarites" if you will. The success of such special rites in a community often relies on the distinctive role of some authoritative persons accepted by the community. The severe or persistent failure of such procedures leads to the fragmentation of a moral community as well as its tradition. Hence, it is not the case that the ritual-constitutive rules of a moral community can never be changed. But they must be changed by following the "metarites" accepted by the community. For the Confucian community, revision of rites may be made by Confucian sages according to the moral virtue of *ren*. Confucius clearly states that the majority view is neither a necessary nor a sufficient condition for making revision. In the *Analects*, we have examples of why Confucius wanted to revise certain rules (*Analects* 3: 4; 9: 3) as well as examples of why he did not want to revise certain rules (*Analects* 9: 3; 17: 21).

Moral disagreements between different moral communities carrying different moral traditions are more severe and difficult than disagreements inside a moral community. In terms of rites, severe cross-community moral conflicts consist in their disagreement about the moral status of certain rites—some rites are held to be evil and should be prohibited by one community, while to be acceptable and should be preserved by another community. Both liberals and libertarians have offered general moral principles to attempt to deal with cross-community moral and bioethical dissensus. In terms of the Confucian view, their strategies cannot succeed because they fail to recognize the ritual-bearing nature of moral dissensus. Either the liberal principle of individual liberty as self-determination or the libertarian principle of individual rights as side constraints is not "thin" enough to handle cross-community moral disagreements because they fail to take different types of rituals seriously. More specifically, they are too "thick" in the sense that they are essentially in favor of the Western *individualist* type of rites over non-individualist types of rites (such as Confucian familist rites). Accordingly, we would need a principle that must be more "thin" than either the liberal or libertarian principle—it should not be biased to any individualist or non-individualist type of rites. It must allow various types of rites to flourish. Of course, at the same time it should not be a relativist principle that grants all rites as equally morally good. It should contain a minimal sense of morality so as to set down a necessary condition for morally acceptable rites. Can Confucianism offer a promising principle in this regard?

A thin principle of *ren* is the hope. The thick Confucian principle of *ren* carries all the important features of Confucianism: its metaphysics, its familism, and its favorite ceremonies, and so on. In order to deal with cross-community moral disputes, a thin principle of *ren* should be abstracted from the thick content of the Confucian tradition and only need to hold a basic moral sense: **humans should treat each other with a sense of love.** I would style this thin principle of *ren* as "the thin principle of love." Although many moral traditions and theories hold a principle of love, this thin principle drawn from the Confucian moral resources contains several special points. (1) Love is an emotion generated from familial relations, cultivated in the family, and extended to other relations through common ritual performance. (2) Love is not only a passion; it is also a virtue—a character that tends to enable one to treat others with love in common ritual performance. (3) Love, as a virtue, is not individual entitlement-oriented, but obligation-oriented. While both liberal liberties and libertarian rights are individual entitlement-oriented, self-centered, and self-regarding, this virtue of love is obligation-oriented, cooperation-centered, and others-regarding. However, as a thin principle, it does not require love in the full-fledged Confucian sense. **It only requires a *minimum necessary* sense of sympathy with others' sufferings, care about others' feelings, or concern of others' expectations in any ritual performance—"a minimum necessary sense" in the meaning that, without it, it cannot make sense to say "treating people with love."** (4) Love is relation-sensitive. It allows differentiation, gradation, and priority. It does not require, although it does not have to conflict with, any claim for universal love without distinctions.[14] It does require universal love—one should treat all humans with love in ritual performance. But universal love with distinctions is normal. (5) The thin principle of love, assuming that performing rituals is essential for human civilization, serves as a minimal condition for the possibility of common ritual performance. (6) The principle suggests that moral disagreements or controversies between moral communities be "solvable" through shared rituals.

Before I turn to point (6), it is necessary to emphasize the "thinness" of this principle again and explain why it is more sensitive and suitable to the moral diversity of contemporary society than other principles. It is thinner than the liberal principle of individual liberty as self-determination because it allows the rituals that do not take self-determination as a central value to be morally good rituals insofar as they exemplify a sense of love of the ritual participants. It is also more thin than the libertarian principle of individual rights as side constraints because it allows local people to decide whether they want an overarching, individual-oriented principle of autonomy or permission to guide their ritual practice as long as the people treat each other with love *according to the local view.* In short, since this principle is unbiased to either individualist or non-individualist type of ritual practice, it is more friendly to actual moral rituals and practices conducted by various peoples in the world and thereby takes moral diversity and epistemological skepticism more seriously than either the liberal or libertarian principle. To apply this principle, one does not have to understand human relations in terms of the Confucian five relations. As long as one accepts that humans should be related to one another in ways that contain at least a minimum sense of love/sympathy, it is sufficient to apply the principle.

This principle is not relativist, though. It sets down a fundamental moral norm for the moral (un)acceptability of actual rituals and practices, while taking moral diversity and epistemological skepticism seriously. It rejects the claim that any ritual is as morally good as others. A morally acceptable ritual must exemplify some relational love to its participants as its moral tenability. Accordingly, under this principle some rituals are not morally acceptable because they do not contain any sense of love in treating the participants. For instance, if a group of people regularly sacks another group of people for their resources, it is hard to see how the former group can meet the basic feature of love/sympathy required by this principle so as to grant its act as a morally acceptable ritual.

However, we should not be overambitious in using this principle to settle controversial rites or rules among different moral communities or districts. For most cross-community or cross-district ethical and bioethical dissensus and controversies, such as those regarding artificial-technology-aided reproduction, stem-cell research, human cloning, abortion, physician-assisted suicide, euthanasia, and homosexuality, this principle cannot be used to show which community or district is performing the morally ideal rituals by maximizing love, because different rituals performed by different communities or districts may exemplify love in quite different ways. Rather, this principle works by treating cross-community and cross-district moral diversity and epistemological skepticism most seriously. In short, the basic moral orientation of this principle is (a) respecting existing local rituals insofar as relational love is exemplified in the rituals *according to the local view,* and (b) appealing to morally acceptable (according to the thin principle) shared rituals among different communities or districts to resolve cross-community or cross-district moral controversies. It is important to recognize the significance of point (a). Here I use "local rituals" rather than "communitarian rituals" because rituals in a local area may be similarly performed by different moral communities even if they interpret the rituals differently. From the eyes of outsiders, some local rituals may seem short of any relational love, but they manifest some sense of love from the local view. Since love is a basic virtue based on a human emotion for common rite-performance, I would contend that the local view should be taken more seriously than an outside view. Accordingly, such rituals would be morally acceptable rituals according to the thin principle of love, even if outsiders find them morally offensive. Respecting local rituals means that one does not attempt to use force to change them, or to coerce local government to legislate a law to prohibit them. We have had many lessons to learn in treating other cultures in this regard in the modern time—the "export problem" in David Solomon's insightful terminology.

Of course, respecting local rituals does not mean that one accepts them as ideal moral rituals. Every moral community or tradition has its own reason to judge which rituals are the best rituals to perform. The thin principle of love is supposed to inform which rituals are morally acceptable, but it is not supposed to inform which rituals are morally ideal—the latter question has to be answered by each community based on its own thick moral views. Then what moral guidance can the thin principle give us in our attempts to improve and alter other people's rituals which, although morally acceptable according to the thin principle, are not best rituals according to the moral standards from our own moral community or tradition? Here point (b) comes to be crucial. Being ritualized animals, humans should attempt to solve their disputes by relying on existent shared rituals that are morally acceptable in accordance with the requirement of the thin principle of love. Just as within a moral community people should appeal to special rites (we called them "metarites" previously) to solve their moral disagreements, cross-community and cross-district people should also appeal to their mutually shared rituals to solve problems. No doubt, there are terribly morally problematic rituals often conducted by people cross-community or cross-district—warfare is a typical example—that violate the thin principle of love.

Fortunately, humans have also had at least four types of well-developed cross-community and cross-district shared rituals that have met the requirement of the thin principle: **dialogue, contract, philanthropy, and the market.** Although these rituals are performed by members of the same moral community or district, they are also shared by members of different moral communities or districts. If we term "first-level rituals" the typical rituals (like Confucian familist rituals or the Orthodox Christian Liturgy) that are shared by members of a moral community or district but are not shared by members of other communities or districts, these special rituals shared by different communities or districts can be termed "second-level rituals."

1. *Dialogue.* At least in small regions, such as villages or towns, people live together and contact each other closely, even if they belong to different moral communities carrying different moral traditions. Indeed, people talk to each other. Some even come from afar to talk to others. So dialogue is a real cross-community and cross-district second-level ritual performed by humans. Dialogue is a ritual in which people sit down to listen to each other and attempt to come to an agreement. It meets the minimal requirement of the thin principle of love—treating each other with love. Just as people base on both argument and procedure to solve their moral disagreements within a moral community or district, people are also doing cross-community and cross-district dialogue, although this latter task is more difficult—arguments are more diverse, procedures are more loose, authorities are more feeble, etc. Still, cross-community and cross-district dialogue is often appealed to and is so important. It may even involve an opportunity of mutual learning, given that people are treating each other with love. Although it is difficult to account for mutual learning theoretically when different, incommensurable religions, metaphysics, and moralities are involved, mutual learning is still possible because dialogue as a second-level ritual is not a self-enclosed, static game. It is by itself living and developing, and may thereby affect the first-level rituals of each community. This might be why Confucius teaches us: "do not entertain conjectures, do not insist on certainty, do not be inflexible, and do not be egotistical" (*Analects*: 9: 4).

Again, people inevitably share dialogue as a second-level rite, which can be very helpful for the resolution of cross-community or cross-district moral controversies. For instance, the Christians may inevitably contact the Buddhists if they live in the same Chinese village, so that they engage in a dialogue with each other. It is naturally up to the Christians and the Buddhists in the same village through a dialogue to make solutions to their moral disagreements. Evidently, each side has its own first-level rites—their favorite rites, acceptable rites, tolerable rites, and prohibited rites. Through a dialogue, their solution to a moral controversy could be some detailed arrangements in which, for all controversial first-level rites, each side can do their own way (including, for example, how they will eat meat when a

Buddhist dines with a Christian). To use the issue of abortion as an example, their agreement could be that abortion is okay for the Buddhists but prohibited for Christians (namely, each side does its only way). But this agreement is only one possibility. They could also reach an agreement that, for all the people in the village (regardless of Christians or Buddhists), only therapeutic abortion is allowed, or only therapeutic abortion and abortion for rape-caused pregnancy are allowed, or no abortion is allowed at all. In short, their solution should simply depend on the outcome of their dialogue. If libertarians want to make the solution of each side doing its own way as a general rule (or right) imposing on these people *a priori,* that is both practically and morally groundless. All rules are rite-sensitive. There is no such a thing as a rite-transcending rule or right. Accordingly, no solution should be imposed on people as a priori requirement transcending their shared second-level rites of dialogue.

2. *Contract.* All people understand the importance of contract. For instance, although Confucians do not like to make formal contracts with their family members or close relatives because they take such formality discounts the intimacy of their relationships, they understand the necessity of making contracts with other people for mutual benefits. One can even use contract to promote the values or ideal rites that one holds. In this way contract can serve as a second-level ritual in handling cross-community or cross-district moral controversies. For instance, if some group of people is really bothered by female circumcision in some African countries, they can offer a deal for those people: we will do such and such business with you if you stop doing circumcision on your female family members. This way not only conforms to the thin principle of love but would work better than a prohibitive governmental law. Similarly, if Confucians really want to promote their familist way of informed consent in medical practice, they can manage to set up a first-rate non-profit hospital in which every voluntarily coming patient is required to be accompanied by a family representative and medical decisions to be made by the family as a whole.

3. *Philanthropy.* Human sympathy can reach beyond one's relatives, neighbors, or friends. We have rich evidence to show that people help each other cross-community and cross-district. Philanthropy is a wonderful ritual for people to perform among different moral communities and districts. It can also be used to help resolve cross-community and cross-district moral dissensus. For instance, infanticide is often a tragic event caused by poverty. Families committing infanticide take such tragic effect as comparatively less harmful to the whole family as well as to the baby. If others can voluntarily donate to such poor families, infanticide as a moral problem can certainly be substantially relieved.

4. *The market.* People exchange things with each other in the market. The market constitutes a special ritual which can be shared easily by all the peo-

ple, no matter to which moral communities they belong and how serious moral disagreements they hold. The market is helpful to the resolution of cross-community and cross-district moral dissensus at least in the two senses. First, by doing business in the market people obtain more opportunities of contacting each other and using contracts to terminate their moral disagreements. Second, a law of the market is that, other things being equal, investments move to regions where marginal cost is low. As a result, if poor regions develop the market, they will receive more benefits than affluent regions. In this way, the market can help poor people so as to relieve the moral problems related to poverty.

In short, it is the basic orientation of the thin principle of love that people should attempt to resolve their moral dissensus via peacefully shared rituals. Cross-community and cross-district rituals (dialogue, contract, philanthropy, and the market) offer the best chances for people to handle their moral and bioethical controversies in following the thin principle of love.[15] In this regard, the Confucian strategy of handling cross-community and cross-district moral and bioethical controversies is neither liberal globalization nor libertarian communitization. It is localization. Liberal globalization wants through state power to impose a particular value of liberty upon all the people who perform different types of rituals from the liberals' so that the liberal aspiration is morally mistaken. From the strategy of localization, the role of the state should significantly be limited. For instance, in respecting people's love with each other substantiated in particular rituals, the state should not impose any egalitarian welfare policy on the people, because such state-created "super-rituals" are not real rituals—they are not shared by people belonging to different moral communities or different districts.

Neither is this strategy libertarian communitization, since it does not impose on all communities or areas an individualism-oriented ethical principle (such as individual autonomy or permission) as a universal procedural requirement as libertarians do. The thin principle of love requires respecting local rituals as long as a sense of love is embodied in the rituals according to the local view. It respects local people in relying on their shared rituals (such as the second-level rituals of dialogue, contract, philanthropy, and the market) to reach specific solutions to moral controversies among different moral communities in the same district. This strategy is fairly called localization because it is most friendly to actual rituals performed by people belonging to different moral communities or holding different moral views in any local areas.

V. Conclusion

The papers by Bayertz and Petroni provide us excellent European experiences and lessons in searching for legitimate approaches to bioethical issues and decisions in the context of moral diversity and dissensus in Europe. Non-Europeans can learn a great deal from these experiences and lessons in order to deal with their moral dissensus appropriately. However, Bayertz and Petroni have not fully recognized the moral defects of the liberal strategy and the serious destructions it is inflicting in the world in general and in Europe in particular, although Petroni enthusiastically argues against centralization, in favor of individual liberty and the free market. With individual fulfillment as a central concern and state-imposed welfare programs as a major endeavor, liberal global ethics is destroying the values of dialogue, contract, philanthropy, and the market as well as the integrity of the family and local culture in society. A super-state institution like the European Union based on the liberal global ethic would make worse come worse in this regard.

Neither liberals nor libertarians have recognized the rite-bearing nature of human civilization. They fail to understand that humans are ritualized beings. In this regard this essay can be taken as providing a Confucian reconstruction of Western moral rationality: the rationality that structures the Kantian community and the contractors in Rawls' original position is not individualistic universalizability or maximin, but is Confucian relational love substantiated in human rituals. That is, Kant and Rawls have the wrong philosophical anthropology, but Confucius has it just right. A thin principle of love is proposed for dealing with cross-community and cross-district ethical and bioethical dissensus by means of people's peacefully shared second-level rituals: dialogue, contract, philanthropy and the market, because these rituals have met the requirement of the thin principle of love. As a result, my proposal in the end is more feasible than is the libertarian cosmopolitan, and is more congenial to diversity and free choice than is the liberal cosmopolitan. It is not committed to an individualist moral principle. It is in tension with state welfare. It is supportive of dialogue, contract, private philanthropy and the free market as special rituals for people to deal with cross-community and cross-district moral controversies and disputes.

Some may want to argue that my thin principle of love contains an intent to impose a substantive Confucian moral view so that it is not sufficiently thin for different moral communities. They may want to stress a libertarian principle of autonomy or permission as a pure procedural norm so that it is more substance-free than the thin principle of love. I concede that my principle contains a substance—love. But I would like to contend that the distinction between substance and procedure can only be drawn in a comparative sense. The libertarian principle of individual autonomy or permission is more procedural (or less substantive) than the liberal principle of individual liberty because the latter sees liberty as a value while it does not. But it is more substantive (or less procedural) than the thin principle of love because it is biased towards the individualist type of moral rituals and practices, while the thin principle of love is not. A context-irrelevant, absolute dichotomy between substance and procedure may be one of a series of the

Enlightenment ideals that, as libertarians correctly argue, can never be well established by reason. It is simply self-deception to believe that a moral norm, no matter how purely "procedural" it is meant to be, could be totally separated from a view of the good and human flourishing. In fact, although the thin principle of love contains a substantive sense of love as an emotion-based virtue, it is maintained in a minimum necessary sense only. It is true that Confucianism offers a profound and full-fledged account of the significance of such relational love for human civilization while other moral traditions do not. But a basic sense of human relational love is universally cherished by every moral tradition—at least it is more universally cherished than the norm of individual autonomy or permission. Accordingly, a minimum necessary sense of love as a moral norm for human relations can hardly be rejected by any moral community with any good moral reason. The burden is on anyone who does not accept this claim to show us why that is not the case.

Notes

1. It is generally accepted that the rebirth of normative political philosophy in the Western world began with the publication of John Rawls' *A Theory of Justice* in 1971, and his theory constitutes the most powerful and representative view of contemporary liberalism. His theory dominates academic debates in the sense that alternative views are often presented as responses to it. Thus, it is appropriate to use his theory as the representative of contemporary liberal political philosophy.
2. For instance, as H. T. Engelhardt observes, "liberal cosmopolitanism finds the significance of sexuality in the free decision with others to achieve common projects of intimacy, satisfaction, fulfillment, and pleasure. This view is often announced in such cliché remarks as 'I hope he is happy in this new relationship' or 'at least she has found satisfaction in her fourth marriage' or 'do whatever makes you comfortable with consenting others.' The focus is not just on permission as a source of moral authority. The focus is first and foremost on autonomous self-fulfillment" (2000, pp. 141-142).
3. For a more detailed explanation of the Confucian view on this issue, see Fan, 1997; 2002. Also see Julia Tao's chapter in this volume.
4. For an insightful discussion of the systematic conflicts among fair equality of opportunity, the autonomy of the family, and the principle of merit within the liberal view, see Fishkin, 1983.
5. For a more detailed argument for this assertion, see Fan, 1999.
6. It is interesting to compare the beginning remarks of Robert Nozick and Tristram Engelhardt in their respective influential books. Nozick: "individuals have rights, and there are things no person or group may do to them (without violating their rights)" (1974, p. ix); Engelhardt: "Moral diversity is real. It is real in fact and in principle" (1996, p. 3). Nozick does not offer argument for why individuals have rights as side constraints. Engelhardt, using moral diversity as an inevitable sociological fact, offers a by-default argument for such rights on the basis of an epistemological skepticism for the moral truth.

7. Chinese *Li* can be classified into different systems. For instance, it can be divided into special ceremonies and ordinary behavior patterns. Special ceremonies include family ceremonies (such as wedding), village ceremonies (such as a drinking gathering), court ceremonies (such as emperor's ascending ceremony). Ordinary behavior patterns include a system of principles and rules about how individuals should treat each other in their ordinary lives (such as how a child should treat his parents). Besides, a system of the five sorts of *li* classified by Qin Huitian (1702-1764) has often been cited: auspicious (*ji*) *li*, propitious (*jia*) *li*, diplomatic (*bin*) *li*, military (*jun*) *li*, and ominous (*xiong*) *li*. See Qin (1994). Importantly, while "rituals" or "rites" only refer to special ceremonies in the English language, the Chinese *li* is a very complicated comprehensive system of behavior patterns, systems, and rules, with family *li* at its core. In short, *li* can be taken as the totality of Chinese ethical rites, norms and rules. In this essay li is translated into "rites" or "rituals"—they are used interchangeably.
8. For an interesting account of the Confucian thought in terms of rites, see Herbert Fingarette (1972). For a useful brief introduction to Confucianism, see Ni (2001).
9. Mencius (327-289 BCE), the Confucian master second only to Confucius, developed this Confucian view by arguing that every human has an original heart of sympathy (*ce-yin*); that is, the heart that cannot bear to see the suffering of others (Mencius 2A: 6). This Confucian sympathy-based view of love may be similar to David Hume's. But a difference is that for Hume, love is only a passion—a simple impression or feeling (1978, p. 329), while for Confucians *ren* as love is first a substance, a potential, or a virtue that must be cultivated and developed.
10. In the West there are two major views of love: one is from the *eros* tradition, comprising the *eros* of Plato's *Symposium,* sexual love, courtly love, and romantic love; the other is from the *agape* tradition, including God's love for humans and Christian neighbor-love. *Erosic* love is property-based and reason-dependent: x loves y because y has some attractive, admirable or valuable properties that give x a reason to love y. On the other hand, *agapic* love is not property-based or reason-dependent. The ground of *agape* love is not in the perceived merit of the object (the beloved), but is in the nature of the subject (the lover). Thus *agapic* love is subject-centric rather than object-centric: x finds the properties that y has attractive *because* x loves y. The structure of *agapic* love is that love is its own reason and is taken as a metaphysical primitive. For instance, the reason why God loves men is not because men have merits deserving love, but because it is His nature to love. Further, individual attractiveness plays no role in the Christian love of one's neighbor, which requires loving the sinner, the stranger, the sick, the ugly, and the enemy, as well as the righteous and one's kin. For a very useful explication of these two views of love, see Soble 1990, pp. 4-13.
11. Some may want to argue that "I love my son" because my son has the property of "being a son of mine" so that parent-child love can still be characterized as *erosic* love. However, this type of property—if we have to call it "property"—is not meritorious, but relational. In such "relational" type of cases I love someone because she holds a particular relationship with me (such as she is my sister, my classmate, or my friend); in the non-relational type of cases I love someone because she holds some meritorious property (such as beauty, wealth, or knowledge). Since these two types of cases carry different moral and practical signifi-

cance, it is necessary to distinguish them. Both *erosic* and *agapic* love covers a clear sense of impartiality—it is agent-neutral, while relational love is agent-relevant. Relational love is closely related to the conception of loyalty or patriotism rather than impartiality. For relevant issues in this regard, see Oldenquist (1982) and MacIntyre (2002).

12. Etymologically, the Chinese character *ren* is made up of the element "human" and the number "two," meaning that the relationship of two humans constitutes the essence of humans. By extension, it also means that a normal human life must be lived with other humans in appropriate relations.
13. Ideally, when people nurture and practice relational love, no one should be a stranger, for he is at least related as older or younger; similarly, no one should be an enemy. See Chan (1963, p. 71). For Confucians, as long as one is a human being, one is related to another human being in one of the five relations that should embody ritualized love. For a recent exploration of the Confucian affective relations, see Chaihark and Bell (2004).
14. The Confucian understanding is that as long as one performs different rituals with different people, he is already practicing love *with* distinctions, because his love is already differentiated among different people in those different rituals. This being the case, even if one claims universal love without distinctions, the claim may simply be empty or even hypocritical.
15. By performing these second-level rites together individuals from different moral communities may become moral acquaintances in a sense that Kevin Wildes identifies: mutual understanding (Acquaintanceship A1). See his 2001, p. 139.

References

Beauchamp, T.L. (2001). 'Internal and external standards for medical morality,' *Journal of Medicine and Philosophy*, 26 (6), 601-619.

Chaihark, H., & Bell, D. (Eds.) (2004). *The Politics of Affective Relations: East Asia and Beyond.* Lanham: Lexington Books.

Chan, W.-T. (1963). *A Source Book in Chinese Philosophy.* Princeton: Princeton University Press.

Confucian Analects, the Great Learning, & the Doctrine of the Mean. (1971). (Trans., J. Legge). New York: Dover Publications, Inc.

Engelhardt, H.T., Jr. (1996). *The Foundations of Bioethics* (2nd ed.). New York: Oxford University Press.

Engelhardt, H.T., Jr. (2000). *The Foundations of Christian Bioethics.* Lisse: Swets & Zeitlingers.

Daniels, N. (1985). *Just Health Care.* Cambridge: Cambridge University Press.

Fan, R. (1997). 'Self-determination vs. family-determination: two incommensurable principles of autonomy,' *Bioethics*, 11, (3/4), 309-322.

Fan, R. (1999). 'Just health care, the good life, and Confucianism,' in F. Ruiping (Ed.), *Confucian Bioethics* (pp. 257-284). Dordrecht: Kluwer Academic Publishers.

Fan, R. (2002). 'Reconsidering surrogate decision-making: Aristotelianism and Confucianism on ideal human relations,' *Philosophy East & West*, 52 (3), 346-372.

Fingarette, H. (1972). *Confucius—the Secular as Sacred.* New York: Harper & Row.

Fishkin, J. (1983). *Justice, Equal Opportunity, and the Family.* Philadelphia: Westminster Press.

Ho, B. (1992). Original Rites (Yuan li). *The 21st Century,* 11 (6), 102-110.
Hume, D. (1978). *A Treatise of Human Nature* (2nd ed.). L.A. Selby-Bigge (Ed.), revised by P.H. Nidditch. Oxford: Oxford University Press.
Kung, H. (1996). *Yes To a Global Ethic.* New York: Continuum Publishing Company.
MacIntyre, A. (2002). 'Is patriotism a virtue?' in I. Primoratz (Ed.), *Patriotism* (pp. 43-58). New York: Humanity Books.
Mencius. (1970). (Trans., J. Legge,) New York: Dover Publications, Inc.
Ni, P. (2001). *On Confucius.* Australia: Wadsworth.
Nozick, R. (1974). *Anarchy, State, and Utopia.* New York: Basic Books.
Oldenquist, A. (1982). 'Loyalties,' *The Journal of Philosophy,* 79 (4), 173-193.
Qin, H. (1994). *A General Investigation of the Five Sorts of Li* (Wu Li Tong Kao). Taipei: Sheng Huan Book Company.
Rawls, J. (1971). *A Theory of Justice.* Cambridge: Harvard University Press.
Rawls, J. (1985). 'Justice as fairness: political not metaphysical,' *Philosophy and Public Affairs,* 14(3), 223-257.
Rawls, J. (1993). *Political Liberalism.* New York: Columbia University Press.
Soble, A. (1990). *The Structure of Love.* New Haven:Yale University Press.
Wildes, K.S.J. (2001). *Moral Acquaintances: Methodology in Bioethics.* Notre Dame, IN: University of Notre Dame Press.
Wong, D. (1989). 'Universalism versus love with distinctions: an ancient debate revived,' *Journal of Chinese Philosophy,* 16(3/4), 251-272.

The Bioethics of Global Biomedicine: A Natural Law Reflection

Joseph Boyle

In this paper I will address several ethical questions raised by the increasingly globalized character of modern biomedicine, namely, how the scholarly conduct of bioethical reflection and discussion are to be informed by the globalization of biomedicine, and how international and other trans-national regulation of health care should responsibly take account of globalization. I will address these questions from the meta-ethical and normative perspective of natural law theory and practice.

I understand "natural law" to be the name of the set of basic principles of moral life. These principles are prescriptive and so constitute a "law." They are accessible to the intelligent reflection of any human being capable of thought and action and in that sense "natural" and "universal." Natural law theory is the elaboration of these principles into a normative account of moral thought and life. Roman Catholic canonists, theologians and philosophers have developed natural law theory within a tradition of moral inquiry since at least the 12th century. The result of this trans-generational inquiry is a developed form of traditional morality.

I propose to address issues of globalized bioethics from the perspective of natural law for several, connected reasons. First, since moral convictions informed by natural law theory and similar moral approaches are common, the assessment of the normative implications of globalized biomedicine in the light of natural law will be instructive both to those who share these

H.T. Engelhardt, Jr. (ed), *Global Bioethics* (pp. 300–334).

convictions and to those who seek to understand them. Second, the capacity of any moral theory or tradition to deal with new conditions that challenge moral thought is an essential part of the dialectic through which the success of a moral approach can be assessed. So, natural law theory, like other moral theories, can be evaluated by its capacity to deal with the realities of modern globalization as they affect the theory and practice of health care and biomedicine. Therefore, although this paper is not an attempt to articulate and defend natural law theory from the ground up, it is an attempt to show that globalized biomedicine does not render it obsolete or incredible.

The increasingly globalized reality of modern biomedicine does challenge moral thought, including the self-understanding of those engaged in bioethical reflection, whether from a natural law or any other perspective. Increasingly, those engaged in health care or in the research on which it depends possess detailed information about the conduct of health care elsewhere. The social and ethical questions have become unavoidable: to what extent should any society imitate, correct or ignore the health care approaches of other societies? To what extent are common global standards for health care and for sharing health care's benefits and burdens (for example, those of pharmaceutical research) appropriate? How are health care transactions that are essentially international to be regulated?

Questions such as these lead naturally to further questions about the character of bioethics itself: how modest or extravagant should the aspirations of bioethics be in the face of the globalized reality of biomedicine? How much significant consensus is possible? How much legislative and public policy regulation deserves support?

In the second section of this paper I will begin to address these questions about bioethics itself. I will do this by undertaking a clarification of the general ways which bioethics can be thought to have become "global bioethics".

In the third section of the paper, I will begin the natural law reflection on the forms of global bioethics distinguished in the second section. I will do this by exploring the structure and some of the content of natural law theory. This exploration will indicate how the ethical universalism of natural law theory can sustain the hope for global consensus about some general moral principles and about some negative precepts. This prospect of consensus can provide one important goal for global discussions of bioethics, and, to the extent it is realized, can provide a limited moral ground for some worldwide bioethical regulation. But this exploration will also show that the universalism of natural law theory does not eliminate moral diversity, since, in order to carry out its job of guiding decisions, moral thinking must take account of the circumstances surrounding decisions. Proper attention to circumstances indicates important limitations on the capacity of moral thought to guide all decisions according to a common detailed code.

In the fourth and last section of the paper, I will consider positive law, which involves the transformation of morality into authoritatively enacted regulations calling for obedient compliance by those governed by them. Positive law is an essential element in a community's efforts to deal with the circumstances of human action. For in enacting positive law, those having responsibility for the welfare of a community specify general moral requirements by reasonable choices, which take these circumstances into account. The result is something both more specific in its direction and less ideal and more embodied in social life than the dictates of reason just as such. Embedded in law and social life, positive law calls for acceptance, but that need not involve a robust moral consensus: obedience and fear of the consequences of non-acceptance are sufficient for the political purposes of fairly coordinating the actions of community members. The application of these jurisprudential generalities to the worldwide regulation of biomedicine reveals the central difficulty in such regulation: there appears to be no worldwide biomedical community of the kind having regulatory powers and so no worldwide authority capable of acting for the common good of such a community.

According to natural law, there is a kind of positive law that significantly escapes the requirements of political authority: this is the *jus gentium,* the law of the peoples, which refers to the common moral customs of humanity. These customary norms govern the interactions between communities lacking a common authority. Modern articulations of human rights share some features of the *jus gentium,* and may, therefore, provide some resolution of the apparent lack of authority to regulate globally. But the strictly moral authority of the *jus gentium* does not seem sufficient for establishing a global regime of human rights, in particular, of welfare rights, since, if these are to be real rights that impose enforceable duties on institutions and persons, they presuppose authority capable of setting priorities in the light of inherently local factors such as wealth, the organization of the economy, the practical control of the government and the level of cooperation of the citizenry, and other aspects of social organization, including the level of corruption.

I. Notions of Global Bioethics

The newly popular expression "global bioethics" can be used to refer to several undertakings, including inquiries, as well as to a cluster of moral aspirations, norms and regulations. I will distinguish three distinct, but related, realities that are sometimes understood as global bioethics.

Before making these distinctions, I will briefly note and set aside from my analysis a group of undertakings, which might be called "global ethics." These are social movements addressing a perceived crisis, or set of crises, in the actions and interactions of communities and individuals that have global impact. Underlying these movements is the belief that technology and modern communications have transformed actions and events that had been of only local importance into actions and events of global significance. This global impact is not necessarily for the better. Globalization, it is thought, is carried on in non-moral, economic terms, and has outstripped humanity's capacity to understand it morally or to deal with the grave dangers it poses (see Kung, 1996, pp. 1-5, 9-11). Since biomedicine is global in its reach, and since the bonds among humans that are threatened by global problems, such as global warming and infectious diseases are biological, "global bioethics" can become the name for part or all of this reformist movement (Macer, 1994, pp. 1-11).

Although the general concerns raised by these reformers deserve to be taken seriously, it is not clear what they have to do with bioethics, whether understood as a clinical profession, an academic discipline, a set of ideal norms, or a regulatory code governing health care and biomedicine. The forms of global bioethics I will address are those more clearly related to bioethics in these senses.

Moreover, the reformers' formulations of the challenges facing the world because of globalization are disputable. The evils that face us may or may not constitute a global crisis or threaten humanity's survival; even if they are as grave as some claim, they may be beyond any human power to fix, or beyond any human power morally to fix. Specific moral recommendations--about who has the responsibility to do which particular acts to resolve the crisis--are wanting. So, I will set aside for other discussions further consideration of this reformist agenda because it is so difficult briefly to deal with on the terms of moral philosophy.

A. The Global Conversation About Bioethics

The first kind of global bioethics I distinguish is the conversation about bioethical matters among bioethicists from around the world. The academics, clinicians and policy advisors who comprise the membership of the bioethical professions and communities plainly have reason to meet together and discuss their common business. There obviously is reason for bioethicists to talk about bioethical questions with colleagues from within their geographical region, from within their political community, and from within other relevant communities, (for example, religious communities) but there is also reason for bioethicists to meet with colleagues from outside their particular communities or locale. Sharing common or analogous problems, facing the challenge of diverse and opposing views, and determining the possibilities for and limits of consensus are among the reasonable goals of professionals whose work is rooted in disciplined conversation and humanistic learning.

Comparative bioethics, critical reflection on the adequacy of the moral principles favored in bioethical discussions in the USA and Western Europe, and reflection on the conditions for free and tolerant debate are usefully conducted in discussions among people from around the world and appear to dominate the global bioethical conversation (Campbell, 1999, pp. 183-190; Sakamoto, 1999, pp. 191-197; Takala, 2001, pp. 72-77). Such areas for discussion and study are much more closely connected to the main themes of moral philosophy and metaethics than to the largely unexplored questions concerning the trans-national global character of the modern practice of heath care and related questions of international political and social philosophy.

This focus of the global conversation among bioethicists suggests that there are ways in which this conversation is not, or not yet, fully global. It is plainly concerned with matters that are of universal human concern even when the problems' formulations are uniquely local in origin, for example, how a given society helps the dependent elderly. Such local matters may have important lessons for bioethicists from far away from the locale in which the issues arise.

But this conversation need have nothing further to do with bioethical questions that are more essentially global. Some problems require the disciplined reflection of bioethics, whether at the clinical or policy level. Such problems are essentially bioethical. The successful results of bioethical reflection are necessarily addressed to some individuals or groups: to health care providers, patients, policy makers and others. When the normative advice of bioethicists' reflection is addressed to those whose arena for action and responsibility is significantly trans-national, then the bioethical reflection is essentially global. Such reflection is called for when the actions about which there is moral question cannot be carried out by persons acting privately or by non-global authorities such as nation states acting alone.

This kind of bioethical reflection has not been prominent within the global conversation. But this does not imply that there are no moral questions calling out for bioethical thought to guide the decisions of agents who have the capacity and responsibility to act internationally. The global problems most often addressed by the actions of such agents do not seem to call for bioethical reflection. Challenges to public health caused by natural events, human actions or cross-border interactions which no single state can directly control, for example, the threat of SARS in 2003, are surely global. Because of the profound effect of such events on peoples' health, there is often need for international cooperation to deal with such challenges, but it is unclear what specific contribution bioethical reflection is required for their resolution.

B. Global Regulation of Health Care and Biomedicine

The regulation of health care decisions by trans-national groups such as the UN and the WHO, and through treaties among states and alliances plainly has become part of modern life. This regulation is bioethical since it deals with health care decisions, even if, as the recent example of the international response to SARS suggests, it does not require the specific reflection of bioethicists. This regulation is also importantly global since those operating under the regulations are global actors, and the regulators are trans-national bodies or states operating through treaty beyond their individual borders by jointly agreeing to protocols commonly established across several or many states.

An example of this kind of bioethical regulation, having potentially global reach, is the Council of Europe's 1997 *Convention on Human Rights and Biomedicine.* This appears to be a treaty the parties to which agree to common regulation of biomedical research and clinical practice. The parties to the Convention are European states, and the Convention emphasizes its European values and culture (Mori & Neri, 2001, pp. 326-327), so it does not pretend to be global. Moreover, some of the Convention's provisions suggest it to be an unlikely candidate for bioethical regulation beyond Europe: Article 13, which virtually prohibits interventions on germ line genes, is certainly controversial and probably ethically indefensible (Mori & Neri, 2001, pp. 327-331); Article 21, prohibiting financial gain from donating human body parts, is one way to address the possibility of the exploitation of vulnerable people in this context. But there are other ways to deal with this prospect that do not prohibit absolutely what sound moral thinking likely allows as sometimes permissible, and what a government might reasonably allow as less than ideal but, all things considered, politically acceptable.

More importantly, however, the Convention is not transnational in an essential way: it contains no specific regulations dealing with biomedical actions that involve crossing borders or lead to effects on several nations. In other words, there is no transnational regulatory content here; each party could on its own have enacted these regulations as law, and the effect of that would seem to be virtually identical to that of the enactment of the Convention as national law by each of them. Sanctions are to be imposed by the parties—that is, by the nations agreeing to the Convention. There may, of course, be some benefit in the agreement of interacting countries to commonly ban and otherwise regulate biomedical activities. Those benefits are not articulated in the Convention.

UNESCO's 1997 *Universal Declaration on the Human Genome and Human Rights* is more fully global in aspiration and reach and more specifically transnational in some of its regulations. Like the *Convention on Human Rights and Biomedicine,* most of its regulations are addressed to states, and prescribe actions within the borders and political competence of the individual states. But Section E, "Solidarity and international co-operation" contains three articles which impose specifically global responsibilities on states, that is, responsibilities towards other states and their citizens: to deal with genetically based disease affecting large numbers of the world's populations (Article 17); to disseminate the relevant knowledge, especially between industrialized and developing countries (Article 18); to take specific cooperative actions with developing countries, so that they may participate in and share the benefits of biological and genetic research (Article 19).

This Declaration, therefore, is global not only in that it is the work of a global agent, the UN, but also insofar as some of its provisions are significantly transnational and potentially global. But even this Declaration is not global in one important way: it does not prescribe or regulate biomedical or health care actions that are robustly transnational or global, that is, actions undertaken not by or under the regulation of a given state acting alone but by the UN or by many states operating cooperatively by treaty.

C. Applying Human Rights to Health Care and Biomedicine

A third form of global bioethics is suggested by the title and by some of the content of the UNESCO Declaration, namely, the application to health care and biomedicine of the human rights agenda of the UN's *Universal Declaration of Human Rights.* This human rights agenda, and the integration into it of bioethical concerns, is pursued differently on several fronts by agents of diverse kinds: for example, by religious leaders, including the Holy See, social reformers, by NGOs and through international conferences. At some points this agenda converges with the global ethics movements mentioned and set aside at the beginning of this section. I will deal with the human rights agenda in only one of its versions: namely, the efforts to implement antecedently accepted human rights by developing specifically bioethical regulations and norms on the part of international agencies having established authority, such as UNESCO, or by treaty.

There is a clear rationale for integrating bioethical issues into the framework of the *Universal Declaration of Human Rights.* The rights to life, liberty and the security of person (Article 3) the prohibition of slavery (Article 4) and the prohibition of cruel, inhuman or degrading treatment (Article 5) have some application or at least relevance to health care and biomedical practice. The Council of Europe's convention makes some of these applications, for example, in protecting those who cannot consent to research or treatment (Article 6, 7 and 14), and does so explicitly in the context of protecting human dignity (Preamble, Article 1). Similarly, the *Universal Declaration of Human Rights* affirms significant welfare rights, including a right to a standard of living adequate, among other things, for medical care (Article 25); the UNESCO declaration goes slightly further and with more specificity, directing states to respect and promote solidarity with those suffering genetic disease or its effects (Article 17). So, the human rights agenda sets a distinctive project of global bioethics.

Here again, however, one can wonder about the sense in which the application of the human rights agenda to bioethical discussions and regulation is or is not *global.* Are there violations of human rights in health care and biomedicine that are significantly global, that is, beyond the power and authority of national political authorities to prevent and remedy?

In this section, I have tried to distinguish, for the sake of discussion, three things that might be called "global bioethics." Two of them are concerned with global regulation of biomedicine and health care by appropriate authority. I distinguish these into two because some global regulation of biomedicine might be justified independently of considerations about antecedent human rights. In practice, of course, appeal to human rights will be essential in any global regulatory scheme. The worldwide scholarly conversation among bioethicists is clearly distinct from these regulatory actions of public authorities. Consequently, in separating out for discussion three forms of global bioethics, I do not mean to suggest three completely isolated social realities.

Questions about the correct balance between the global and the universal on the one hand and the local and the particular on the other are central to the global conversation about bioethics. They must also be central to the deliberations of international authorities seeking to devise fair and workable global regulations for biomedicine and health care. Related questions about moral consensus and disagreement and their significance in moral life and social cooperation must also be part of these conversations and deliberations.

My suggestion is that these questions will take different forms for those differently engaged in global bioethics: authorities having responsibility to regulate cross border biomedical actions should, of course, attend to what the bioethics professionals say, but to carry out this responsibility they hardly need to resolve all the epistemological, ideological and metaethical debates of the bioethics community. Thus, it may be that some robustly transnational regulation of biomedicine is called for in some areas, perhaps global public health measures to control infectious diseases or perhaps limitations on drug companies' influence on research. Although such measures might depend in some ways on established human rights, it would nevertheless remain *ultra vires* or just silly for international actors to tell a state how it should set up its health care system. Likewise, the global conversation might well continue for the benefit of many people, even if bioethical regulation were left entirely to states, and the human rights agenda were to be set aside as empty or imperialist.

II. The Limitations of Moral Reasoning

As I noted in the introduction, natural law theory underwrites the hope of consensus in moral matters, supports the existence of universal human rights that are pre-contractual and favors regulation to insure such rights and other aspects of the common good. These aspects of natural law thinking suggest to many—within and without the tradition of natural law thought—that this moral approach is unequivocally on the universalist side of the universalist/particularist debate in ethical theory, and unreserved in its support of global regulation of biomedicine. Both these suggestions, while pointing in the right direction, are in need of significant qualification.

In this section I will deal with the qualifications of these suggestions that are implied by the natural law account of ideal moral reasoning. In the next section, I will deal with the qualifications implicit in the natural law account of positive law and public authority.

Natural law theory includes an account of how moral reasoning functions and of the results, in sound moral judgments, of its proper working. Aquinas provided the classical account. Sound moral norms and correct judgments of conscience are the results of practical reason working fully and correctly. "Right reason" is the canonical general formula Aquinas used to refer to the principles that rectify our practical thought, and to that thought itself when it is made "right" by those principles.[1]

As this dual reference suggests, right reason serves to perfect and correct the practical reasoning people do as they formulate goals and seek to realize them through deliberation, choice and action. Consequently, the moral norms which, when recognized, can render a person's actual practical thinking an instance of right reason, are not deontological constraints imposed on a person's pursuit of the good, but implications of the full, rational demands of the full human good.

To explain: a person's reasoning in formulating goals and in deliberating is based on his or her judgment about what is good, what is desirable to pursue for personal or social benefit. Ultimately, these judgments identify intelligible goods, which are the grounds of the rational desirability of prospective goals. These goods are the good-making features of the concrete purposes, which constitute a person's goals. Some of these goods are basic or ultimate, in the sense that instantiating them is desirable without reference to instantiating further goods. Since there are several dimensions to the reality of human beings, there is a plurality of basic human goods, that is, there is not a single ultimate property or feature in virtue of which what humans have a reason to pursue is desirable; rather there is an irreducible plurality of such goods.

Aquinas provides a generic list of such goods: maintaining one self in being, mating and having and raising offspring, knowing the truth, knowing and relating to God and living in society (*Summa Theologiae* 1-2, q. 94, a. 2). Health would presumably be also on a more articulated list, since it is the part of the good functioning of humans as biological realities—an aspect of the full being of humans as animals.

Since these goods are the intelligible grounds underlying the goals that are the actual purposes individuals and communities pursue in choosing and acting, in many situations they are not by themselves sufficient for the moral evaluation of choices. They are sufficient for moral guidance only when the alternative to an action for the sake of a human good is motivated only by the promise of pleasure or satisfaction—that is, by the appeal of what one knows is not really good even though it has an appeal sufficient to motivate action. The other kind of choice calling for moral guidance arises when one must choose between courses of action all of which are motivated by the appeal of genuine goods.

The direction of such choices by right reason involves rational considerations not provided by the goods supporting the conflicting actions, since these are the motivational basis for the conflict. Such choices are directed ultimately by moral principles, which Aquinas illustrates in several unsystematic formulations, including his identification of the basic moral principle as the twofold Love Commandment (*Summa Theologiae,* 1-2, q. 100, a. 3, c. and ad 1). These principles direct us not only to avoid actions directed towards merely apparent goods, but also to be fair in considering those who will benefit and suffer harm as a result of one's action, and to promote goods in a way compatible with a community of love that potentially includes everyone.

The second love command—love your neighbor as yourself—makes reference to other people, neighbors, and extends to any human being the possibility of being one's neighbor. The extension arises because there is no rational basis excluding from the set of one's neighbors anyone who can be affected by one's actions or decisions.

Embodying the moral principle, which can be formulated as the Love Commandment, and giving it specificity, are the very general norms enjoining and prohibiting some generally defined kinds of acts. These immediate implications of the basic principle are understood to be captured in the precepts of the Decalogue. As Aquinas holds, the self-evident principles of the natural law imply, by easy inferences ("*modica consideratione*") these precepts (*Summa Theologiae* 1-2, q. 100, a. 3).

A. The Universalism of Natural Law

As noted at the start, "natural law" refers in the first instance to the set of common moral principles, knowable in principle to all humans capable of thinking and choosing, which is the normative foundation for the precepts and virtues that comprise a moral life. These are the human goods and the principles ordering choice among them. This conviction that the principles of the natural law are naturally knowable—that is, knowable to any competent human—makes natural law a form of universalism. These principles are naturally knowable because of their accessibility to common human reason, and so those addressed by them are addressed as human beings, not as members of any smaller community. In its foundations, moral truth is the common property of humanity.

Moreover, it is clear that the universalism of natural law has another aspect, based on the content of its principles. The second tablet of the

Decalogue, spelling out the second part of the Love Commandment, contains some precepts governing actions affecting any human being whatsoever; for example, those not to be killed comprise all the innocent, and the property of all owners is to be respected; no one is to be harmed by false witness.

The two sides of this universalism—common awareness of moral principle and some common responsibilities reaching to any person—points to a common morality for humankind, a morality in principle knowable to all and including responsibilities to all. At the very least this universalism implies that meaningful consensus about moral principle and some general norms is possible, and that this consensus can include recognition of responsibilities having global reach.

This implication of natural law theory provides a ground for one of the most compelling aspirations of the conversation about global bioethics. Plainly, that conversation can be conducted without hope of significant consensus, and even as part of a relativistic agenda affirming the irreducibility or incommensurability of moral perspectives. But many who engage in this conversation hope for more than this, that is, they aspire to some lessening of normative misunderstanding, or even for some common moral judgments backed by reasons that are not in conflict, or at least for that mutual understanding that will enable further discussion to move towards agreement. Natural law theory implies that these aspirations, difficult as they may be to realize in practice, are not vain. Those, like natural law theorists, who believe that there are common moral truths, some of which can be attained only a dialogue that includes a clash of divergent views, and many of which can be better formulated by such discussion, can enter this conversation profitably and honestly.

Of course the account of the global moral conversation which I have sketched in the preceding paragraph would not be credible if natural law implied that those who accept it must cognitively stand above all moral traditions and communities with a capacity to formulate moral issues as only God could formulate them. Acceptance of the natural law implies no such pretensions, nor have those who accept natural law and have developed its theory held such a view (Boyle, 1992, pp. 3-30). Natural law theorists ordinarily recognize that the intelligibilities that ground their moral beliefs can be articulated in more than one way, and have been given practical effect in a variety of social forms. Thus, for example, the medieval and Neo-Scholastic formulations of natural law propositions have proved useful in articulating the implications of moral principle, but they are not the only ways to express moral truths, nor are these formulations immune from criticism. The moral realism of natural law does not imply the truth of all the claims in the natural law tradition of moral theorizing, nor does it imply that the preferred formulae of that tradition are beyond criticism and the possibility of revision.

Thus, there is nothing about accepting natural law that prevents those who do so from recognizing that their formulations of moral principle and conduct of moral reasoning are subject to correction and improvement by discussion with those who approach moral issues very differently. Consequently, on natural law grounds the global bioethical dialogue, understood as an attempt at mutual understanding and at achieving such reasoned consensus as is possible, is not vain but indeed worthwhile, for themselves as well as others.

The universalism of natural law also implies the normative existence of some natural human rights, that is, that some people and institutions have duties to people rooted in the welfare of those people, prior to contracts or other covenants among them. Although the preeminence of the language of rights is modern, on natural law grounds there are rights in the sense just specified if there are duties to people generated by sound moral arguments from considerations primarily about their welfare. And there surely are such duties within natural law theory's traditional morality: it is the harm to neighbor that makes killing, stealing, false witness and adultery wrongs; and we violate the victim's rights when we do such things.

This conception of rights suggests a reason why Roman Catholic teachers and natural law theorists have affirmed some of the principles and some of the rights—although certainly not all of the alleged rights—of the human rights agenda, and have given them application beyond any national borders. For those who accept the natural law affirm a common, though multifarious, human good which makes some moral demands all can recognize, including demands of significant forbearance in our dealings with others. That affirmation leads quickly to affirming those rights that are, as it were, reflexes of the prohibitions of the Decalogue. Some of these rights certainly have application in bioethics—in the ethics of killing, for example.

Other rights, whether welfare rights or those protecting autonomy, are not so immediately read off the natural law; if they are normatively justifiable, the reasoning is more complex. In the case of the liberties and forbearances so central to modern conceptions of rights, natural law plainly provides for the legitimacy of property rights and the discretion they provide to owners. It does this without any modern presumption that autonomy, as such, is intrinsically good, although it does seem to suppose that some aspects of owners' acting with reasonable discretion is an aspect of virtuous living. Recent natural law expands the area for personal discretion, particularly in respect to religious liberty (John Paul II, 1995, pp. 2104-2109).

Natural law arguments for welfare rights are even more complicated, since the underlying duties to help those in need are duties to perform and not simply to forebear and responsible people reasonably must situate these duties into their larger set of duties. Wealthy and functionally differentiated societies can provide some forms of help to those in need by taxing citizens and publicly supporting and coordinating the help. When the help is better provided in that way than by individual action and if the supporting taxation is held to levels compatible with citizens having discretion over their own lives, the duties to help others become rights that are appropriately enforced and guaranteed by public authority (Boyle, 2001, pp. 206-226). In a word, natural law supports the concern for human rights found in Catholic social teaching and provides a rationale for the global application of that concern.

B. The Limits of Universal Moral Judgments

The implications of universalist moral conviction, as specified in the preceding section, both for the success of the global bioethical conversation and for the human rights agenda are significantly limited. These limitations follow from the limited extent to which sound moral reasoning can go in creating a common bioethics for the communities of the world. Moral sensibility, public virtue and decent political decision making may perhaps go far in creating a common bioethics; but *moral reasoning* alone—the combination of moral principles and general precepts with the morally relevant characterization of human actions—cannot generate a set of informative and directive norms that could begin to be sufficient to address the entire set of questions of global bioethics.

I have already suggested that there are some common generalities, common human goods, common rights, and a potential for consensus on some general moral precepts. To understand how much of the content of moral life and of virtuous action can be rationalized into something common by these unifying factors we must take a closer look at how moral thinking works and what, beyond the common and universal, it must consider.

Some of the precepts of the Decalogue have obvious relevance to the conduct of health care and biomedicine, but they cannot, without careful interpretation, be of much use in resolving many of the particular questions that arise within the health care context. For example, it is true that some doctors, like other people, sometimes maliciously kill their patients and so obviously violate the prohibition against killing. The prohibition violated in this scenario is not specifically bioethical. By contrast, the detailed application of the universal prohibition of killing to bioethical questions is often complex. For example, euthanasia and physician assisted suicide are neither malicious killing nor obviously killing that is unjust; consequently, application to them of the prohibition of killing requires reasoning not required in paradigm cases of unjust killing. The difficulty is greater in cases of withholding medical treatment necessary for life. Withholding treatments necessary to preserve life causes death, in one widely understood sense of causing death. But this is not, at least in ordinary language, killing. Again reasoning and interpretation are needed.

The bioethical complexities in the area of killing and letting die are no greater than those involved in applying other basic precepts. Consider the precept prohibiting bearing false witness, understood broadly as prohibiting not only lying in legal proceedings but also all harmful and malicious lying. The applicability of this precept to well intentioned ("officious") lies by doctors and family members to patients requires considerable reasoning. And even more reasoning would be required to apply or extend the precept forbidding adultery to issues of artificial and assisted reproduction.

This complexity in applying to bioethical issues the precepts of the Decalogue and the principles underlying these precepts suggests that many clinical bioethical judgments and much of the policy advice provided by bioethicists fall among the most epistemologically complex and controversial of moral judgments. As noted above, Aquinas maintained that moral principles are self-evident to all capable of understanding their terms. He also held that some specific moral norms (including the precepts of the Decalogue) are immediate implications of moral principle and so relatively easy to recognize as true. But he noted a third category of moral judgment, judgments based on reasoning that must take into account a variety of moral circumstances. Judgments in this category are bound to be controversial and only those learned in moral thinking can be expected to know that they are true (*Summa Theologiae,* 1-2, q. 100, aa. 1, 3).

Aquinas's example is the classic Platonic case of the "exception" to the general rule that goods should be returned to their owner upon request. The general rule is a requirement of right reason which holds for the most part, but right reason will warrant a different judgment when the goods requested are to be used for seditious purposes (*Summa Theologiae,* 1-2, q. 94, a. 4). Other examples might include the right to kill in self-defense (*Summa Theologiae,* 2-2, q, 64, a. 7), or to take for one's own use in conditions of necessity what ordinarily would rightfully be another's property (*Summa Theologiae,* 2-2, q. 66, a 7).

In short, it seems that moral judgments in bioethical matters tend to fall along a continuum between the immediate implications of moral principles and the detailed casuistical judgments that require the analytical expertise of a trained casuist. To the extent such judgments fall closer to the end of this spectrum in which many diverse circumstances need to be considered, the prospects grow dimmer that we might have the capacity to articulate a body of bioethical norms that is at the same time circumstantially more nuanced than the Decalogue and useful for guiding bioethical decision making—that is, providing the guidance without complicated casuistical inquiry into circumstances.

The recognition of universal norms that follow from the application of moral principle to generally described actions is important in several ways for the moral life and thought of individuals and communities: for example, as warnings against temptation, as a basis for dialogue, as premises for further moral reasoning, and in the case of moral absolutes, as markers of the boundaries within which good moral reasoning must remain. But this recognition, plainly, is not the whole of moral thinking, which must move into the fuller consideration of circumstances if it is adequately to do the job of guiding choice. Consequently, the common recognition of universal moral standards cannot remove controversy about complex cases. When the full details of the circumstances of troubling decisions come to light, controversy and disagreement are to be expected as a result of the complex structure of moral reasoning, and no bioethics, global or other, can remove that. Therefore, those thinking ethically about global biomedicine must not aspire (or be "set up" for refutation as aspiring) to remove all moral ambiguity, diversity, and disagreement.

The recognition that disagreement is to be expected in the difficult cases of bioethics does not imply that there are no correct answers to difficult moral questions, or that those thinking about such questions can never be confident that they have discovered the correct answers. But epistemological modesty is in order in such judgments since missing or misunderstanding a morally relevant circumstance is often more than an abstract possibility.

C. The Moral Irreducibility of Individual Discretion and Local Authority

In addition to the morally significant circumstances, which require careful attention in casuistry, there are conditions of people's lives, which they alone can assess in balancing the entire set of their moral responsibilities. Many moral responsibilities involve initiatives to carry out commitments, to improve one's life, to carry out a vocation, or to help others. Such initiatives form much of the fabric of moral life, and define a good person's concrete character. The moral tensions that arise between and among these initiatives are addressed by appealing to a sense of what is reasonable, proportionate or fitting. People can rationally determine what is proportionate or fitting, as is clear from the fact that they can be criticized by friends, and they repent of failures to be reasonably responsive to one or another of their commitments, but it is very difficult for outsiders to make this determination, and impossible to formulate general rules for such things as how many children to have, how intensely to pursue a career, or how much time and money to give to charity.

There is, in short, an important element of a person's or a community's responsible and reasonable living that defies general formulation and relies upon the discretion of responsible moral agents. This characteristic of upright and reasonable living places an important limit on appropriate expectations for uniformity and detailed agreement in moral matters. These limits should be noticed in the global bioethical conversation, since some solutions to global health care and biomedical challenges may overlook the human importance of such discretion, especially in understanding the content of human rights.

These limits are important in two ways for understanding human rights. On the one hand, autonomy rights, at their best, protect the discretion of people to determine what is fitting in their pursuit of the good, and so have a principled justification in the natural law conception of moral life. Indeed, the natural law justification of private property includes just such a protection of discretion.[2] But that discretion will be removed if what Catholic social teaching calls "the principle of subsidiarity" (from the Latin subsidium, meaning support or help) is ignored: whatever the scale of social coordination, authorities coordinating more action from a greater social distance should defer to and support those closer to and more involved in concrete actions.

On the other hand, welfare rights limit the area of personal and social discretion, since they involve social organization in which there is determination backed by taxation concerning such matters as how much health care will be universally available, how much support will be given to the poor, and so on. As noted above, such rights can be justified in societies that are both rich enough to allow their existence without removing people's discretion over their lives, and organized enough to provide help more effectively than private actors (Boyle, 2001, pp. 215-225). The general affirmation of welfare rights is warranted whenever these conditions obtain. And since countries meeting these conditions are rich and capable enough to help those beyond their borders, reminding them of the grounds of their duties in the welfare of those far away also justifies talk about the rights of nations and peoples too poor or undeveloped to cooperate politically to help themselves. The emphasis in Catholic social teaching on these rights claims against the richer nations by the poorer seem to me to refer to this aspect of rights—the grounding of duties in others' welfare—and not to any pretense that there is a world-wide organization in which welfare rights are actually funded and guaranteed.

Indeed, natural law theory does not underwrite a proposal that seriously compromises the discretion of the leaders of the distinct political societies that exist in the world. Setting world wide standards for what constitutes, for example, equitable access to health care, or the level of health care to which people in a given country are entitled, would make impossible the proper discretion of leaders who must serve their common good in the actual conditions in which their society exists. They know, or are more likely to know than outsiders, both the economic and social opportunities for biomedicine in their nation, and the needs of their citizens and the priorities for actions to meet them.

As noted above, according to natural law wealthy nations have significant duties to help people in poorer countries; but the former are in no position to set health care standards that are within the latter's proper discretion. Indeed, neither are other bodies in a position to tell the wealthy nations how much, and in what form, they should help outsiders, or to tell the poorer nations how much they should allocate for health care and other welfare needs.

D. Recognizing Moral Error

The preceding sections show ways in which, according to natural law theory, the hope for a common worldwide code for global bioethics must be a vain one. The irreducible complexity and difficulty of casuistry indicates one important limit to the capacity of moral principle to render generally applicable judgments; and the ethical importance of individual and local discretion in determining what is ethically proportionate indicates an area where prudence and discernment, not general norms, should have the final say. Failing to attend to these limits of moral reasoning will lead to mistakes about what norms apply and how they come to bear concretely.

But natural law theory also contains an account of moral error, of how individuals and communities can fail to know even fairly general and fundamental moral truths. Aquinas thought that people are often ignorant of, or mistaken about, the norms which should guide their choices. The norms about which ignorance and mistakes are possible include some fairly straightforward implications of moral principle. The cause for such ignorance and mistakes is not limited to individual moral fault, which, of course, does explain much moral ignorance.

However, individuals' culpable ignorance cannot explain the ignorance of communities and other groups of people, and communities can be ignorant of fairly obvious moral norms. Aquinas's example was drawn from Caesar's report that the *Germani* did not know that brigandage was wrong. This ignorance was attributed to bad custom or bad formation of nature ("*ex mala consuestudine seu ex mala habitudine naturae*"). Aquinas did not speculate as to how much responsibility for this ignorance is attributable to any individual (*Summa Theologiae* 1-2, q. 94, a. 4).

Aquinas's account needs, and has not yet received, the amplification it needs to respond to the forms of relativism and ethical particularism that have developed in the 19th and 20th centuries. It seems fair to say, however, that the "bad customs" of the *Germani* cannot be limited to exceptionally deprived or impoverished groups but infect humanity generally. By the standards of the natural law, all societies, Aquinas's medieval Christendom included, fail to see implications of moral principle that are objectively there to be seen, for example, the immorality of the institution of slavery and the right to religious liberty. The ethical point about moral error is not, therefore, an imperialist or colonial point. All can be affected by the factors, moral and otherwise, that cause us to miss the implications of moral principle.

Any account of moral diversity and disagreement, whether universalist or relativist, rationalist or emotivist, must recognize the possibility of moral blindness on the part of some or all the individuals and groups who hold different or conflicting views. That moral blindness can also affect efforts to overcome moral conflict by reaching a consensus or an accommodation. When moral disagreement blocks necessary cooperation, something must give, and that might well be the moral conviction or integrity of some or all those seeking to cooperate. But a person in this situation can be quite confident of the moral truth of his or her conviction and unwilling to surrender the conviction or act against it. Sometimes such a person will see that some compromise or accommodation is possible that will preserve his or her moral conviction and allow the needed cooperation.

Such accommodations will often involve the belief that the others are morally mistaken, and perhaps culpably so, but that toleration is in order (Boyle, 1994, pp. 183-200). The results of this kind of accommodation hardly comprise a robust moral consensus. The norms agreed upon by such a process have little tendency to be understood by those involved as more than results of accommodations, perhaps based on unjustified compromises, and perhaps based on compromises or deals that are immoral. In other words, a consensus recognized simply as the outcome of a modern political process hardly can count as morality. Nor could the outcomes of such deals realize what the global bioethical conversation reasonably aspires to achieve—such things as the clarification of ideas and differences, and the achievement of consensus that has a chance of reflecting moral truth.

So, global bioethics, if it is to be ethics and not accommodation, must aspire to a consensus based on morally relevant considerations. Overlapping consensus about the moral questions raised by global health care issues is worth seeking, but not any consensus will count as a moral consensus. Bioethical regulation based on accommodation should be recognized for what it is–political decision that should, but often fails to, embody moral principle.

III. The Authority Needed to Regulate Biomedicine Globally

In the previous section I elaborated some pertinent elements of the natural law account of how moral reasoning works. The structure discussed there is that of practical reason, and the norms it justifies are those that exist ideally in the judgments of those who see their truth. Those who judge these norms to be true can do so because they see how they follow from undeniable principles. From this ideal perspective, a person judges that a specific moral norm is what should direct his or her action when the person is confident he or she has considered all that is morally relevant in the action, including the fact that other rational persons may disagree with him or her. The natural, rational character of the results of good practical thinking is contrasted by natural law theorists with positive law: divine and human, customary and enacted, civil and *jus gentium.*

This distinction was not originally drawn nor is it maintained to demean positive law or the established, lived morality of a community. For positive law completes in several essential ways the process of directing individual and social choice that begins with the principles of the natural law. This completion is essentially connected to the fact that the varieties of positive law are promulgated concretely within the social space of human communities and interactions in ways that the ideal norms of the natural law, just as the rational dictates of right reason, are not. This positivity of human law applies not only to law in the narrow sense but to authoritative customs, institutional regulations, moral practices, professional codes of ethics and so on.

Global bioethical regulation, whether or not strictly codified as law, is plainly on the positive side of the positive/natural distinction. Indeed, much of the effort to apply the human rights agenda to bioethics on a global scale is a movement to establish positively certain bioethical implications of rights already positively established in some jurisdictions or ideally held. Global regulation of global biomedicine could not usefully address the issues raised by the global scale of the moral questions raised by modern health care and biomedicine unless its rules and guidelines were readily available, and widely understood and accepted—unless, in other words it were positively established among the societies of the world. Indeed, it is difficult to imagine any strictly rational set of norms that could achieve these goals without positive enactment, without existing as a social reality in the social world of globalized health care and biomedicine. Therefore, even the global conversation among bioethicists has positive aspirations.

A. Positive Morality and Social Authority

As in the discussion of practical reason, Aquinas provides the classical natural law account of human positive morality. In this account, Aquinas took political society as the paradigm for a community and law as the paradigm for positive regulation. Aquinas recognized, of course, the existence and importance of other communities, most importantly families, the Church and the society of nations. And he recognized the existence of authority within those communities.

Authority for Aquinas is a form of service to the common good of a community. It serves that by directing and coordinating the actions of community members so that the common goals of the community can be promoted and realized by actions made common through this coordination. The limits of authority are set by the common good of the community in whose service the authority is justified.

Consequently, although legislation in the political sense is a paradigmatic exercise of social authority, what Aquinas said about positive law specifying or determining the natural law has application, mutatis mutandis, for other communities, their authorities and their regulations. What Aquinas called "*determinatio*" is the specification of moral norms by the reasonable choices of those in authority. His example is the determination of the moral norm that evildoers are to be punished by social decisions specifying on various punishments for various crimes (*Summa Theologiae,* 1-2, q. 95, a. 2).

Aquinas's treatment of property perhaps provides another, more pertinent example. Following the canonists and Christian authorities, he did not regard personal ownership as a matter of the natural law but of morally justified convention. But there exist good reasons, which have force in most conditions of human life, for dividing up responsibilities for things among different persons; this division of responsibility is meant to serve the just goal of making good use of things to satisfy human need (*Summa Theologiae,* 2-2, q. 66, a. 2). Many aspects of the division of useful things into the property of different individuals and groups are likely to be settled by custom, itself influenced by the level of social and technological organization of a society. The presumptions about property are likely to be very different among hunter-gatherers, farmers and industrial and post-industrial groups. Aquinas's account preserves this diversity. And his account also allows that political society can change such customs, and specify property arrangements so as better to serve in the circumstances their basic human purposes.

These examples from Aquinas illustrate the proper working of authority. The requirements of moral principle within a society—including how to cooperate for common goods—remain indeterminate, or have been determined in ways that are not appropriate. Authority makes reasonable decisions to specify principle. The outcome need not be simply an accommodation but ideally is a proper part of the morality of the community. It is part of the community's morality if it reflects what that community can do in the circumstances it faces, including the disagreements and moral limitations of its citizens, to realize its common good. By becoming enshrined in law and custom because of its authoritative sources, the outcome of the responsible exercise of authority becomes positively embedded within the lived morality of a community, and since authoritative rulings have propositional content, they have implications that can be drawn by inference and analogy, logical relationships with other elements in the normative system, and so are open to critique, refinement and creative development.

B. A Worldwide Biomedical Community?

Applied to global bioethical regulation, this natural law idea of the determination of ideal moral norms by the choices of legitimate authorities raises the question of who might be the appropriate authority to develop and set the regulation. The biomedical community itself, the researchers, physicians, policy makers and so on might be thought of as a kind of global community. I will argue that this view of worldwide biomedicine is false, at least for the present. There is no worldwide health care or biomedical community, which pursues an integrated set of common goals (its common good) by coordinated action.

Moreover, the regulation of biomedicine, whether within a state or across the world, cannot be simply the internal regulation of its own internal authorities such as professional organizations. Because of the impact on the life and welfare of so many people of those involved in health care, its regulation inevitably includes a substantial legal and political element. Proper political authorities are those with the responsibility and power to regulate health care because of its relationship to their communities' common goods—including the cooperation with other communities in respect to their mutual interests.

In saying that there is no global community pursuing health in a coordinated way, I am not denying the health is a basic human good. Quite the contrary: health is something in which all people have a rational and legitimate fundamental interest. But basic human goods, as I indicated in section three above, are the intelligible features underlying purposes. Those purposes also include particular goals, in the case at hand, the health one can get by taking advantage of one's resources to protect or promote health. Ancient people pursued the same good of health as we do, but their goals, given their knowledge and technology, were vastly different than ours.

The difference between the actual goals pursued by health care in wealthy nations today and those pursued in former times is greater than the difference in the goals of health care in wealthy and in poor nations today. But the difference remains, not only because of the differences in the health care challenges presented in different places, but also because of cultural and economic differences. As the world is now organized socially and economically, the health care goals of authorities in third world countries are necessarily different from those in North America—even if North American and European health care provides a wishful horizon for others around the world. And because these Western countries differ among themselves in political structure and history, their health care goals will likely remain significantly different among themselves.

The denial that the modern organization of health care and biomedicine is a community with common goals and authorities is not a denial of the many features that unify health care and biomedicine around the world. These are real: the science on which modern health care and biomedicine is the result of international research; the many interactions of scientists and clinicians from around the world are global; the medical professions are importantly trans-national organizations; and the health care and other markets unite people across the globe. Moreover, abstractly considered, the benefits of the most advanced biomedicine may seem to be exportable around the world. These global aspects of the modern biomedicine surely give rise to some global bioethical questions, and may generate some limited common goals of a global nature, for example, in respect to the standards for biomedical research, including research on human subjects, and in respect to public health threats that are transnational in character.

In a word, the practices which comprise modern biomedicine, particularly when understood as a set of interrelated scientific, technological and economic undertakings reaching around the globe, are less of a community and more an intersection of scientific knowledge, technique, professional expertise and commitment that allows the members of many communities to cooperate more or less robustly to provide health benefits for their own communities and others. But like the peoples of the world more generally, these do not pursue a common good in the way needed for common authority to regulate–that is, there is no common goal or set of goals around which the many undertakings are unified and properly coordinated by common authority.

The organized practices of health care and biomedicine do not come to be or stand free of the local, national and transnational communities who create them, or of the projects and goals of the people who create and sustain them. Those projects and goals are distinct. Consequently, there is no single project or goal that could unify these diverse undertakings into the common action of community working for its worldwide concrete health goals. What is common besides the human good of health is limited to the science, the common understandings, technique and markets, and to diverse and often uncoordinated collaborative undertakings by biomedical professionals.

This fragmentation of the pursuits of health around the world implies that no authority within any health care or biomedical community such as a medical association or expert group could qualify as having global bioethical authority—even in those areas in which appropriate political regulation of biomedicine might allow such authority. So until the world is much more integrated and unified, there will be no properly bioethical legislature or Supreme Court for the whole world.

It is important to note, however, that this fragmentation is based on the diversity of the goals and projects for pursuing a common human good—health. And since it is this common, human good that is pursued in these fragmentary ways, the relevant universal moral responsibilities towards persons and their health are not put in question. Therefore, this fragmentation complicates carrying out responsibilities to help others, including those in different countries or communities, in health care as elsewhere. But it does not render them null.

As noted above in section three, natural law implies a right to health care, and significant duties to help those in need, as we can. Their being members of morally and politically distinct communities may limit our capacity to help, but it does not mitigate the underlying obligation (Boyle, 2001, pp. 216, 225). The combination of this normative consideration with the growing interdependence of human beings is, I believe, the sense of the Catholic teaching about a "universal common good" for humankind (John Paul II, 1995, n. 1911). The underlying obligations are general human responsibilities of individuals and communities. These responsibilities point to the requirement to develop mechanisms appropriate to the reality of interdependence. As John Paul says: "The good calls for an organization of the community of nations able to provide for the different needs of men" (1995, n. 1911). But the existence of such responsibilities does not imply the actual existence of worldwide communities capable of pursuing goals they justify.

C. Political Leaders have Final Authority in Regulating the Global Aspects of Bioethics

There are bioethical issues with global aspects, and some of these may require regulation. There may even be some particular health care or biomedical goals that require global action—action no private party or state or local alliance can effectively pursue. Political authority is needed here, and the right kind—global authority—may seem altogether lacking. But natural law theory supports the view that the authority of the leaders of states, acting alone internally, and acting externally in concert through treaty and by delegation through organizations such as the UN, is sufficient for this set of purposes. In other words, the fragmentation of the pursuits of health around the world does not preclude the political authorities of states from regulating transnational aspects of biomedicine by cooperating by treaty with authorities of other countries.

Many bioethical issues having global dimensions fall completely within the jurisdiction of a state, and are appropriately subject to the various officials having authority in its health care system. In modern multi-cultural societies there are many morally defined communities within the larger society, and the differences among these communities, are often important for bioethics. For example, issues with a global dimension arise regularly in Toronto hospitals--not only issues of translation narrowly conceived, but also of expectations about candor, concerns about terminating treatment, religiously based objections to organ donation and so on. The fact that groups whose plurality within a given political society defines it as multi-cultural are in important ways transnational does not lessen the responsibility of that polity's authorities to make pertinent regulations.

A consideration of the various authorities within the health care system of a state, and of the limits and interrelationships among these authorities reveals the decisive role of political authority in health care generally, and in the global dimensions of biomedicine in particular.

Plainly there are many authorities within the health care system of a developed society, and many authorities directing patients and families who make use of health care. For example, religious leaders have obvious authority over health care institutions sponsored by their religion and over the health care decisions of their members, not only in matters having to do strictly with morality or religious practice. They have a responsibility for the spiritual welfare of their members, which often looms large in health care decisions. Any regulatory regime for health care and biomedicine that ignored this authority would involve a straightforward violation of the natural law norms concerning religious freedom.

Similarly, the organizations and professions upon which modern health care depends are not narrowly national organizations, and they surely should have an irreducible say in the proper formulation of concrete bioethical norms. What physicians and nurses will do, the nature of the evidence required for medical knowledge, and so on cannot be decided independently of the expertise and experience of these professions. To ignore it beyond some threshold is destructive of health care, and to refuse it proper consideration violates political respect for voluntary associations. Therefore, the principle of subsidiarity implies that bioethical regulation attends to this legitimate authority, and a global bioethics must respect this professionalism.

But political authority itself has a proper responsibility for health care and biomedical decisions. In addition to obvious matters of criminal law, public health, guaranteeing professionalism and so on, political leaders must make decisions about governmental spending for health care, including decisions about helping foreign countries and people, rationing health care and so on. Hospital and health system administrators have responsibility to specify and carry out these political choices.

These areas of responsibility overlap and potentially conflict: policy makers' and hospital administrators' responsibilities affect physician professionalism—as physician concern about managed care (and its politicized near relative in Canada). Both of these exercises of authority are likely to limit the proper exercise of religious authority within health care.

But fairly sorting through such conflicts with the authority of law when necessary is one of the chief tasks of political authority and the law. So, the authority for providing necessary regulation for bioethical issues within its jurisdiction—including those having a global dimension—is that of the government.

It is difficult to justify on natural law grounds institutional arrangements that obscure this governmental responsibility, by handing it over to a regional alliance or international organization. That would make sense if there are issues that need regulation but cannot be regulated by the law of any single polity, and require states to act in concert. The need to operate in concert in actions that are primarily the responsibility of cooperating states is perhaps based on the greater effectiveness of coordinated action in dealing with agents, like researchers, who can operate in any of several countries. However, as the Council of Europe's Convention's (1997) prescriptions strongly suggest, clear cases calling out for such coordinated regulation are wanting. Thus, protecting the vulnerable poor from exploitation by drug companies or from rich people seeking body parts is better done, and only effectively enforced, by a local government. More generally, in the absence of clear cases calling for internationally coordinated action, it is the more local authority, which necessarily has much to say about its own health care system and biomedical organization that can best attend to the circumstances of its health care arrangements.

Still, I do not exclude the possibility that there are or may be issues in health care or biomedicine that can only be handled by global action. As Papal teaching on globalization generally has emphasized, one of the key moral challenges raised by globalization is the effective regulation of markets to prevent the abuse of the people of poorer countries (John Paul II, 2003; Martin, 2000, pp. 86-88). Natural law theory respects private property and the discretion it brings; it also respects the utility of markets in serving human needs and expanding wealth. But markets can be driven by greed and abused. Natural law reasoning by itself cannot settle the balance of factors necessary for generally preserving the benefits of markets and preventing the unjust treatment of some affected by them. But sometimes people can confidently judge that the working of markets has results that are unjust, and when that judgment is publicly established, regulation of markets is in order. This concern to regulate markets for the sake of protecting the vulnerable has bioethical application, for example, the prevention of the use of the poor guinea pigs or organ sources; and here cooperative action by the states of the world may be more effective than unilateral action by a nation; it is possible that such action is necessary.

On the view I have been developing in this section, the authority to deal with such issues also falls to the leaders of states, who can cooperate by treaties or by delegating their agency to an international actor such as the UN (cf Martin, 2001, pp. 90-92). On the conception of the world as a group of interacting sovereign polities, they can operate normatively in their interactions by the consent of treaties and covenants. Such cooperation is a part of the common good of each, and so properly within the authority of the political leaders of a state. So, justified international agency to regulate health care and biomedicine is possible; however, its moral force seems more like that of a contract among authorities than like an exercise of social authority. The agreeing states are the locus of authority; the agreements are promises, having the moral force thereof, and the sanctions of international law.

Of course, this natural law assignment of authority to national leaders would not hold in all possible political organizations of the world. It is certainly possible that global interaction and the mutual cooperation of all the people on earth will develop to the point that the community of communities that comprises the world will in effect become a single community, at least for some purposes such as security. The leaders will have the responsibility legally and politically to coordinate the actions of all insofar as they have global impact. That possible world, I am assuming, is not the real world. The openness of Catholic social teaching to the development of such a world does not imply that it is committed to its existence; the Church's natural law based concern is that nations address the implications of the much greater level of interaction between the peoples of the earth (Martin, 2000, pp. 90-92).

An important implication of the contractual nature of international agreements concerning global bioethics should be noted here: such agreements by some states have little normative force against states not consenting to them, and would likely have moral force only if one nation's refusal to consent were so harmful to other nations or to the non-consenting state's own citizens as to constitute a *casus belli* for the consenting states. A member of the UN, for example, which had reason to reject the duties imposed on it by Article 19 of UNESCO's *Universal Declaration on the Human Genome and Human Rights* (concerning cooperation in sharing with developing countries information about the human genome and the benefits of research on it), might be given pause, but hardly an exclusionary reason, to set aside this refusal by the fact that this UN body approved the declaration. Similarly, a European nation whose leaders judged that regulating a market in human body parts was more appropriate for its overall situation than the outright prohibition of the Council of Europe's 1997 Convention (Article 21) is given no decisive reason to reorder its priority in virtue of the Council's action. It would be an extravagant legal fiction for an international court to hold that a nation not consenting to a bioethical covenant was in fact bound by it.

D. A Bioethical *Jus Gentium*?

In the previous sub-section, I reasoned that there is no worldwide community in respect to health care, because there is no global goal that could unify the various health care and biomedical undertakings around the world. Therefore, there is no global bioethical authority, only the authority of the leaders of the nations of the world. It seems, therefore, that we should not pretend that there is a world wide health care community, or community of communities, whose leaders rightly specify for the entire globe the bioethical implications of moral principle.

Nevertheless, since people from many nations and from diverse human communities interact on health care matters, it would be useful if, over and above treaty based agreements, there were some positive directions for the bioethical interactions of nations and of people from distinct communities.

Groups of people in situations that are significantly different in ways that affect the working out of moral principle can discover some moral practices—or at least effective accommodations—to govern their interactions, particularly when each group makes use of common resources and technology, for example, when primitive groups walk the same paths and use the same watering places, or when traders use the same overland or sea routes, or even more robustly, when they trade with each other. This capacity of groups to develop moral standards that apply across the boundaries of morally defined groups such as nations or civilizations need not be limited to bilateral agreements between groups. Such standards can potentially embrace the relationships between many morally distinct communities, and perhaps between all such communities that interact—the entire globe.

There appears to be—or to have been—a set of such standards with global or nearly global reach; this is what ancient and medieval lawyers called the *jus gentium,* the law of the nations, or the justice or right of the nations. These standards were understood to apply to the interactions between nations and their citizens on the one hand and, on the other hand, other countries and their citizens in the absence of treaty agreements governing the interactions. For example, rules of war and standards for respecting the rights of alien travelers were part of the jus gentium. Gratian, a 12th century codifier of canon law, provides a standard list of the subject of the *jus gentium*:

> The law of nations deals with the occupation of habitations, with building, fortification, war, captivity, servitude, postliminy, treaties, armistices, truces, the obligation of not harming ambassadors, and the prohibition of marriage with aliens. This law is called the law of nations because almost all nations make use of it (Gratian, 1993, p. 7).

This "law" was understood to be a form of positive law, because of the wide acceptance of its standards. But it was not understood as capable of competing with or replacing the local customs and legislation, which were thought to be the proper source of direction of the interactions of community members within their community.

Since the social forms, knowledge-base, technology and markets of modern life are much more common around the world than the interactions between groups in pre-modern times, there is reason to expect some set of norms similar in function to those of the *jus gentium,* including norms to govern actions that involve crossing the boundaries of groups having morally significant differences. Of course, we would not expect a modern form of the *jus gentium* to be rooted in customs reaching back to pre-historic times, because of the relative novelty of modern markets and technologically based interactions. Nor would we expect the norms of the *jus gentium* to remain customary in our globalized social reality, but reasonably anticipate their becoming embodied in international law and accepted by treaty.

In other words, the social reality in earlier times of a *jus gentium* does not provide a blueprint for modern interactions among states and peoples, but it does suggest that there may be positive norms with sufficiently wide acceptance to allow them, without further authority, to direct the interactions of people and communities having significant moral differences. Of course, the diversity in positive law and morality among the interacting peoples of antiquity was likely far less radical than the diversities of moral outlook obtaining today. But the idea remains promising: there may be some things on which we agree normatively, and that could provide some resolution of troublesome moral conflict, a fact that moral theories can explain and justify in different ways.

Michael Walzer's discussion of the rules of war, their application to some recent wars and the debates and rationalizations about these applications, strongly suggests that there are some norms meeting these conditions (Walzer, 1977). The overwhelming presumption against aggressive war, applied in the presumption against border crossings, the almost indefeasible immunity of non-combatants and other such norms certainly exist today in what Walzer calls the "moral world." This is a social world in which even belligerents can explain themselves to each other, debate moral issues, give excuses and so on. Like other positive norms the rules of war have a logic; they have implications and logical relationships to themselves and to other positive norms. As Walzer admits, this body of positive moral doctrine certainly can be abused to provide cover for immoral activities, but, since it is a world governed by ordinary logic and rules of evidence, casuistic rationalizations can be–and sometimes have been—exposed for what they are (Boyle, 1997, pp. 83-98).

So, the precedent of the ancient and medieval *jus gentium* is met in one important realm of international affairs. The diversity of moral communities and principles does not destroy this social world. Rather it provides a context within which at a very practical level, the incommensurabilities that may exist among moral outlooks and practices can be discussed in a common language and possibly diminished or overcome on particular matters.

Modern health care is an area of human interaction in which some norms of a present day *jus gentium* might exist. The shared values and the similarities in the goals of the health care professions and the similarities in expectations of those seeking and paying for health care around the world create a presumption that some common moral standards will unite a social world that seems now to embrace so much of humankind, and to cross so many otherwise morally significant boundaries.

Two candidates suggest themselves as the bioethical inheritors of the *jus gentium*: the four principles of Beauchamp and Childress (2001), and the natural rights of the *Universal Declaration of Human Rights* as applied to bioethics.

The principles of bioethical "principlism" are widely accepted within Western bioethics; they serve usefully to stake out important areas of bioethical concern that must be taken into account in moral thinking. But, they are not specific enough to direct action, and indeed appear so general that they can be interpreted in contradictory ways (Takala, 2001, pp. 72-77); for example, the principle of justice might be understood to provide justification for solidarity often affirmed in international ethical pronouncements, but surely this principle is also understood as excluding solidarity to fairly respect liberty and property (Knowles, 2001, p. 256; Mori & Neri, 2001, pp. 325-326). This objection—that the principles are too general to exclude or imply anything—seems decisive. For as Walzer shows, the norms of the common moral world maintain a function within the social space of human intercourse only by having some definite logical implications.

Moreover, there is another opposite objection: that the generality of the principles is not so complete as to remove all contradiction; for example, the principle of respect for autonomy raises objections from many quarters, for example, from traditional moralists who hold it justifies immorality in the name of freedom, and from non-Western moralists who are likely to object to its individualism (Sakamoto, 1999, pp. 192-195).

The other possible source of globally accepted norms is the enacted body of affirmations of natural and universal human rights. Although there is ongoing debate about the exact meaning of human rights, and their implications for people in different social arrangements, they seem more widely accepted than the four principles of principlism, and more definite in their content. As noted above, natural law accepts some of these rights as reflexes of the prohibitions of the precepts of the Decalogue, some as protections for the exercise of morally necessary discretion and some as the implications of the common responsibilities to help others.

Rights of the first kind are essential for human well-being, but their contours are likely to be unclear and disputed. Rights of the second kind—such as religious liberty, property rights and other protections of autonomy—are also socially basic, but, it is not clear how they are immediately or directly relevant to bioethical interactions between morally distinct communities, which may reasonably protect human discretion in diverse ways.

Rights of the third kind are widely recognized, at least at minimal levels. But except as important general principles to be affirmed by all—both by outsiders who should help and by members of a state who should cooperate to provide fairly for the welfare of all—these welfare rights cannot be concretely established within a polity except by its authorities. The authority of the moral law itself, or of widespread consent to parts of it, cannot override this local authority. In short, human rights may be important elements in the common moral world, but are not obviously of help to global bioethics.

Some rights, however, might be part of a contemporary bioethical *jus gentium.* A comparison of health care actions with those in a marketplace helps specify which rights they might be. The value of markets is not tightly tied to the community values of those who use them; strangers, even those disliking one another and their ways, can trade and make deals. Yet people can make use of markets only if certain positive moral expectations are in place. People will not cooperate willingly in markets they think will increase the chances of their being killed or enslaved, or in markets in which the exchanges undertaken are as likely as not to be systematic frauds. Preventing fraud and putting some checks on possibilities for exploiting weaker parties in deals seem to be necessary moral conditions for markets to work—and those requirements appear to point to the need to regulate markets.

Hospitals and other health care facilities are similar in several respects: one seeks help there for health problems; one's moral community and that of the health care facility need not be the same, but one reasonably expects competent advice and assistance based on medical science, truth in diagnosis, respect for one's decisions and so on. There must be positively established and enforceable norms to guarantee that at least some of these expectations will be met. Indeed here the moral presuppositions are if anything more robust than in a marketplace. The person seeking health care trusts his or her health care providers, their honesty and their professionalism. One then often puts oneself in a position of significant dependence on the health care providers. *Caveat emptor* is a lot more tolerable in a market than in a hospital.

So, it seems that the moral preconditions under which people are willing to make use of health care, particularly when that use takes them outside the moral community with which they identify, justify norms that are common and potentially global in reach. But formulating such norms and providing evidence of their widespread acceptance is easier said than done.

Consider the very basic issue of professional candor in interactions with patients. This seems to be not only an implication of ideal moral principle but also one of the most elementary requirements of the relationship of trust needed for patients rationally to seek health care. However, it is very difficult to formulate this requirement as a crisp, positive norm that directs anything more than not lying to patients. "Always communicate with patients with candor" provides a standard that it would be difficult for a health provider to be confident he or she has met. The casuistry for applying this norm would be as complex of that of omissions generally. Established legal requirements aside, we might wonder whether such a positive norm would ever be specific enough to provide the confidence patients need to put themselves in the control of health care professionals. This appears to be one of the norms whose practical application involves discretion as to what is appropriate, and, therefore, accepting the norm is of limited use in structuring the expectations of those who do not share with providers—and often know they do not share—a common sense of what is fitting.

The norm "never lie to patients" removes this discretionary element, but too many people in health care, as elsewhere, seem to think that some lying to patients is morally permissible. So, the widespread acceptability that is needed for norms to function as elements of the *jus gentium* is likely to be lacking here. Since there is no authority behind the norms of the *jus gentium* in addition to the consensus reasonably held to reflect or approximate moral truth, only the continuing discussion of the implications and possible legitimacy of some lying to patients could make this norm what it now is not: a part of a widely accepted set of norms.

I suspect that many of the norms that would spell out the preconditions for people's cooperation in modern health care are in the same predicament as the norm requiring candor: either one has a prescription, the practical content of which depends on discretion guided by the agent's sense of what, all things considered is morally proper, or one has a definite prescription that does provide guidance but fails the requirement of widespread acceptability or consent.

So, it seems that the preconditions for entering into modern health care are harder to formulate as non-discretionary, positive precepts than one might expect. In general, defensible presumptions rather than absolute norms seem sufficient for the trust most of us require to seek the benefits health care practice can provide. Believing that others sometimes break promises, for morally good and for morally questionable reasons, and sometimes lie, whether out of weakness or to be helpful, does not appear to be sufficient to destroy trust.

These difficulties may suggest that there are no norms capable of directing health care and biomedical actions involving crossing morally important community boundaries, and not likely to be any. But that suggestion goes too far.

First, the vague and discretionary norms needed for cooperation are not emptied of normative content by their discretionary elements. Patients' expectations of helpful treatment and truthful communication can include the recognition that health care professionals' interpretations of the relevant norms are likely to diverge from their own. And this awareness need not undercut the expectations, or their understanding of the expectations as structured by the professionals' adherence to the moral norms.

Second, one of these norms does seem to meet the conditions for being a norm of global bioethics: it is precise, widely accepted, and not a mere accommodation. This is the norm requiring that health care professionals refrain from treating competent adults without their consent. In effect, this norm allocates the responsibility for an important class of health care decisions, namely, those to treat competent adults. It establishes an authority for an area of human cooperation.

Plainly, there are vague terms in this norm, especially the notions of "competent adult" and "consent." These do not make the norm empty. The practical force of the norm is independent of the difficulties that sometimes arise because of this vagueness. For there are many cases where the application of the norm is not affected by the vague boundaries of these terms, and where the application of the norm, nothing else, settles what decision will be made about treatment. This happens when the health care professionals and patients share a community's particular values and when they do not. But invoking this norm serves a practical purpose: when there is a conflict of opinion about treatment, however grounded, the competent patient has the final say as to what will be done to him or her.

Likewise, although rationalizing casuistry can be invoked to remove the practical authority of the norm, this can be exposed and rejected as can similar abuses of the rules of war.

It might be objected that, like my example of lying to patients, the right to refuse medical treatment is specific enough to qualify as a norm of positive ethics, it is not widely accepted. I concede that if the right to refuse treatment was understood as essentially intertwined with modern western ideal of personal autonomy, then this objection would be well taken. For many people around the world, including defenders of natural law, do not accept the blanket appeal to autonomy, which is often understood as meaning that if an action is based on an exercise of a person's freedom or autonomy, then it is morally justified.

But modern autonomy is only one account of this norm and not the norm itself. Indeed, it is sometimes confused with the norm by those who would like to use the right to refuse treatment as a precedent for euthanasia or assisted suicide. But the right to refuse treatment leads there only if its logic is taken to be that of modern autonomy. The allocation of responsibility and authority for health care decisions to competent adults need have no such basis. This allocation need be based on no illusions about the wisdom or moral rightness of a person's decision, but rather on the belief that some allocation of responsibility in this area is needed and that this particular allocation is reasonable, perhaps because of the impact health and health care have on every patient's life.

It is significant that very different practical authorities affirm this norm or something very close to it. Justice Cardoza, still a judge on the New York bench in 1914, stated the following:

> Every human being of adult years and sound mind has a right to determine what shall be done with his own body; and a surgeon who performs an operation without his patient's consent commits an assault for which he is liable in damages (Schloendorff vs. Society of New York Hospital, 211 N.Y. 125, 105 N.E. 92)

Pope Pius XII affirmed this norm several times, most notably in his famous 1957 allocution on prolonging life:

> The rights and duties of the doctor are strictly co-relative to those of the patient. The doctor in fact has no separate or independent right where the patient is concerned. In general, he can take action only if the patient, explicitly or implicitly, directly or indirectly, gives him permission (Pius XII, 1957-58, 395-396.)3

The wide acceptance of this right is suggested by the fact that it is taken by Pope and Justice as an established right (contrary to the suggestions that it was invented by bioethicists in the 1970s as a development of the consumers rights movement). Not everyone and not every community accept this right and some try to keep it narrowly limited. But many of these communities have sufficiently internalized the common law or the Catholic or the modern secular judgments about this matter, to allow reasoning internal to the community to allow for the acceptance of this norm. Thus, for example, many of Toronto's Southern Europeans (mostly Catholics) do not share North American values in relation to candor in discussing a patient's prospects with him or her. But they can come to accept the idea that there must be sufficient candor to allow for consent to treatment—if not from the common sense of the practice then from authority they accept. Similarly, the most paternalistic doctors can recognize this constraint on their paternalism

If I am correct in thinking that the right to refuse treatment is in fact sufficiently widely accepted to be part of a global bioethics, then there is a foothold for a global bioethic—global at least insofar as it addresses a bioethical problem that arises in all health care contexts and constitutes a solution that has very wide acceptance. This right has a logic and so can be extended by casuistical reasoning. As already suggested, the current efforts to extend it to issues such as euthanasia are too ideological to command widespread consent. But other sorts of extensions are not so obviously ideological and may, like this right, extend the areas where there is agreement about who is in authority, for example, in decision making for children and other non-competent patients, or in providing directives for one's possible non-competent future self.

All these are examples of allocating responsibility for decisions; they are not examples of taking a robust value or moral concern as an object of potentially widespread bioethical agreement across communities. Perhaps norms based on such robust moral concerns could become part of a widespread bioethical consensus. If, for example, Pope John Paul II's "Culture of Life" came to be accepted as an element of the many cultures of the world, then such pro-life norms might become part of the new *jus gentium.* But the example suggests how unlikely that is.

I finish by underlining that this attempt to assess the possibilities for a global bioethics is carried out from a natural law perspective in which practical reason can recognize the existence of significant universal norms. On this moral view, there are moral absolutes and universal affirmative duties–duties whose reach is extended by the successes of globalization. But these principles and responsibilities give shape to moral life only by application and specification that takes full account of morally important circumstances. Positive morality gives a community its unique moral shape by addressing those circumstances pertinent to its social life and common action; in positive morality, universal and ideal obligations are specified through responsible decisions of appropriate authorities. Thus positive morality introduces the local, not ordinarily the global, and local authority has the responsibility and capability to deal with most of the global aspects of biomedicine. The more universal part of positive morality, the *jus gentium,* is necessarily thin, since the only authority behind it is widespread agreement, and the belief of many that that agreement can reflect moral truth; but even widespread agreement can be suspect in its sources and fragile in its positive status.

Notes

1. For a recent interpretation of Aquinas' moral theory supporting my reading of Aquinas, see Finnis (1998). Most of what I say about Aquinas does not depend upon the controversies concerning the interpretation of Aquinas favored by Finnis and me.
2. The Thomistic text is *Summa Theologiae* 2-2, q. 66, a. 2; the concern to protect discretion is tacit, but I believe present; see Boyle, 2001, 208-214.
3. See Boyle, 1981, 80-94 for references and this and other statements of Pius XII. He makes these statements as if they are not controversial or novel.

References

Beauchamp, T., & Childress, J. (2001). *The Principles of Biomedical Ethics* (5th ed). New York: Oxford University Press.

Boyle, J. (1981). 'The patient/physician relationship,' in D. McCarthy & Morascewski, A., O.P. (Eds.), *Moral Responsibility in Prolonging Life Decisions,* (pp. 80-94). St. Louis: The Pope John Center.

Boyle, J. (1992). 'Natural law and the ethics of traditions,' in R. George (Ed.), *Natural Law Theory: Contemporary Essays,* (pp. 3-30). Oxford: Oxford University Press.

Boyle, J. (1994). 'Radical moral disagreement in contemporary health care: a Roman Catholic perspective,' *Journal of Medicine and Philosophy,* 19(2), 183-200.

Boyle, J. (1997). 'Just and unjust wars: casuistry and the boundaries of the moral world,' *Ethics and International Affairs,* 11(1), 83-98.

Boyle, J. (2001). 'Fairness in holdings: a natural law account of property and welfare rights,' *Social Philosophy and Policy,* 18(1), 206-226.

Campbell, A. (1999). 'Presidential address: global bioethics--dream or nightmare?,' *Bioethics,* 13(3-4), 183-190.

Europe, Council of. (1997). *Convention for the protection of human rights and dignity of the human being with regard to the application of biology and medicine: convention on human rights and medicine.* [Online]. Available: http://conventions.coe.int/treaty/en/treaties/html.

Finnis, J. (1998). *Aquinas: Moral, Political, and Legal Theory.* Oxford: Oxford University Press.

Gratian, (1993). *The Treatise on the Laws (Decretum DD. 1-20) with the Ordinary Gloss,* (A. Thompson, O.P. & Christensen, K., Trans.). Washington DC: Catholic University of America Press.

John Paul II. (1995). *Catechism of the Catholic Church (with modifications from the editio typica).* New York: Doubleday.

John Paul II. (2003). *Governance of globalization.* [Online]. Available: www. zenit.org.

Knowles, L. (2001). 'The lingua franca of human rights and the rise of a global bioethic,' *Cambridge Quarterly of Health Care Ethics,* 10(3), 253-263.

Kung, H. (Ed.). (1996). *Yes to a Global Ethic.* New York: Continuum.

Macer, D. (1994). *Bioethics for the People by the People.* Christchurch: Eubios Ethics Institute.

Mori, M., & Neri. D. (2001). 'Perils and deficiencies in the European convention on human rights and biomedicine,' *The Journal of Medicine and Philosophy,* 26, 323-336.

Martin, D. (2000). 'Globalization in church teaching,' in L. Sabourin (Ed.), *The Social*

Dimensions of Globalization (pp. 82-93). Vatican City: Pontifical Academy of Social Sciences.
Pius XII. (1957-58). The Prolongation of Life. *The Pope Speaks,* 4, 395-396.
Sakamoto, H. (1999). 'Towards a new "global bioethics,"' *Bioethics,* 13(3-4), 191-197.
Schloendorff v. Society of New York Hospital, 211 N.Y. 125, 105 N.E. 92.
Takala, T. (2001). 'What is wrong with global bioethics? On the limitations of the four principles approach,' *Cambridge Quarterly of Healthcare Ethics,* 10, 72-77.
Thomas Aquinas. (1988). *Summa Theologiae.* Milan: Editiones Paulinae.
United Nations, General Assembly. (1948), *Universal declaration of human rights* [On-line]. Available: http://www.un.org/Overview/rights.html.
UNESCO. (1997). *Universal declaration on the genome and human rights, 1997* [On-line]. Available: http://www.unesco.org/human_rights/hrbc.htm.
Walzer, M. (1977). *Just and Unjust Wars.* New York: Basic Books.

Domestic Disarray and Imperial Ambition:
Contemporary Applied Ethics and the Prospects for Global Bioethics

David Solomon

It is generally regarded as one of the major political advances of the last half of the twentieth century that, during this period, the political and economic imperialism that had dominated the relation of industrialized North Atlantic nations to their third world neighbors largely disappeared. Former colonies of European nations won their independence and did so largely by appealing to political values they had drawn from the cultures of the masters themselves. The largely "western" values of autonomy and self-determination were used to good purpose in making the defeat of imperialism in many ways a self-inflicted wound. Insofar, however, as the political slogans under which anti-imperialist forces marched were drawn from the foreign culture whose dominance they were opposing, the battle against imperialism acquired a paradoxical air. Wasn't the very act of rebellion at the same time a form of acquiescence? Like the tar baby, some might say, the imperial powers frustrated every effort of their colonial clients to escape their domination by rendering their efforts at genuine independence as additional means of attaching them to the cultures they so despised. By convincing their colonial peoples to use the moral rhetoric of the imperial powers to achieve their

H.T. Engelhardt, Jr. (ed), *Global Bioethics* (pp. 335–361).

independence, the imperial powers assured their continued hegemony in one form or another.

The danger that movements dedicated to freedom and independence might in fact function as new forms of oppression in the global context is surely a real one. It raises the specter of a kind of *ethical imperialism* that might threaten the cultural integrity of ethically colonized peoples every bit as much as political and economic imperialism. This threat would be a particularly insidious form of oppression in that it would infiltrate a culture by providing for it the arguments precisely against oppression. Ethical imperialism, of course, might take many different forms, some more benign than others.

A particular instance of the worry about ethical imperialism generally is the question of how we are to think of exporting medical ethics to distant countries and peoples given the vast differences—culturally, technologically, spiritually, morally and economically—that exist in our pluralistic world. Part of what lies behind this question (which I will call the "export problem") is the recognition that contemporary medical ethics is to a very large extent a western invention (and largely an invention of the academic culture of the United States in the last 35 years.) Part of the worry, too, involves a widespread skepticism about the credentials of much contemporary medical ethics. There are problems in this area, then, from the point of view of both the consumer of ethics and the producer. The potential (world-wide) consumers of medical ethics, it might be thought, share too little in common (especially of the cultural background of contemporary western academics), and are too different both from us and from each other to be addressed by a single universal message. The (largely Western) producers of medical ethics, on the other hand, may seem too embedded in the particularities of a broadly technological approach to the world and too committed to a broadly liberal and individualistic political theory to produce ethical materials of genuine relevance to patients and doctors nurtured and socialized in more traditional societies.

The goal of the research project of which this paper is a part is to examine the prospects for a global bioethics. I will argue that a necessary preliminary to this project is an examination of the manner in which philosophers have dealt with ethical disagreement and debate within our own culture. This examination, in turn, will require a careful look at the peculiar situation of applied ethics generally in contemporary Anglophone philosophy, and much of the central part of this paper will be taken up with a critical look at the recent history of Western applied ethics. The larger project we are undertaking focuses on the imperial ambitions of bioethics and seems to presuppose that we understand the culturally authoritative role of academic ethics within the domestic arena of the western democracies. The presupposition is, that is, that problems only arise when we attempt to export ethical understanding to distant cultures. Things are just fine on the home front. I want to examine the domestic situation then in medical ethics (as well as applied ethics more generally) in order to see if this presupposition is justified. Secondly, it seems important to determine what lessons are to be learned about the export problem if it proves to be unjustified.

I begin then with a cursory discussion of the different varieties of the export problem with the hope of loosening the grip on us of the picture that portrays global ethics as involving problems quite different from local ethics. I turn next to a selective account of the recent history of applied ethics in the United States and Western Europe and its current state as I understand it. This history, while sketchy, is intended to suggest that the recently acquired cultural authority of applied ethics may be problematic in more than one way. This discussion in turn leads to an examination of a number of techniques developed by moral philosophers to deal with the problems of local disagreement. I will suggest that all of these techniques fail, and for more than one reason. Finally, I ask how the conclusions of this discussion might be relevant to the ambitions of global bioethics with which this paper begins. In this final section I will pay special attention, although surely not enough, to the question of the implications of my discussion for questions of liberty.

I. Forms of the Export Problem

The export problem, as we have defined it, is the problem of how ethical insights central to western ethics can be exported to cultures quite different from ours. As defined, however, it suggests that export considerations only arise between cultures that are quite different from one another in moral practices and moral beliefs. We might envision the export problem then as a problem about the relevance of Kennedy Center Bioethics to the situation of Nigerian, Filipino or Afghanistani health care workers. Or as a problem about the relevance of western ideas emphasizing the importance of personal autonomy to ethical discussions within a more traditional culture that takes the authority of family elders more seriously than do we. One can imagine, however, that there might be other problems of exporting ethical insights that do not involve radically different contemporaneous cultures. Three other versions of the export problem come readily to mind: the problem of exporting ethical insight across time in historically continuous cultures, i.e., **the temporal export problem**; the problem of exporting ethical insights among persons in the same culture, i.e., **the local export problem**; and the problem of translating ethical insights within the ethical viewpoint of a single person, i.e., **the personal export problem.**

Consider first the temporal export problem as a problem about appropriating the moral insights embodied in the moral past of our own culture.[1] Many of the most important issues in contemporary ethics turn precisely on questions about how ethically different our past was and what measures might be taken to make that past available to contemporary moral reflection. Some questions that exemplify this problem are these: How strange is Aristotle anyway? Did Aristotle even have the concept of the moral ought?[2] Or is the moral itself, as Bernard Williams has suggested, an invention of modernity—and late modernity at that?[3] Is the concept of a right a mere survival (like the 18th century notion of taboo in Polynesian culture) as Alasdair MacIntyre argues so that those who use the notion of "right" to translate key political notions of Aristotle or Aquinas are guilty of gross misunderstanding of the texts they are trying to make accessible to us?[4] Does the contemporary "cult of authenticity" in ethics involve a distortion of certain earlier moral ideas ripped from the contexts in which they made sense?[5] All of these questions are being raised in contemporary ethical discussions and seem to exemplify difficulties similar to those involved in the global export problem. The problem of bridging the gap between Aristotle and contemporary culture certainly seems no less daunting than bridging the gap between John Rawls and a Taliban warrior, although the latter may be more dangerous.

Of course, one need not turn to such philosophically sophisticated issues as the problem of appropriating Aristotle's thought in modernity or questions about whether the ancient Greeks had a term properly translated by "morally ought" in order to encounter the temporal export problem. How can we today understand the moral sensibility of our great grandfathers who defended the morality of slavery or the morality of executing the mentally disabled for what we would today regard as trivial crimes. In many cases our ancestors and their moral practices can seem as strange and distant to us as the moral practices of those who live in contemporary but distant cultures. And it can be as difficult for us to learn moral lessons from our ancestors as for third world doctors to learn from medical ethicists trained at the Kennedy Center.

The difficulties contemporary citizens of the advanced western democracies have in communicating their ethical ideas to their neighbors also seem similar to the global export problem in many respects. This local version of the export problem arises when one considers the possibility that we might live (even in our own neighborhoods and cities, surrounded by person watching the same evening news programs) in a world made up of moral strangers. Is it more difficult for an ordinary American physician to discuss bioethics with health care workers in a traditional Islamic culture or one immersed in African animist traditions than it would be for a Mormon farmer in northern Utah to discuss bioethics with a secular, Jewish, feminist pro-life attorney, raised in Manhattan, educated at Harvard, and working full-time for the ACLU? The problem here is surely not physical distance since if the farmer takes a tour to New York City he might sit next to the attorney, just as she might sit next to him in the Utah airport while on her way to her skiing holiday. Even Rawls in attempting to develop an overarching theory of justice suitable for our culture, finds it necessary to emphasize that one of the primary facts about our culture is "the fact of pluralism"—the fact that inevitably we will live in a culture of diverse "reasonable comprehensive religious, philosophical, and moral doctrines"(Rawls, 1993, p. 36).[6] This fact of pluralism might of course be taken to be the natural condition of reflective persons who have moved beyond the pull of traditional culture.[7] One might, however, regard it, as MacIntyre does, as a particular, historically conditioned state of contemporary people—a feature of modernity. But either way it seems to raise export problems even within particular cultures. Indeed, if MacIntyre is right, there is the interesting consequence that pluralism itself may be something that the west is engaged in exporting. Export problems would then be nested like Russian dolls.

Finally, there seems to be a kind of export problem implicated even in the conflict or incommensurability among the ethical ideas that might be contained within the ethical viewpoint of a single modern person. The modern self is often portrayed as a kind of meeting place of various ethical ideas and traditions, deeply fragmented by its participation in the myriad cultures that converge in modernity. MacIntyre, indeed, identifies this fragmented nature of the self as one of the primary features of modern men and women. In speaking of a certain kind of typical modern person he says:

> ...they tend to live betwixt and between, accepting usually unquestioningly the assumptions of the dominant liberal individualist forms of public life, but drawing in different areas of their lives upon a variety of tradition-generated resources of thought and action, transmitted from a variety of familial, religious, educational, and other social and cultural sources. This type of self which has too many half-convictions and too few settled coherent convictions, too many partly formulated alternatives and too few opportunities to evaluate them systematically, brings to its encounters with the claims of rival traditions a fundamental incoherence which is too disturbing to be admitted to self-conscious awareness except on the rarest of occasions. This fragmentation appears in divided moral attitudes expressed in inconsistent moral and political principles, in a tolerance of different rationalities in different milieus, in protective compartmentalization of the self, and in uses of language which move from fragments of one language-in-use through the idioms of internationalized modernity to fragments of another. (The simplest test of the truth of this is as follows: take almost any debatable principle which the majority of members of any given group profess to accept; then it will characteristically be the case that some incompatible principle, in some form of wording, often one employing an idiom very different from that used in formulating the first principle, will also receive the assent of a substantial fraction of that same group.) (MacIntyre, 1988, pp. 397-398).

If this is right, the export problem is to be found even within the souls of individual modern men and women. Our moral idiolect itself exhibits the fact of pluralism. And each of us may have as much difficulty understanding ourselves and building a coherent and integrated life as the diverse cultures in the world may have in building a common language in which the most profound ethical issues can be discussed reasonably and with some hope of moral understanding and progress.

The export problem, then, seems not to be confined to interactions between distant cultures. Or if it is we have to refine the notion of distant cultures in such a way that any number of them can live within the ethical viewpoint of a single modern agent. Rather, we should think of the problem of global bioethics as just a species of a more general problem of ethical understanding that can arise in ethical conversations conducted across time, across space, across neighborhood fences or even across the different moral perspectives that might inform the activity and practices of a single agent. If this is right then we might suspect that light can be shed on the global form of the export problem, by looking at recent vigorous attempts to promote moral consensus within our local culture. Indeed, the drive for a kind of global bioethics is frequently fueled by a sense that we have successfully dealt with many of the problems of local bioethics and we are now ready to conquer the world for goodness. The high prestige of academic medical ethics in contemporary western cultures, especially among the cultural elites, might suggest that we have a product worth exporting. This sense of ethical manifest destiny often draws either explicitly or implicitly on an alleged analogy with the great goods associated with the export of western science to "nonscientific" cultures.[8]

This is a suggestion, in any event, that I would like to pursue. I suspect that we can learn much about the prospects for global bioethics by examining the recent history of local bioethics, and to do this it is necessary to discuss, again briefly, the remarkable renaissance in applied ethics more generally within the American academy in the last three decades. I will suggest that this history is surprising in more than one way and that a proper understanding of it will be instructive for those eager to pursue the imperialist path of global bioethics. The tale I will tell is a largely cautionary one, but I will turn to more constructive suggestions at the end of this paper.

II. The Recent Prominence of Applied Ethics in the Academy

The prominence of discussions of relatively concrete ethical issues in contemporary universities and colleges involves in many respects a revolutionary change in academic culture. It is also a quite recent change. Up until the 1960s and 1970s, practical deliberation about ethical matters tended to be left to centers of cultural authority that operated quite independently of the academy. Religious bodies, the family, the professions, and other intermediate institutions made authoritative pronouncements on ethical issues, and also provided the main social vehicles for inculcating "values" in their constituents.

In the late 1960s, however, the direct involvement of institutions of higher learning, and professional philosophers in particular, with practical ethics increased dramatically. There is a renewed interest in research in ethics, new ethics institutes and centers are founded, large numbers of textbooks in "applied ethics" are published to supply an increasing number of applied ethics courses, and new journals in medical ethics, business ethics, feminist ethics and environmental ethics appear.[9] The new and well-funded ethics centers which appear at this time symbolize this new professional interest among philosophers. Although the new ethics centers and institutes all have an academic character, they are situated in quite different ways relative to universities and colleges. Some, like the Hastings Center (founded in 1969), are free-standing, foundation-supported research centers with no direct university connections. Others, like the Kennedy Institute at Georgetown University (founded in 1971), are free-standing within a university setting. Still others, like the Center for Clinical Medical Ethics at the University of Chicago Medical School, are located within particular colleges or professional schools within a larger university.

Although there are major differences among these centers with regard both to focus and methodology, they share a number of features. They all aspire to contribute to ongoing discussions within the culture concerning concrete ethical dilemmas. Although they frequently draw on highly theoretical academic resources the origins of which are quite distant from questions of concrete practice, they focus on real-world problems. Among the problems addressed by early discussions in applied ethics were the moral permissibility of abortion, the allocation of scarce medical resources such as kidney machines and bypass surgery, the moral character of affirmative action programs, and the requirements for being a conscientious objector. The new centers also tend to draw primarily on the same academic specialties. The social sciences make some significant contributions to these ethical discussions, but the primary contributors are theology and philosophy. Finally, these centers are, for the most part, unrelentingly secular. Even though many of the major figures at these centers are Catholic, Protestant and Jewish theologians, they aspire to carry on ethical discussions free of the presuppositions or the moral commitments of particular religious traditions. And this secular character is certainly no historical accident. It is clear early on in the "ethics revolution" that the very point of such centers is to provide a forum for discussing difficult dilemmas about human conduct independently of the competing religious frameworks which seemed to the founders of these centers to make such dilemmas intractable. The new ethics centers thus aim to provide a religion-free zone for talking about human problems. And the reason for this secular emphasis is surely the desire to speak to an audience that is as wide as possible. The particularity of religious discourse tends to conflict with the universalistic ambitions of these ethics institutes, thus creating export problems.

The causes of this "ethics revolution" in universities and within philosophy departments in particular, are no doubt complex and they have certainly been the subject of much discussion among scholars. (But not, I think, as much discussion as this phenomenon deserves.) But some appear obvious. The 1960s were a time of deep cultural dislocation in this country. Many formerly respected institutions lost their cultural authority, an energetic and market-driven youth culture thumbed its nose at its elders, the professions (e.g., law, medicine, and the clergy) lost power and authority within their institutional settings, and the family with its interlocking set of obligations and rights among parents and children was transformed almost beyond recognition. And, unlike some earlier cultural revolutions, the revolution of the sixties involved not merely the elites, but everyone. The powerful influence and ubiquity of television and pop music insured that these cultural changes were felt not only among the anointed in the centers of large cities, but in Peoria, too. The hairstyles, the lifestyles, the clothes and the moral attitudes central to the sixties were soon commonplace among even relatively young children and working class men and women.[10]

The two most prominent public debates about ethical issues in the sixties concerned the struggle to end racial segregation in American public schools and the ethical propriety of the actions of the United States military in Vietnam. Both debates spawned discussions of many other related ethical problems about equality, rights, justification of state authority, and social justice. There were other cultural phenomena, however, which, while not as prominent as the civil rights debate and the Vietnam debate, were formative in bringing about renewed academic interest in ethics. The affluent U.S. population of the post-war years was transformed in many ways by new technologies, many of which had grown out of the opportunities provided by the war for financing technological innovation. Many of the changes in sexual mores, and the consequent changes in attitudes toward family life, were the result of possibly the most significant technological development in the second half of the twentieth century, the development of cheap, safe, and effective contraceptive devices. Within medicine, new devices like kidney machines, new therapeutic settings like the intensive care unit, new procedures like bypass surgery and transplant surgery and new drugs like the unprecedentedly effective antibiotics introduced after the war were making medicine simultaneously more expensive and more effective. The great revolution in the financing of medical care which came about in 1965 with the passage of the Medicare and Medicaid bills under the Johnson administration had as its goal to ensure that these great new advances in medicine would be equally available to all segments of our population, including especially the most threatened segments, the elderly and the poor. It soon became obvious, however, that medical technology was developing faster than the federal budget was growing, and the struggle of American health care policy since the second Nixon administration has largely been to find ways of containing medical care costs. The problems of cost containment in turn gave rise to an entirely new set of ethical issues.

While many of the problems of ethics arose from technological innovations and social change in the post-war years, they were also related to radical changes in citizen attitudes toward traditional loci of moral authority. The decade of the sixties was characterized by an emphasis on individualism and autonomy, which called into question many received moral beliefs and the institutional settings and supports for those beliefs. Individuals were empowered to "make their own choices" about fundamental ethical issues, and self-fulfillment was increasingly understood in terms of emancipation from restricting and suffocating traditional norms. This new emphasis on individualism and autonomy found expression both in popular culture ("do your own thing", "different strokes for different folks") and in academic moral and political thought–the work, for example, of such influential social theorists as David Riesman with his criticism of "other-directed" persons, and the philosophical work of such continental thinkers as Jean-Paul Sartre and Herbert Marcuse.[11]

These various movements led to a kind of "privatization" of moral opinion, which had implications for the whole culture. In the schools, for example, the fashionable model for moral education came to be "values clarification," in which the emphasis was on encouraging each student to work out his or her own "value system," free from coercion or authoritative pronouncements by teachers. In the courts, the most significant decision of this period was the *Roe v. Wade* decision, which invalidated virtually all of the restrictive abortion laws in this country.[12] What was remarkable about the Roe decision was not just its dramatic overthrow of legal prohibitions at the heart of Jewish and Christian culture, but also that in overthrowing them the court felt no need to comment substantively on the nature of the moral controversy associated with abortion. The decision rested rather on an interpretation of a constitutional right to privacy which had been recognized by the Court for only a few decades, and its argument was based almost entirely on the claim that the state has no right to interfere with the private decision of a pregnant woman to have an abortion. The courts too, then, along with philosophy, popular culture and fashionable educational theory licensed a kind of privatization of moral judgment. This trend toward privatization reached its apex with the much discussed "mystery passage" in the Casey decision rendered by the Supreme Court in 1992.[13] In its decision, the Court wrote, "At the heart of liberty is the right to define one's own concept of existence, of meaning, of the universe, and of the mystery of human life" (O'Connor, Kennedy, & Souter, 1992).[14] The radical autonomy of each person was thus found to be another constitutional guarantee.

These aspects of the great social sea-change of the 1960s add up to a kind of ethics revolution. The social dislocations associated with the civil rights movement and the Vietnam debate, the new technologies, and the rise of individualistic approaches to human life and the consequent pressure on traditional loci of moral authority led to significant changes in the way our culture deals with ethical issues. Instead of relying on traditional centers of ethical authority distributed across such diverse institutions as the family, the church, and the traditional professions, there was a turn to specialists in ethics and the academic settings in which such specialists made their home. In particular, philosophers and theologians were called on to bring their expertise to bear on what was increasingly perceived as a crisis in our culture.

Although it was not entirely clear what the agenda should be for such specialist forays into ethics, they were clearly responding to the demand that some ethical expertise be deployed in dealing with particular moral quandaries in our culture. Who is entitled to have his or her life saved by a kidney machine if there are too few kidney machines to go around? Are we required to use all of the medical means at our disposal to save the lives of seriously disabled children? Is it sometimes permissible to shorten deliberately the lives of infants whose continued life promises nothing but pain and slow decline? How do we decide how to attend to the interests of nonhuman species, e.g., the snail darter or the spotted owl, when their interests conflict with human needs or wants? Do corporations have a moral obligation to attend to the larger interests of the communities in which they operate even when they have no statutory obligation to do so? These practical moral questions, and our culture's inability to provide compelling and authoritative answers to them, provided much of the impetus for the revival of academic ethics.

It is important to emphasize that the ethics revolution we are here discussing is one that takes place not simply in the philosophy departments of American and European universities. This revolution is culturally significant in any number of ways: academic philosophers (or those speaking in the name of academic philosophy) have assumed a number of prominent and publicly visible roles in dealing with some of the deepest moral and existential conflicts in contemporary culture. They have given ethical guidance to hospitals, corporations, government bodies at federal, state and local levels, and educational institutions. They have addressed these groups on a number of different topics, including ethical issues having to do with the environment, gender relations, bioethics, racial matters, corporate etiquette, and social responsibility. They have given expert testimony at trials and exercised influence in criminal appellate decisions, even at the highest level.[15] They are regularly asked to appear on the nightly news and on the front page of the *New York Times* where they render moral judgment on every new piece of technology.[16] Certain philosopher/ethicists have become public intellectuals whose views on particular issues transcend "ordinary ethics." Some of the most prominent are Peter Singer on infanticide, animal liberation and radical giving; Daniel Callahan on abortion and health care for the aged;

Ronald Dworkin on jurisprudential issues; and Art Caplan on a wide range of issues in bioethics. The competition for space on the national media is keen among ethicists, and newcomers work hard to get a leg up.[16]

III. Some Puzzling Features of the Applied Ethics Revolution

The discussion in the previous section was intended to demonstrate both that there was a kind of revolution in moral philosophy some decades ago and that this revolution has a kind of cultural significance that reaches far beyond the academy. I now turn to some puzzling features of these changes. The principal irony of the turn to the ethical in the 1960s was that the academic disciplines of theology and philosophy were called on for help at precisely the moment in their history when they were least able to provide it. At the time this revolution took place, academic moral philosophy, at least in the English-speaking world, had been engaged for most of the century in the discussion of a number of technical issues about the meaning of central moral terms and about the nature of moral knowledge. This focus on semantics and epistemology in ethics had been accompanied by an almost complete neglect of more practical issues. Indeed, moral philosophy in this period was dominated by two dogmas. The first, the thesis of moral neutrality, claimed that the conclusions of moral philosophy, properly done, will always be neutral with regard to concrete normative issues. A sharp distinction was drawn between metaethics—the investigation of abstract conceptual issues in ethics—and normative ethics, the investigation of the truth of particular moral judgments or the rules, principles or set of goods that might entail particular moral judgments. The argument for moral neutrality alleged that the proper work of moral philosophers is confined to metaethics and, in accord with the thesis of moral neutrality, that the results of metaethical inquiries have no relevance for normative conclusions.[18]

The second dogma, associated with what was called the fact-value problem, claimed that there was a logical barrier between factual investigations and value investigations, preventing anyone from drawing legitimate conclusions about what ought to be done from premises about the way things are. According to this dogma, which had proponents as far back as the eighteenth century, no set of factual claims such as the conclusions of the natural sciences, the social sciences, or history, taken alone, can entail any normative claims. To put it more bluntly, in the twentieth century, most Anglophone moral philosophers concluded that moral judgments could not draw any meaningful support from an account of the way the world is.

The practical effect of these two widely shared commitments of twentieth century moral philosophers was devastating for those who turned to philosophy for a response to the moral crisis of the 1960s. The first dogma, the thesis of moral neutrality, ensured that the work of moral philosophers themselves would be irrelevant to practical moral issues. The second dogma, the sharp separation of facts and values, went further and seemed to imply that no other discipline anchored in "factual" investigations could be relevant either. Moral philosophers in the late 1960s were confronted then with demands that, according to their own principles, they were unable to satisfy. It was not only that there were within the curriculum of philosophy departments in this country and England very few courses in applied ethics, and very few textbooks for such courses besides. Nor was it simply that there was no tradition of training graduate students in moral philosophy to deal with normative issues. It was much more serious than this. The methodological heart of moral philosophy, as it was understood and practiced in England and America, was hardened against the very investigations moral philosophers were being asked to undertake. Of course, it was open to moral philosophers to use their technical skills to "clarify" the ethical issues and the moral quandaries that bedeviled the surrounding culture; and if one were optimistic, one might expect such clarification to move us in the direction of well-grounded consensus in response to these issues. But such optimism seemed ill-advised. Given the cultural confusion and deep disagreements that prevailed, such clarification was just as likely to deepen conflict as it became clear what the debate was all about.

Moral philosophy, then, if it was to respond to the culture's demand for ethical assistance, would have to change—and beginning in the early 1970s it did so. Although there had been a number of challenges to the reigning orthodoxy of the two dogmas in the 50s and 60s (especially by a brilliant triumvirate of British philosophers, Phillipa Foot, Elizabeth Anscombe, and Iris Murdoch[19]), it was the publication of John Rawls' remarkable work, *A Theory of Justice,* in 1971, that marked a sea-change. Rawls abandoned the exclusive attention to conceptual issues that had characterized most moral theory in the first half of the century, and revived the older Enlightenment tradition of foundational ethical theory which attempted to ground substantive moral and political principles in rational procedures.[20] Rawls and his students such as Thomas Nagel, Onora O'Neill and Thomas Hill developed their normative theories out of the classical German rationalist theory of Immanuel Kant.

But the revival of normative theory did not proceed in any unified fashion. Rawls' book was followed quickly by a number of books in the utilitarian tradition of Bentham and Mill—the great modern alternative to Kantian rationalism. Richard Hare of Oxford University, who had also been a significant contributor to the metaethical debates of the first half of the century, came eventually to the conclusion that his metaethical views did have normative consequences: specifically, that analysis of key moral terms revealed an underlying commitment by anyone who used these terms to satisfy as many people's desires as possible.[21] Hare and his students, Derek Parfit and Peter Singer, together with a number of other ethical consequentialists, quickly produced a body of literature to rival that of the neo-Kantians.[22] But this did not exhaust the explosion of normative theory.

As early as 1958, Anscombe had argued that the differences between Kantian and utilitarian alternatives were insignificant—that they were guilty of similar errors which could only be avoided by returning to a classical, Aristotelian vision of ethics emphasizing virtue. Beginning in the mid-1970s, a number of thinkers, liberated by the Rawlsian revolution but drawing inspiration from Anscombe, began to develop neo-Aristotelian theories. Alasdair MacIntyre's 1981 book, *After Virtue,* was the most influential contribution to the neo-Aristotelian revival, but important contributions were also made by Martha Nussbaum, Charles Taylor, and Julia Annas.

Finally, there was a reaction, beginning in the 1980s, against normative theory itself, a reaction which proceeded by way of theorizing about normative structures. Inspired by Nietzsche's skepticism about the very possibility of sound ethical theory, traditional analytic philosophers such as Bernard Williams and Annette Baier, together with post-modernists such as Richard Rorty in the United States, and François Lyotard in France, argued in different ways that ethical theory is itself dangerous to living a genuinely ethical life. Although these thinkers hold vastly different views in many respects they share the view that ethical theory distracts us from aspects of our lives which are morally important, but which, in their particularity and concreteness, escape the grasp of abstractive theories. They also contend that ethical theory frequently serves as a disguise for self-deception and self-centeredness on the part of the theorist.

In sum, the cultural ascendancy of academic ethics is puzzling because of its deeply contested nature. At exactly the moment that academic ethics came to have an important cultural role, it was least able to speak authoritatively. It had its own house least in order. And despite the revival of normative ethical theory, mainline Anglophone academic ethics in the last half of the 20th century continues to be beset with three quite different kinds of deep disputes which continue to dominate in-house discussion among moral philosophers, although they tend to play down this domestic disharmony when dining out with physician or corporate clients. The first major kind of disagreement involves a continuation of many of the metaethical disputes about the cognitive status of moral judgments, only now the discussion has taken on more of an ontological tone and the main disputants are labeled ethical realists or antirealists. Some of the main protagonists in this dispute have been John Mackie, Gilbert Harmon and Simon Blackburn on the one hand, who have vigorously defended versions of moral anti-realism, and the views of John McDowell, John Finnis and Alan Gewirth on the other who are among the leading defenders of anti-realism.

Secondly, there are the deep disputes within normative theory which we have already noticed. The last half of the 20th century has seen the revival, as we have seen, of broadly Kantian, broadly Benthamite and broadly Aristotelian ethical theories. All of these theories have their leading figures, their acolytes, their set of disputed research problems and their summer camps. They even have their own mannerisms. Utilitarians are certainly the most laid-back and are mostly men. The neo-Kantians are the most confident and imperious, as befits advocates of a theory born in the heart of Harvard yard. The neo-Aristotelians have been on the losing side of these debates for the better part of the last millennium, and now seem cautiously optimistic that their time may have come. The most diverse group is the neo-Nietzscheans, whose main tactic is to belittle ethical theory itself and call into question the epistemological standing of the whole enterprise. Even they, however, are prepared to write columns in our leading cultural journals advising the rest of us how to live.

The third level of disagreement is at the heart of applied ethics itself. Applied ethicists who work in hospitals or corporations frequently disagree fundamentally about their conclusions in practice. Among leading practitioners of applied ethics one finds vigorous defenders of abortion rights and vigorous opponents. And there is similar deep disagreement about, for example, the morality of affirmative action, capital punishment, war, and human cloning. Some applied ethicists argue that it is always wrong to eat animals, while others argue that the final end of a pig is to be eaten. And, of course, disagreements in applied ethics are not only at the level of substantive conclusions, but also at the level of method. Do we proceed foundationally, defending and applying principles in a traditional way? Or do we proceed in coherence fashion, juggling intuitions and hoping that in the long run, our clipping and adjusting of our moral sense will lead to convergence in the moral beliefs of the individual as well as the group? Just as there is little consensus among applied ethicists on their conclusions, there is similar disarray with regard to their method.

The world of academic ethical theory became a very complicated place, then, divided and divisive, following the breakdown of the metaethical research program of the first half of the century. This only deepened the predicament, already severe, over how to adjudicate the cultural disputes and dilemmas which helped give rise to the revival of normative theory. Recall, the culture had turned to moral philosophy in the late 1960s, seeking a culturally authoritative response to the social dislocations of the postwar period, but Anglophone moral philosophy was at the time largely unable to respond to this challenge because it had given up its normative ambitions. Substantive moral theory was revived in the 1970s, but its long failure to address normative questions authoritatively resulted in confusion over where and how to begin; consequently, a variety of competing theories arose, and philosophers had no clear idea how to adjudicate the differences among them. In practice, philosophers largely reproduced the disagreements found at the level of cultural practice at the level of normative theory. Whereas initially the problem with Anglophone ethics had been its impotence, caused by its commitment to moral neutrality and the alleged gap between facts and values, now the problem was (and is) different: there are too many rival approaches to ethics, and no clear way to adjudicate among them. The academy cannot respond authoritatively to the cultural crisis, because it has no sense of how to ground such an answer, or even how to pursue an appropriate ground.

In view of this crisis at the very foundations of ethical theory, the recent turn to applied ethics with its proliferation of ethics centers and institutes—and its global ambitions—looks problematic. If applied ethicists and their institutions admit that they are unable to provide authoritative moral guidance of a definitive and universal sort, they undermine their *raison d'être.* If they don't admit this, they are guilty of deception. In any case, they are badly equipped indeed, on their own terms, for the job they have been asked to do.

IV. Responses to the Problem

This problem has not, of course, gone unnoticed by the world of applied ethics. Several strategies have emerged for dealing with deep, foundational disagreement in ethical theory, strategies which allegedly allow applied ethicists to present their conclusions to the public in good conscience. These strategies are diverse and defy easy and clear formulation, but the following list attempts to capture crudely some of the main varieties:

1. **Strategies of assimilation**—This strategy suggests that what appear to be deep disagreements (especially at the normative level) are really not. Utilitarians, Kantians and Aristotelians, according to this view, are analyzing different parts of the ethical arena, and what appears to be deep disagreement is simply division of labor. This strategy has appeared in both sophisticated and intellectually challenging forms in the work of Shelly Kagan and Barbara Herman, among others, and sometimes in overly simple and unpersuasive forms.[24]
2. **Minimalist strategies**—This strategy though often closely related to assimilationist strategies does allow that there might be genuine disagreement at the deepest levels of normative theory. It claims, however, that the areas of disagreement do not (at least for the most part) lead to disagreement at the practical level. It is possible to identify a set of mid-level principles consistent with all reasonable normative theories and substantive enough to produce genuine ethical arguments powerful enough to settle at least a broad range of concrete ethical disputes. This strategy has been enormously influential and is most closely identified with the work in bioethics of Childress and Beauchamp.[25]
3. **Casuistry**—The casuistical strategy counsels an abandonment of normative theory altogether (or almost altogether) in favor of a relentless focus on particular cases. The applied ethicist on this view must acquire highly developed Aristotelian phronetic skills and exercise them in the analy-

sis of particular cases. This strategy does not deny that there might be deep disagreement at the level of normative theory but, like the moral minimalist, attempts to avoid any kind of moral argument that engages this moral disagreement.

4. **Triumphalism**—Triumphalism is not so much a strategy for overcoming foundational disagreement within normative theory as a strategy for denying that the disagreement is inevitable. It claims that one or another of the contending normative theories really can prove its rational superiority to the others. Indeed, in its strongest form, it claims that one already has (the preferred theory of a particular triumphalist), and that the arguments are available for all to inspect. In recent philosophy, where the standards for having confirmed a normative theory are set very high indeed, there are not, of course, many triumphalists, but Alan Gewirth, Bernie Gert and Jim Sterba seem to me to come as close as any major figures in ethical theory. They all believe, as I understand them, that they are in possession of an argument (or arguments) which provide to those who fully understand them a rationally compelling argument for a comprehensive moral conception. There are, of course, many weaker forms of triumphalism, most importantly the weakened forms which argue (or at least hope) that although we presently lack compelling arguments for any particular comprehensive moral argument, there is reason to believe that we will at some time in the future have such rationally compelling arguments. Both Thomas Nagel and Derek Parfit, among contemporary moral philosophers, have defended such weakened forms of triumphalism.[26]
5. **Rising above the ruins**—This strategy is adopted, I believe, in the latest version of John Rawls' account of his own approach to the incommensurable disagreements within ethical theory. Since Rawls' *A Theory of Justice* did so much to solidify the cultural respectability of applied ethics, it is not surprising that we find in his work one of the most sophisticated accounts of how to approach the deep disagreement and fragmentation of comprehensive moral conceptions which he thinks is inevitable even in the best community. Rawls' view, as I understand it, is that it is possible to develop a political account of a democratic regime which will provide a kind of constitutional framework for dealing with disagreement about the most fundamental human problems.[27] Such a political account will not be just one more comprehensive doctrine, but will rather rise above such doctrines (hence, the image of rising above the ruins), and will make stable, decent and reasonable human cooperation possible in a morally divided world. As Rawls makes clear, his proposal is not just enlightenment liberalism which is, according to him, just another comprehensive doctrine. It is rather political liberalism, which is a set of reasonable arrangements that normally constituted persons can find it reasonable to follow.[28]

My account of these strategies is obviously oversimplified, but this taxonomy at least gives some idea of the lay of the land. This is not the place to engage in detailed arguments about the merits of each of these strategies, but for our purposes such argument is not really necessary. It is sufficient here to notice only that there is no agreement within applied ethics about which of these strategies might succeed. That is why, of course, there are so many. Although none of these strategies has secured anything like general agreement, some have a kind of local notoriety. There is certainly much talk about the Beauchamp-Childress minimalist strategy in medical ethics, but I suspect that has more to do with bureaucratic control than philosophical argument. The Kennedy Center has trained through its summer seminars many doctors and nurses who have carried these doctrines back to many local hospitals. Many medical ethicists use the Beauchamp-Childress method, but certainly no one has been able to give a philosophically compelling argument in its favor. And, of course, many medical ethicists have been severely critical of their approach to medical ethics.[29] Recall that these strategies are put forward as a way of making philosophical expertise authoritative even in a world in which there is fundamental disagreement at the deepest level of normative theory. If that same disagreement is reproduced at the level of the strategies, then they fail as strategies of reconciliation even if we don't criticize each one of them individually. They are intended to deal with the fact of philosophical disagreement, but they simply reproduce philosophical disagreement.

This description of the state of recent applied ethics inevitably raises questions about why philosophical ethicists have the cultural cachet that they now have. A careful look at the state of contemporary ethics, as we have seen, suggests that it is driven by disagreement and discord. This fact of disarray within ethics mirrors in a sense Rawls' fact of pluralism. Although the disagreement in the ranks of moral philosophers and theologians is rampant and fundamental, they nevertheless are invited into the citadels of public policy, jurisprudence, medicine, corporate America, educational bureaucracies and scientific practice, and they are treated as if they possessed expert knowledge derived from well-ordered and rationally based methodologies. Nothing, as we have seen could be farther from the truth.[30] In the next section, we will turn briefly to look at the upshot of this state of affairs.

V. Prospects for Solving the Export Problem

The conclusions of the previous section of this paper are disappointing. We suggested in the second section of this paper that the global export problem was not different in any important respect from local export problems that arise frequently in complex pluralistic cultures like our own. We had hoped, as a consequence, to discover clues for assisting us in formulating strategies for thinking about global export problems by examining the procedures of applied ethics in local contexts. But our examination of the current state of applied ethics in our culture in turn suggested that the local applications of applied ethics are, to put it somewhat over simply, part of the problem and not part of the solution. The field of applied ethics is in a state of disarray, we have suggested, reproducing within itself most of the conflicts in the wider culture which it was intended to resolve. It is as if the medical profession was constituted by persons and agencies which simply exhibited the range of diseases they were intended to cure.

Does this result have any implications for the global export problem with which we began? Someone might think that the conclusion to be drawn is a relativistic one. If the current state of applied ethics—and of normative theory more generally—is as fragmented and filled with apparently irresolvable disagreement as we have suggested, then doesn't it follow that there is no hope for an objective, non-relativistic account of the ethical?[31] And if ethical relativism is true, then surely the export problem is beyond solution. But this problem at least can be put aside. The fact of disarray as we called the current state of applied ethics in our culture lends no support to the claims of ethical relativism. There may perfectly well be a non-relativistic truth about ethics, and perhaps this truth is even known and savored by, say, an Orthodox monk living in a cave on the Holy Mountain. Perhaps we don't have access to the truth because he doesn't want to tell us or because he knows we are not yet able to understand it as he is. Or perhaps he has already told us and we haven't understood him. The point is that no evidence about the ubiquity of disagreement and disorder within normative theory and applied ethics will have any implications for questions about whether ethics is objective.[32] Just as the deep disagreements in certain areas of mathematics or physics don't show that physics and math are "relativistic" but only that they are difficult, no relativistic conclusions about ethics can be drawn from the current pervasive disagreement in the field.

This pervasive disagreement does show something important, however, about the capacity of contemporary applied ethics to actually resolve ongoing disputes about health care policy (and other disputed areas) involving the conflicting interests and moral beliefs of institutions, agencies and persons. Recent conflicts about the creation and use of human embryos for experimental purposes, for example, involve disagreements about the deepest ethical issues. They also involve large financial interests, powerful scientific ambitions, the fears and hopes of countless sick people hoping desperately for a cure, and the voracious appetites of educational institutions and other research centers for the prestige associated with scientific breakthroughs. "Ethicists" have been arrayed on all sides of this issue, surely creating, by their sharp, acrimonious and persistent disagreement a kind of cynicism (where it was not already present) about the pretensions of academic ethicists to bring consensus to these contested public policy areas. The "fact of ethical disarray" is relevant then to the prospects of ethical theory helping to resolve ethical disagreements associated with the "fact of pluralism." Academic ethics cannot be what Bernard Williams has called "a force" with the capacity for wrenching moral consensus out of a divided and disputatious culture.[33] There may be pockets of consensus developing around particular moral perspectives (like that pocket of agreement among the readers of the New York Review of Books which allows Ronald Dworkin to publish an article called, "The Philosopher's Brief.") But the agreement among such groups, and their influence, however privileged and powerful they may be, is likely to be precarious and short lived in contemporary culture. In any event, surely our goal in ethical investigation is not simply consensus, but rather consensus converging on the truth.

What do we do then? Shall we close the book on the aspirations of ethics and attempt to cobble together mutual protection treaties with our neighbors? It is surely impossible, at least, to give up on ethics altogether. If ethics is, as it seems to be, merely sustained and rational reflection on the best way to live our lives both as individuals and as members of communities, nothing recognizable as human life could survive the disappearance of ethics. A more promising path, I think, is to attempt to re-conceive the nature of ethical enquiry in such a way that it simultaneously promises less and delivers more. What seems most striking about contemporary applied ethics is the contrast between its heady pretensions to a universal authority and its utter inability to provide compelling arguments of relevance to contemporary issues.

An alternative conception of the task of the moral philosopher, and indeed of the whole of moral inquiry, is provided in the recent proposal of Alasdair MacIntyre's that we adopt a picture of moral inquiry as tradition-constituted. Although MacIntyre's proposals on this matter are far too detailed and rich to be explored in detail here, his central ideas are readily accessible and provide a stark alternative to the contemporary way of conceiving the ethical. In tradition-constituted inquiry, inquirers do not attempt to stand outside of particular moral positions (or rise above the ruins) and speak to all parties; they rather speak from within the traditions within which they live their lives. In one brief description of this approach to practical rationality, MacIntyre says:

> The conclusion to which the argument so far has led is not only that it is out of the debates, conflicts, and enquiry of socially embodied, historically contingent traditions that contentions regarding practical rationality and justice are advanced, modified, abandoned, or replaced, but that there is no other way to engage in the formulation, elaboration, rational justification, and criticism of accounts of practical rationality and justice except from within some one particular tradition in conversation, cooperation, and conflict with those who inhabit the same tradition. *There is no standing ground, no place for enquiry, no way to engage in the practices of advancing, evaluating, accepting, and rejecting rea-*

> *soned argument apart from that which is provided by some particular tradition or other* (MacIntyre, 1988, p. 350).

By abandoning the pretense of speaking authoritatively on matters of ethics and practical reason from outside any socially constituted tradition, ethical inquirers are able to more seriously engage their audience. By trying to speak from nowhere, they end up speaking to nobody. By learning to speak from somewhere, they might end up having something to say to everybody. Or as MacIntyre puts it:

> Genuine intellectual encounter does not and cannot take place in some generalized, abstract way. The wider the audience to whom we aspire to speak, the less we shall speak to anyone in particular (MacIntyre, 1988, p. 398).

If ethical inquiry were conceived as tradition-constituted in this manner, its relation to cultural disputes and its public role generally would be quite different from their present state. And, the global export problem would be transformed almost beyond recognition. Instead of being a problem about how we export ethical expertise to the ethically needy or deprived, it would rather raise issues about how conversations between competing traditions would take place.[34] What kind of political situation might be required as a setting for this kind of ethical dialogue?

Here we come finally to questions of liberty. If the kind of rationality appropriate to ethics is tradition-constituted rationality characteristic of thinking and arguing out of thick communities held together not only by shared beliefs but also by shared practices and attitudes, then one important political question is: What political arrangements are best suited to promote and enrich this kind of rationality? How much liberty is enough? More particularly, (and reminiscent of the export problem) how do we settle questions about restrictions on the practices central to traditions foreign to us but with whom we are in dialogue? Are those of us formed and expressive of traditions, for example, which reject the direct killing of the innocent, prepared to allow other communities the liberty to violate this proscription on a regular basis? Should communities expressive of traditions alien to us be free to practice female circumcision, to discriminate against homosexuals, to force women who are pregnant through rape or incest to forego abortion, to practice infanticide, to promote the burning of widows or to slaughter endangered species? And if we are not prepared to allow these practices, what grounds can we give for our refusal to allow them and from what perspective do we speak when we appeal to those grounds.

These questions, difficult enough in their own right, are complicated by what we might call the *doubling-back* phenomenon. The amount of liberty to be allowed for the dialectical development of competing ethical views depends at least partially on the content of these particular competing views. Put more abstractly, the question of which social and political arrangements are most conducive to constructive dialogue between divergent tradition-constituted moral perspectives is itself one of the points at which these perspectives diverge. Here again, we begin to look for some thin commitments shared by all of these perspectives that can provide the basis for agreements on the "best" arrangements for housing disputes among them. The Kantian tradition, as we have seen, suggests that the appropriate thin commitments are found in very basic political agreements about the fairness of certain procedures. The natural law tradition would surely argue that something more substantive and less political is shared. Once again, however, we encounter the problem of doubling back. There are internal commitments of many moral perspectives which will make either this Kantian approach to this problem of conflict or the Natural Law approach more attractive. And we begin looking, once again, for some shared thin commitments that will provide a basis for agreement about the social arrangements for housing disputes between the Kantian proposal and the Natural Law proposal.[35]

Is there then any end to this regress or is it finally, in the terms of James' famous anecdote, turtles all the way down? This in many ways is the question left for those of us struggling in the twilight of the Enlightenment, a twilight in which the Enlightenment's particular ideas of universal reason and foundational arguments no longer shine so brightly. We long for methods, themselves based in reason, to resolve disagreements among moral perspectives each of which claims to be based in reason. And when we disagree about which methods are most rational, we seek further second-order methods, again based in reason, to resolve disagreements among first-order methods each of which again claims to be based in reason. The stakes seem too high for us to settle for anything less than rational procedures. Perhaps, though, this ambition is just one more residue of those Enlightenment ideals which seem impossible to sustain. We hold on to these ambitions, I suspect, because we fear that without them, all hope of living distinctively human lives will be lost.[36] We would have to think of ourselves, in the absence of these ambitions, as mere playthings of technology, or of our natural endowments, or of our personal attitudes based in the barest contingencies of our personal history. We would simply be what the thinnest kind of scientistic naturalism says we are.

But, of course, perhaps this is all wrong. There might be other ways to think of ourselves which fall somewhere between the unsustainable ideals of Enlightenment rationalism and the despair of scientistic nihilism. Some have found such ways in religious belief, others in immersion in the particularities of local culture or in the practice of the arts and sciences. These alternatives, one must admit, promise little in the way of a *general* solution to the export problem (in any of its forms), and some of them have seemed to many moderns to be retreats into self-deception or irresponsible self-indulgence. But perhaps they are the best we can do right now.

VI. Global Bioethics

The conclusions of this investigation are depressingly negative with regard to our resources for resolving the export problem in any of its forms. Recall that our hope was that by examining attempts to solve the export problem among particular groups within our community we might find resources for thinking about strategies for resolving the global export problem. If matters are as unpromising as I suggest, however, with regard to the local export problem, we are not entitled to much hope in the global case. Much ingenuity has been invested, as we have seen, in devising strategies to overcome the local export problem, but there are finally just too many strategies in conflict with one another, and we merely reproduce the normative disagreements at the level of methodological disagreement in developing these strategies.

When one examines the arguments advanced by the proponents of a global ethics generally or of a global bioethics more particularly, we find many of these same strategies being recommended. The minimalist strategy is particularly popular among advocates of a global ethics. We find Hans Kung saying for example in his brief for a global ethics that we need to "emphasize the minimal ethic which is absolutely necessary for human survival" (Kung, 1996, p. 2). But surely this particular minimalist argument must acknowledge the fact that many persons (including many of the most religious whom Kung hopes to recruit to his cause) would reject the notion that human survival is the trump in the ethical game. Christians and Jews with their rich traditions of martyrdom can hardly regard a commitment to human survival as the nonnegotiable bare minimum of an ethical approach to the world.

Other advocates of a global ethics rely on forms of the triumphalist strategy. In the *Declaration Toward a Global Ethic,* produced by the Parliament of the World's Religions, appeal is made to a version of the Golden Rule. The document says, "There is a principle which is found and has persisted in many religious and ethical traditions of humankind for thousands of years: what you do not wish done to yourself, do not do to others…This should be the irrevocable, unconditional norm for all areas of life, for families and communities, for races, nations and religions" (Kung, 1996, p.17). Perhaps this principle should play this foundational role, but its longevity will surely not give it the authority required if it is to do so. This principle when developed in a more formal way in the moral philosophy of Kant has not met with universal acceptance and indeed its claim to a foundational role in a global bioethics would be widely disputed by a number of moral traditions as rigorously developed as the Kantian tradition from which it is drawn.

In many of the defenses of a global ethics, the fact that things would go better if there were universally shared fundamental ethical norms is put forward as if it were a reason for believing that there are such norms. In the document, *In Search of Global Ethical Standards,* it is claimed, for example that "human beings need rules and constraints. Ethics are the minimum standards that make a collective life possible. Without ethics and self-restraint that are their result, humankind would revert to the jungle." (InterAction Council, 1996). While this may be so, it gives us no reason for believing that there is a global ethics which can in turn provide the foundation for a global bioethics. It is surely false that a global consensus on just *any* ethical view would be better than lack of consensus. Presumably, it is important that the global ethics be the true view. But if so we must seek arguments to establish the truth of some particular ethical view with enough substance to guide action determinately. Insofar as we lack such arguments, we are surely not in position to defend the project of global ethics.

The case for a global bioethics has been put powerfully recently by a number of different advocates and organizations. It is difficult to see, however, how any of these arguments can be successful as long as the local disputes within North Atlantic bioethics continue to be as deep and apparently irresolvable as they presently appear to be. Some might claim that even if arguments cannot be sustained for a relatively determinate conception of global bioethics, the *rhetoric* of a global bioethics will be useful in rallying persons to a common banner, and hence make the cooperation of these persons on common medical tasks more effective. Even this, however, seems unlikely. The rhetoric of a global bioethics is more likely to raise expectations about what kind of global agreement we require to work in concert as a global community. Raised expectations are likely to be followed by frustration and disappointment when the hopes for a widely accepted bioethics are dashed. This, in turn, may actually hamper common efforts based on more fragmentary ethical overlaps we may have with our fellows. Holding out for too much may lead to our getting too little.

None of the arguments in this paper, of course, should be taken to demonstrate that the aspiration for a global bioethics is misguided. Perhaps, just as the Peircean notion of truth might guide scientific inquiry, the ideal of a global bioethics might guide bioethical inquiry. What we have raised questions about in this paper is whether programs of global bioethics containing substantive moral principles and goals can be reasonably promulgated in the current context of deep and apparently incommensurable disagreement among the moral conceptions available to modern men and women. This question must surely be answered in the negative.

Notes

1. There are notorious difficulties, of course, in identifying "our" culture, but for purposes of this discussion it should be sufficient to understand "our" culture as our current culture and the past and future states of culture which are "sig-

nificantly" continuous with it. I realize how many problems this leaves unanswered.

2. As Miss Anscombe famously argued in "Modern Moral Philosophy."
3. For Williams' discussion of these issues, see especially the last chapter of *Ethics and the Limits of Philosophy* entitled, "Morality: The Peculiar Institution."
4. MacIntyre discusses this issue in a number of places, but the discussion in Ch. 9 of *After Virtue* is probably the best.
5. Charles Taylor discusses the historical entanglements of moral ideas of authenticity in a number of places, but especially in *The Ethics of Authenticity and Sources of the Self.*
6. Rawls, 1993, p. 36, *Political Liberalism.* Rawls distinguishes between the fact of pluralism and the fact of reasonable pluralism. Although this distinction is important for the development of Rawls' constructivist account of justice, it is not important for our discussion here.
7. As Rawls clearly sees it.
8. I don't here want to quarrel with the claim that exporting the tools and conclusions of modern science to "pre-scientific" cultures is a great good, although I have many reservations about what is frequently being exported in the name of science. In the next section, however, I will aim to undermine this analogy by suggesting that the epistemic position of contemporary natural science is quite different from that of contemporary ethics. Although, the doyens of applied ethics have often adapted the trappings of the natural sciences, there is nothing in the world of academic ethics like the well-organized hierarchy of expertise that one finds today in the natural sciences. And there are many other salient differences as well. I will suggest, indeed, that the contemporary world of applied ethics is socially more like a group of warring Protestant sects, than like the well-ordered social machine of the natural sciences.
9. This story is told in detail in a number of places. One of the best is in Al Jonsen's *The Birth of Bioethics.*
10. As a sixties saying had it, "After Elvis, *everyone* can be cool."
11. Charles Taylor's discussion of autonomy in *The Ethics of Authenticity* is a particularly good guide to these developments.
12. *Roe v. Wade*
13. *Planned Parenthood of Southeastern PA. v. Casey*
14. The full text of the judgment of the court in the *Planned Parenthood of Southeastern PA. v. Casey* is available online at: http://www.tourolaw.edu/patch/Casey/Judgement.asp.
15. The influence of the work of bioethicists like Daniel Callahan on the Roe v. Wade abortion decision has been widely acknowledged. The more recent attempt by Ronald Dworkin and a small group of his philosophical allies to influence the Supreme Court's decision on whether there is a constitutional right to physician assisted suicide failed but was widely discussed. It was unclear whether "The Philosophers Brief", as Dworkin hubristically called his piece, failed to convince the Supreme Court because of its consistently condescending tone or because of its bad arguments, but either would surely have been sufficient.
16. Devries and Conrad in their article, "Why Bioethics Needs Sociology" say, "Publicists of medical ethics do not train for that capacity; they aspire to it, and

if they are industrious, clever, and lucky enough, they become 'known' (which is to say, called upon regularly) in the most diffuse forms of media such as television, radio, newspapers, and magazines. A host of lesser 'knowns' crowd the corridors of new-class institutions, including various think tanks, special offices of federal agencies, hospitals, universities, and other strategic sites that now afford occasional, if not regular, opportunities for public visibility. Those outside these spheres of public influence on medical ethical matters generally teach or practice medicine in the clinical trenches." They go on to point out that Arthur Caplan has encouraged bioethicists to participate publicly as much as possible in bioethical matters. They quote him as saying, "The challenge is for bioethicists to position themselves to be on panels, boards and other decision making bodies where public policy positions will be established--where the exploding changes in health care that are now underway will be addressed."

17. See again the Devries and Conrad quote in footnote 16. But anyone who has ever organized ethics conferences, especially in medical ethics, will be familiar with the phenomenon of being showered with requests to "present" at the conference. (At applied ethics conferences, one never gives papers; one always "presents.") Sometimes quite exorbitant fees are asked (in line with the corporate culture to which many of these experts aspire), but sometimes applicants explain in a kind of plaintive way that they will work for free because they are "trying to get established" in the business.
18. For more detail on these matters, see my article, "Normative Ethics" in the *Encyclopedia of Bioethics.*
19. The most important essays by Foot are "Moral Beliefs" and "Moral Arguments" both collected in her book, *Virtues and Vices.* The most important statement of Elizabeth Anscombe's views is in her magisterial article "Modern Moral Philosophy". And Iris Murdoch's views are best stated in the essays collected in her book, *The Sovereignty of Good Over Other Concepts.*
20. Rawls abandonment of the older theory was a bit abrupt and caused, one suspects, more than a few bruised feelings. He dispatched the life's work of R.M. Hare, the leading moral philosopher in the older metaethical tradition, in a few sentences (*Theory of Justice,* p. 51). For an illustration of the bruised feelings, see Hare's two part review of *A Theory of Justice in Ratio.*
21. This new turn in Hare's thinking is fully on display in *Moral Thinking,* although Hare would not characterize the change in his views quite as I have.
22. Of special importance in the revival of utilitarianism was Parfit's *Reasons and Persons.*
23. I say a good deal more about these strategies and why I think they fail in an article, "Virtue Ethics: Radical or Routine" which will appear in an anthology forthcoming from Oxford University Press on moral epistemology edited by Linda Zagzebski.
24. As developed in their enormously successful textbook in medical ethics, *The Principles of Biomedical Ethics.*
25. See Nagel's remarks on pp. 185-188 of *The View from Nowhere* and Parfit's remarks on pp. 453-454 of *Reasons and Person.*
26. This view is first fully introduced in his article, "A Theory of Justice: Political, not Metaphysical" and receives its full elaboration in Political Liberalism and The Law of Peoples. A similar approach to the problem of moral pluralism is found, I believe, in Rorty's "The Priority of Democracy to Philosophy".

27. It is important to point out that although applied ethicists have helped themselves to this Rawlsian strategy for purposes of applied ethics, Rawls himself does not introduce it for that purpose.
28. See, for example, many of the articles in *A Matter of Principles? Ferment in U.S. Bioethics.* Edited by DuBose, Hamel and O'Connell.
29. Once again, I am going to pass lightly over some treacherous philosophical territory. There are many kinds of ethical relativism and many more difficulties in formulating clearly each of these kinds. I will proceed here as if these complications can be ignored—as I think they probably can for our purposes.
30. This point is frequently put by saying that the truth of descriptive relativism is irrelevant to the truth of normative relativism. I agree with the conclusion, but I would prefer not to lean on such a sharp distinction between the descriptive and the normative.
31. In this sense, I agree with Nagel and Parfit that we should not foreclose genuine optimism about discovering the truth in ethics. Indeed, I have difficulty knowing what human practical life would be like if that possibility were genuinely foreclosed.
32. See his discussion in the last chapter of *Ethics and the Limits of Philosophy.*
33. And on this topic MacIntyre has a vast amount to say, especially in the last quarter of *Whose Justice, Which Rationality?*
34. Notice the similarity here to the problem that dominated much of mid-century analytic epistemology: the problem of the criterion.
35. This is a fear most ably articulated, of course, in Kant's moral thought and felt strongly by his heirs in contemporary philosophy.

References

Anscombe, E. (1958). 'Modern moral philosophy,' *Philosophy,* 33, 1-19.

Beauchamp, T.L. & Childress, J.F. (2001). *Principles of Biomedical Ethics* (5th ed.). New York: Oxford University Press.

Blackmun, H. (1973). *Roe v. Wade* [Online]. Available: http://www.tourolaw.edu/patch/Roe/

DuBose, E.R., Hamel, R.P., & O'Connell, L.J. (1994). *A Matter of Principles? Ferment in U.S. Bioethics.* Valley Forge, PA: Trinity Press International.

Foot, P. (2002). *Virtues and Vices.* New York: Oxford University Press.

Hare, R.M. (1982). *Moral Thinking.* New York: Oxford University Press.

InterAction Council. (1996). *In search of global ethical standards.* [Online]. Available: www.asiawide.or.ip

Jonsen, A. (1998). *The Birth of Bioethics.* New York: Oxford University Press.

Kung, H. (1996). *Yes To a Global Ethic.* New York: Continuum Publishing Company.

MacIntyre, A. (1988). *Whose Justice, Which Rationality?* Notre Dame, IN: University of Notre Dame Press.

MacIntyre, A. (1994). *After Virtue.* London: Duckworth.

Murdoch, I. (1967). *Sovereignty of Good Over Other Concepts.* Cambridge: Cambridge University Press.

O'Connor, S., Kennedy, A., & Souter, D. (1992). *Planned Parenthood of Southeastern PA. v. Casey* [Online]. Available: http://www.tourolaw.edu/patch/Casey/Judgement.asp

Parfit, D. (1984). *Reasons and Persons.* New York: Oxford University Press.
Rawls, J. (1971). *A Theory of Justice.* Cambridge: Harvard University Press.
Rawls, J. (1993). *Political Liberalism.* New York: Columbia University Press.
Solomon, W.D. (1995). 'Normative Ethics,' in W.T. Reich (Ed.), *Encyclopedia of Bioethics,* Vol. 2 (pp. 736-748). New York: Simon & Schuster MacMillan.
Taylor, C. (1992). *The Ethics of Authenticity.* Cambridge: Harvard University Press.
Taylor, C. (1992). *Sources of the Self.* Cambridge: Harvard University Press.
Williams, B. (1986). *Ethics and the Limits of Philosophy.* Cambridge: Harvard University Press.

Global and Particular Bioethics

Kevin Wm. Wildes, S.J

I. Introduction

Globalization has become a common expression in contemporary life. People talk about it, write about it, and argue about it. Globalization has also been the target of numerous street protests and demonstrations and yet it is championed by other people. The use of the term globalization has even become part of bioethics.[1] There is, however, a danger that in the widespread use of the term globalization the term will lose significance and become a meaningless slogan. We must ask what does the term mean when it is used in bioethics?

At first glance the use of the term globalization presents a paradox for bioethics. While there is talk about global bioethics there is also a greater discussion of "multi-culturalism" and "diversity" in bioethics and a concern that the field be more than "American" bioethics.[2] There is an emphasis in the field on the particular, cultural, or religious ethics while talking about global bioethics. Yet, few people seem to grasp that the calls for globalization and multi-culturalism may not fit together easily. The desire to have a global ethic may not coincide with a respect for local or community norms.

H.T. Engelhardt, Jr. (ed), *Global Bioethics* (pp. 362–379).

As a field, bioethics highlights this tension more than most other fields of inquiry. The field brings together medicine and ethics both of which struggle with the tension of the universal and the particular, the global and the local.

The essays in this volume by David Solomon and Joseph Boyle[3] make some of the problems of globalization very clear. In examining the field of bioethics, and philosophical ethics generally, Solomon raises the "export problem." He asks: If we hope to develop a global bioethics is there anything to export to the rest of the globe? In the export problem Solomon raises very fundamental questions about both globalization and the substance of bioethics. His questions call to mind an article in the *New York Times* that took a critical look at the growing role of bioethics in public policy debates and health care practice (Stolberg, 2001). The article was prompted by the debate about President Bush's policy on federal stem cell research. The *Times'* article used the specific question as a way to thoughtfully, critically explore the field of bioethics and the roles that people in the field have come to play. Bioethics has, at the moment, taken on an aura of expertise in American life. Bioethicists are sought after for television appearances, commentaries, and news shows. Their counsel is sought on public commissions at federal and local levels. They are employed by hospitals, universities, research firms, and health care organizations for their expertise. They are also used in courts of law (Wildes, 1997). The *Times'* article not only noted the roles for bioethics but it also raised important questions about the content of the field and how it is practice. The articles asked fundamental questions about the substance of the field. The *Times'* article raised the question, to borrow from David Solomon's essay, of whether or not the field has anything, really, to export. The article also raised the question of whether or not the field is aware of these limits and problems. Later in this essay I would like to raise the corollary to Solomon's export problem: the import problem.

In his essay Joseph Boyle raises another key set of fundamental questions for global bioethics. Though rarely articulated, an examination of the literature of bioethics demonstrates that there are different understandings of the field and different expectations about what the field can accomplish. Boyle thoughtfully examines the different aspects of the field of bioethics. Bioethics not only has differences about method and content but there are also has very important differences about how the field is defined and differing expectations about what the field can do.

Boyle identifies an important tension that exists between particular moral judgments and universal moral norms. This distinction is important since the field attempts to speak on both the levels of particular judgments and on the general level as well. Often, in areas of policy and clinical ethics, bioethics in involved in particular judgments. At the same time, the field needs to be able to articulate general principles. The field of bioethics is often caught between the level of general principle and particular judgment. Boyle's exploration of bioethics and natural law raises important questions for the possibilities of a global bioethics. He argues that the natural law can give broad moral guidance. But, the general level does not, however, lead to particular moral judgments. This exploration by Boyle raises fundamental questions about how much guidance a global bioethics will yield. It is the tension between the multi-cultural and the universal.

This essay will argue that, in a sense, the new is old. In debates about globalism bioethics finds itself caught in a dilemma that has always been a conundrum for ethics whenever particular moral cases are addressed. On the one hand, many of the issues and questions in bioethics are particular and they need to be addressed within the context of particular morality and locally cultural. Today such efforts are often captured under labels like "multi-culturalism" or "moral pluralism" and we champion respect for diversity in views and cultures. On the other hand, there is a desire to articulate an ethic that transcends local boundaries and establish global bioethics. This dilemma is not new. The Romans faced a similar dilemma in administering an expansive empire. Within the empire there were many cultures with differing, particular moral views. At the same time, there was a belief that there was a natural moral law which transcended particular cultures (Boyle, 2006). But the natural law worked at a general level and one needed some type of casuistry to address particular cases. The "bio-politics" discussed by Kurt Bayertz identifies an important element in how the field of bioethics works.

II. Defining Bioethics: The Emergence of the Field

To scrutinize claims that are made, positively and negatively, about global bioethics it is important to understand both how and why the field of bioethics has emerged. Understanding the field will be helpful in evaluating claims for a global bioethics. In recent years there has been a good deal of reflection on the development of bioethics as a distinct field (Reich, 1994; Jonsen, 1998; Walter & Klein, 2003; Stevens, 2000). These reflections, though diverse, can serve as a basis for understanding bioethics.

If someone knew nothing about the history of medicine or bioethics that person might wonder about the relationship of ethics and medicine before the emergence of bioethics in the late 1960s.[4] Contemporary discussions in bioethics can sometimes leave the impression that there was no ethical reflection in medicine before the emergence of bioethics. Of course this is a false impression that is easy to correct. There has been long association of philosophy, ethics, and medicine dating to the ancient Greek schools of medicine and many of these associations have been about ethics. In the ancient world there were several different school of philosophical reflection about medicine. One thinks of some of the works of Hippocrates, Galen, Democrates,

Plato, and Aristotle (Carrick, 2001), as examples of ancient philosophical reflections on medicine. However, these schools, though they differed in many respects, were primarily concerned about the physician's conduct in a paternalistic relationship. Ancient writings shape the beginning of philosophical reflections on medicine in the west. In addition to philosophical reflections there have also been extensive theological reflections on ethics and medicine in many religious traditions (Fletcher, 1960; Healy, 1956; Jakobvits, 1958; Ramsey, 1970; Gustafson, 1975; McCormick, 1984).

In light of this long history of ethical reflection involving medicine, one might ask: Why was there a need to develop a new area of ethical reflection that has been named bioethics? Why not simply rely on the various traditions of medical ethics which already existed? There are at least three developments that encouraged the emergence of bioethics as a field distinct from the traditional medical ethics. One can argue that traditional medical ethics was really physician ethics.[5] It focused on the conduct of physicians and the virtue of obedience for others like patients and nurses. Bioethics emerged in response to the new choices and challenges brought out by the development of medical knowledge and technology

A key influence in the development of bioethics was the development of scientific medicine. The nineteenth and twentieth century witnessed the grounding of medical epistemology in the basic sciences. The modern understanding of illness is rooted in anatomical, physiological, bacteriological, and—now—genetic, causal factors. Changes in medical epistemology in the modern age have been tied to new, scientific standards for the acquisition and validation of knowledge. One could argue, more accurately, that modern medicine was born when the clinic and the laboratory became conjoined (Engelhardt, 2000). The union of the clinic and the laboratory provided a basis for the development of scientific medical knowledge and related technological interventions. Laboratory research became essential to clinical practice and research.

In the contemporary world of medical miracles we often forget the profound impact of the scientific model on medical epistemology and medical practice. The joining of the laboratory and the clinic led to a transformation of medical knowledge and to the development of medical technology and interventions. From the development of effective surgery to the manipulation of human genes, the physician, as medical scientist, has been transformed from an observer to a manipulator of nature and the body. These scientific possibilities have led to the transformation of expectations and goals of medicine.[6]

For most of its history there was very little that medicine could actually do very little to help patients. Gradually, with each success, the social expectations of medicine have changed. In contemporary first world nations, people have come to think of medicine as curative (Cassell, 1991). In the past people looked to god, or the gods, primarily for a cure. Cures often were thought to be miraculous. Medicine was looked to alleviate the suffering of patients but not, necessarily, to cure them. With the development of a knowledge base that is scientific and the development of technology to use this scientific knowledge medicine has been radically changed. Today, in first world medicine, we expect medicine to cure patients. Some have argued that with the development of knowledge and technology the very purpose of medicine has changed.[7]

The changes that have taken place in medicine have not come exclusively from the development of medical knowledge and technology. These developments have also been driven, in part, by development of other technologies, like the automobile or the computer, or sociological developments such as the urbanization of society. These types of changes are important factors as they have made these new medical technologies accessible to men and women in society.[8]

While the development of medical knowledge and technology are necessary conditions to understand bioethics, these developments alone are not sufficient to explain the emergence of this field. These scientific and technological developments are only part of the story. The creation of real choices and alternatives is a major element in the emergence of the field. To understand why neither of these sources is sufficient for contemporary medicine one must, I think, take the phenomena of moral pluralism and cultural diversity into account. What I mean by moral pluralism is the phenomenon in which people hold, not only different moral views on an issue (e.g., abortion), but also that they work out of different moral frameworks and methodologies (Wildes, 2003).

The development of medical knowledge and technology creates real choices and decisions for people; especially patients. Traditional medical ethics had been focused on *physician* ethics and judgment about what was good for a patient (Veatch, 2000, 1981). The development of scientific medicine gave patients choices and options about the course of treatments to be pursued or refused. If the physician and patient shared the same moral values and way of thinking, such choices may not be all that problematic. However, when patients and physicians hold different views, the understanding of medical ethics needs to be transformed beyond the judgment of the physician alone.[9] Determining what is in the patient's best interest can not be judged by the physician alone. The physician may speak to the medical best interest of the patient but not, necessarily, the overall best interest of the patient. To make such best interest judgments the patient needs to be involved. Furthermore, in secular societies there are likely to be different religious views that shape people's judgments about what is morally appropriate. That is why procedures like informed consent has come to play such a central role in both clinical and research ethics. Such procedures allow people to exercise judgment about what is in their best interest.

Moral pluralism not only affects the relationship of patients and physicians. It also affects the profession of medicine itself. A key part of the classical notion of a profession was that there was a moral dimension to the profession. Many people still assume that professionals act in ethical ways and that it is reasonable to have fiduciary expectations of professionals. However, with a more widespread moral pluralism, there will be a different view about what is appropriate or inappropriate professional conduct. If one studies codes of professional ethics in health care one will find a move away from a particular content to more general procedures. In issues such as abortion, physician assisted suicide and conflicts of interest one finds a wide range of opinions, among physicians, about what is appropriate behavior. There is moral pluralism within the profession as well as from others such as patients and nurses. So, it becomes more and more difficult to sustain claims based on an internal morality of medicine which had been a cornerstone to traditional medical ethics. The internal ethic of physicians becomes less and less tenable.

At the same time one cannot assume, in a secular, pluralistic society, that theological ethics will supply the type of guidance that is needed. In several religious traditions there have been long, well developed reflections on medicine, its uses, and its ethics. In light of these traditions it is not surprising that theologians played such an important role in the development of bioethics. Many who first grasped the profound impact of developing medical knowledge and technologies were theologian. They were often the first voices to raise broader social questions that transcended traditional physician ethics. As the field of bioethics began to emerge it is not surprising that many theologians, working out of faith traditions that addressed questions of medical care, would be interested in these questions. These traditions had long standing reflections on medicine and health care. They were able to easily engage the changes that were taking place in medicine. Yet, fairly quickly, theology came to play less and less of a public role in bioethics. The role of theology and religious commitments has been a difficult question not only for bioethics but for many areas of public life in the United States. But, as ethicist Daniel Callahan has argued, bioethics became acceptable in America because it "pushed religion aside" (Callahan, 1993, pp. 8-9). Callahan does not argue that religious thought became irrelevant to these questions. Rather that as bioethics became a form of "public" discourse (Caplan, 1993, pp.14-15) it moved to more the more "neutral" languages of philosophy and law and away from the closed language of the medical profession and theological discourse.[10]

Cultures and communities often embody a common moral vision which helps bind a group together. In secular societies, where there are often many cultures, moral pluralism is very likely. In turn the two traditional sources of ethical reflection for medicine—professional ethics and theological ethics—are much less helpful. The two sources of moral knowledge are limited in their effectiveness in a secular, pluralistic society. They are very helpful within communities that share the same basic views and commitments. Religious traditions will have far less claim on the lives of men and women in general in such societies. Furthermore, traditional professional classes will be more limited in their moral authority.

It is also important to understand that the field of bioethics emerged at a time where there was a greater awareness of individual rights, choices, and the protection of individual freedoms and liberties. This has been particularly true in the United States. Bioethics emerged in the era of civil rights in the United States. It was a time when minorities and women were arguing for, and achieving, greater and greater legal protection. At a time when there were more and more options for medical treatments, patients were more and more aware of their liberties and protections. It was a time when many groups, such as women and minorities, found a voice in society and in their lives. It was also a time when patients found a voice.

Bioethics then emerges as the result of several developments in contemporary secular societies. First there is the development of medical knowledge and technology which expands options and creates real choices in medical care. With these choices the question arises of who is the appropriate authority to decide what is or is not appropriate treatment. Such choices involve more than medical judgment. Second, bioethics emerges, in part, as a response to the multi-culturalism and moral pluralism in secular societies like the United States. The emergence of different moral voices and views means that there will be differing views on *appropriate* medical care. Again this judgment about what is appropriate care is more that a strict medical judgment. Third, the field emerges as a way to help people from different moral views navigate these choices and cooperate together. In studying the emergence of the field one can make the claim that bioethics provides an insight into the life and practices of a society.

The tension of global and cultural ethics is a new version of an ancient problem. It was a problem faced by the Romans with their multi-cultural empire. Multi-culturalism and moral pluralism represent a challenge for a global ethic. The difficulty will be to avoid a complete relativism where only power wins the day or the simple assertion of a global ethic.

III. Bioethical Consensus in a Secular Society

In the midst of moral pluralism bioethics has sought some common ground—in reason, affections, and intuitions—to help address difficult moral issues. Often, the language of "consensus" has been used as a way to find a common ground in bioethics. In trying to understand the claims that are often made for a global bioethics it is essential to understand the claims that are often made in the name of "bioethical consensus."[11] The notion of consensus is important for those who want to claim a global bioethics. The claims about consensus are something like a bioethical "jus gentium." But the claims about consensus also illustrate that bioethics is closely related to bio-politics, as Kurt Bayertz argues in his essay.[12] The relationship of ethics and politics articulated by Aristotle is evident in many areas of bioethics.

A. Pluralism and Consensus

Consensus can take place at a number of different levels: at the level of belief, it affects theory and cognition; at the level of action, it is pragmatic and practical; and at the level of values, it enables coherence and motivation. For consensus to play an important role in bioethical method one needs to understand which of these levels is being asserted. Thus, it becomes important to ask why a consensus exists (Rescher, 1993, p.15). Is it mindless conformity? Is it about a submission to, or support of, existing power structures? Or is the consensus driven by the weight of appropriate evidence? Nicholas Rescher suggests that one should ask whether the consensus being appealed to is an idealized version of consensus or one that is practically attainable. Philosophers tend to use the former while social scientists deploy the latter. Understanding what is meant by consensus when it is used in bioethics is important for exploring the extent and nature of normative claims. Also it is important to understand at what "level" consensus attributed. As I will argue, there are a number of judgments that are embedded in moral judgment and understanding where the consensus actually occurs is important. It could take place on a very general, broad level (e.g., do good and avoid evil). But as a field bioethics often addresses much more particular, specified judgments. So when people appeal to a "bioethical consensus" it is important to probe and understand what is being appealed to.

One way to understand the complexities of moving from general to particular judgments is to examine moral judgment. The nature of agreement, disagreement, consensus, and dissensus can be understood through an analysis of moral judgments. Boyle's essay examines, in part, the complicated questions surrounding moral judgment. Of course the questions of judgment take us back to the assumptions people make about the field of bioethics. Is the field to function as the clinical "answer person" or the clinical Solomon when there are moral disputes? Moral judgments should be understood not simply as choices about what should be done in a particular situation, but as involving logically prior judgments about how one justifies such choices. One's assumptions about moral rationality are a priori judgments that commit one to a particular view of the moral world. For example, those in the natural law tradition understand moral rationality in a different way from those who deploy an instrumentalist view of reason. Charting the geography of judgment reveals a number of points where agreement can be reached and help understand when a breakdown of agreement occurs.

The reality of moral pluralism in a secular society illustrates that there are many ways in which to construct the categories of the moral world. By distinguishing the three levels or types of judgment (object, justification, foundation) involved in moral argument, the spectrum for possible moral agreement and disagreement is greatly increased. It ranges from a strong sense of agreement, in which we are of one mind on how and why to proceed, to a weaker sense of proceeding together but only for a specific, limited venture.

The complex spectrum of relationships that lies between complete agreement at the levels of object, reason, and foundation to complete disagreement on those levels can be summarized under eight headings.

1. Object level agreement with agreement on justification and foundations.
2. Object level agreement with agreement about justification and disagreement about foundations.
3. Object level agreement with disagreement about justification.
4. Object level agreement with agreement/disagreement in part on the levels of justification.
5. Object level agreement with disagreement about both justification and foundations.
6. Object level disagreement with agreement on justification and foundations.
7. Object level disagreement with justificatory agreement/disagreement in part.
8. Object level disagreement with disagreement about justification and foundations (Wildes, 2000).

The possibilities and the limits of each genus of controversy resolution in bioethics can be analyzed under these eight headings. To reach agreement regarding justification there needs to be prior agreement on what counts as a relevant moral appeal and what is a proper set of moral reasons to which one could turn. Unless moral agents stand within the same foundational framework, they will not reach agreement on how moral judgments are justified.

Boyle's essay raises the difficulties associated with moral judgment. The more carefully one examines the complexities of moral judgment the more cautious one should become about the possibility of a global bioethics. Even if there is significant agreement on a global level, which there often is not, it is hard to grasp how such agreement will help on the level of judgment which so often at the heart of bioethics.

The different levels of judgment point out the fragility of any claim for consensus. The levels should make anyone skeptical of the depth of any consensus.

B. The Sociology of Agreement and Consensus

The field of bioethics has been marked by the work of international and national commissions, hospital ethics committees, Institutional Review

Boards, and Data Safety and Monitoring Boards. The work of these groups has been important to establishing the credibility of the field. The work of various bioethics commissions and committees provide examples of moral agreement in a secular, morally pluralistic culture. Given that commissions have played an inspirational role in the development of bioethics, it is important to examine how such committees and commissions achieve agreement. The sociology of such commissions raises important and interesting questions about what conclusions can be drawn from their work. The first question bears on the composition these committees. Usually people who are selected for such work are, at least, moral acquaintances. One rarely finds individuals with strongly different views, like a Pat Buchanan or a Rev. Al Sharpton, appointed to the same committee or commission. In the selection of members, the committee's agreement is already being managed. A second question focuses on the committee's process. Such groups are shaped by a dynamic toward reaching a consensus.[13] The expectation, before the commission begins work, is that the committee will reach consensus on certain recommendations. A third question focuses on the establishment of the agenda of the committee. Insofar as the committee is mandated to act in certain questions (and not in others) the possibility of disagreement is reduced.

Notice how the work of such groups contrasts with the exchanges between individuals with great moral differences. One can imagine Cardinal Ratzinger and Peter Singer agreeing in a chance meeting in the John Paul II Hospital that the treatment of a PVS patient in the MICU should not be continued. However, as they discuss the mission of the hospital and the practices it should or should not countenance, the limits of their agreements emerge. They do not agree, for example, about the question of whether or not John Paul II Hospital should distribute condoms as part of its care for HIV infected patients. As individuals are apt to have wide ranging discussions of issues, their disagreements often become apparent very quickly. Unlike Cardinal Ratzinger and Peter Singer the committee will not, officially, wander from its topic. The agenda of such committees gives directions to, and sets limits for, their moral reflections.[14]

The control of the agenda is a crucial point often overlooked in the heralding of agreement by committees. A necessary condition for resolving a moral dispute is consensus regarding the essence of the dispute. So often in bioethics the most difficult problem is the lack of a common description of a moral controversy (e.g., abortion, assisted suicide). Is abortion about rights of choice or the killing of an innocent human being? Is physician assisted suicide an act of mercy or an act of murder? If an agenda is established before a committee or commission begins its work, then the mapping of a general moral geography has already begun. The agenda not only identifies the problem, but also provides a way whereby differences are confined and minimized.

Understanding these sociological elements should lead philosophers and ethicists to be cautious about how one should evaluate the claims of "agreement." It is helpful to remember that agreements and disagreements can be found at a number of points in bioethical discussions. We simply need to be clear on what is being agreed to and not make extravagant claims.

Excluding thinkers like Buchanan or Sharpton from commissions means that fundamental questions about the agenda or agreement will not be asked. Consider Sharpton and Buchanan's participation on a national commission evaluating federal research and the funding of reproductive technologies. Conceivably they may agree that such research should be stopped yet they may reach their conclusions from very different reasons. Buchanan may see the research as an immoral tampering with the natural order and an unjustified use of state authority and resources while Sharpton may regard such research as unjust because its results cannot be distributed equally to all and because it takes necessary resources from the poor. While they agree on a policy recommendation, few would see this as a hopeful sign for future moral deliberations. One has only to think of recent examples to see how important controlling the membership of commissions is to achieving a consensus.

There are a number of interesting examples of consensus ethics and statements in public bioethics. One recent contrast is the work of President Clinton's National Bioethics Advisory Commission (NBAC) and President Bush's President's Council on Bioethics (PCB). Both groups examined the question of stem cell research. While there were similarities of opinions, each group reached differing conclusions about the direction, and ethical justification for, federal policy on stem cell research. When President Bush did not renew the terms of two members of the PCB who had dissenting views on embryo research (Smallwood, 2004; Blumenstyk, 2004), it provided an interesting example of managing bioethical consensus. James Childress gives an older, though very insightful account of ethical consensus in the public forum.[15]

Childress's observations remind us that when people claim agreement, it is important to know what types of questions were asked and agreed to. His account raises anew the question of how and what kinds of agreement are possible in a secular, morally pluralistic society. Contrary to the Jonsen-Toulmin experience in the work of the National Commission, Childress cites agreement on the level of principle.[16] It is possible that different methods of bioethics may be appropriate to different activities. For example, issues of public policy, or institutional policy, may be better articulated as principles insofar as principles give broad guidelines for actions. At the same time, particular clinical issues may be better addressed by the agreement of cases. Since method and content cannot be separated it is clear that different methods reflect different moral views.

Committees and commissions have come to play a central role in bioethics. From local hospitals and nursing home ethics committees to national policy commissions, committees have taken on important roles in moral deliberations. As one examines the work of such groups, one becomes aware, however, of the importance of power and control in guiding the resolutions of such committees. The power to set the agenda, membership, and timetable are crucial to reaching any agreement. The Childress account helps us to understand how the agreement of such commissions is managed. It relies on both the agenda of the commission being set and the members of the commission not dissenting in bad faith. That such agreements are managed should not be surprising. Governments, like the people who run them, often seek the opinions of others to support a desired policy or to suppress an unpopular one. The Health Care Task force of the Clinton Administration assembled an ethics task force. Members of the task force shared some common assumptions about society and health care that were important for their deliberations (Daniels, 1994). It is not hard to imagine how the conclusions of the committee would have been very different had its membership been altered in substantial ways.

Again a good example of such managed solutions in the *presidential bioethics* of stem cell research. The Clinton Administration's NBAC made recommendations about the use of embryos for stem cell research which were more open and liberal than those made by President Bush's Bioethics Commission, it is clear from the guidelines that he set out that the recommendations will be much more conservative and restrictive.[17] The Commission will reach very different conclusions from the last presidential commission because the membership is decidedly different and the contours of the questions have been set in very different ways.

Members are selected and agendas are set so that a desired result may be achieved. The members of the commission, unlike the Senate (in its role to advise and consent), are bound to the agendas given them. What emerges from this account is a picture of agreement that is often carefully managed and crafted. The result may be an agreement that is more causally achieved and less rationally justified than we craved. This confusion about the nature of agreement occurs often in bioethics. The tendency is to draw principled conclusions when the conclusions are more sociological in nature.

The article by Kurt Bayertz in this volume gives another example of this point. Bayertz analyzes the fragile nature of "European Bioethics." It is clear from his article that the challenges of moral pluralism are not limited to the United States. Furthermore, he also highlights the political nature of many of the claims for such a consensus in Europe (Bayertz, 2006). His essay illustrates the political dimension of bioethics.

Just as there has been a great deal of emphasis in bioethics on respect for persons, and their judgments, the phenomenon of global bioethics raises important questions about respect for cultures and cultural diversity. It is not often clear, and seldom explored, how a global bioethics does not degenerate into some form of cultural imperialism.

IV. Possibilities and Limits for Global Bioethics

As one examines the controversies in bioethics it seems that the potential for a global bioethical consensus is limited. This ought not to be surprising in a morally pluralistic, secular society. Rescher notes that any talk or use of consensus must also investigate dissensus (Rescher, 1993). Consensus and dissensus, like health and disease, dissensus are dialectical terms, and one cannot be understood without the other. In general the over emphasis on consensus has led to an over emphasis on agreement and not enough attention being paid to disagreement.

That there should be dissensus in bioethics is not surprising. If morality is part of a way of life and ethical reflection is grounded in moral experience, then different experiences will lead to different views of what is or is not morally appropriate behavior. One way to understand these different bioethical views is by using a moral relativist view. Often, when people use terms like "moral pluralism" they are employing a relativist position. The relativist view is that it really does not matter which position one holds on any matter. However, a problem with this view is that if one holds it, he or she will have no incentive to reach a consensus with anyone who holds different views. There is no reason for anyone to negotiate a consensus if he or she has no reasons to hold any position whatsoever. Furthermore, the relativist view also leaves us with no intellectual or moral argument against the use of power simply to impose a position. We are left in a position where might makes right. An alternative argument would be that in a secular world, which may have many differing moralities, the only source of moral authority will rest with the human person. People are able to work together, morally, by consent and agreement. It is the web of agreement and consent that becomes the basis of moral authority in a secular world filled with many gods and commandments.

In thinking through the language of global bioethics it might be helpful to make some distinctions about ethical consensus and dissensus. Elsewhere I have argued that morality is part of a way of life (Wildes, 2000). It is often tied to particular cultures and communities. If one thinks about global bioethics from this perspective it does not seem very useful. But, if one views the question in terms of respect for persons as moral agents, then one can talk about a thin sense of global bioethics in terms of respect for persons and cultures. In such a view of the world one can talk of moral friends, who live in a moral community and share a thick moral world view, moral strangers who have differing world views but who can cooperate in moral endeavors by using public, agree upon procedures of agreement and consent, and moral acquaintances who rely on proceeds but share some overlapping moral views. In such a world of respect and moral pluralism a person, and a community, needs to understand his/her moral commitments. In such world a person and community will often face a question of cooperating with others in different moral enterprises. To maintain their integrity they will need to know their moral values so they can understand what can and cannot be compromised.

An alternative approach, articulated by Rescher and helpful for bioethics, is "perspectival pluralism" (Childress, 1994, p.105). This position holds that a person needs to have the "courage of one's convictions." One needs to know the positions she or he holds and how they differ from other positions. Such knowledge is crucial to compromise and consensus. These are essential to living out a notion of integrity. Any meaningful practice of global bioethics will involve a respect for these differences, often significant, in a multi cultural world.

V. Conclusions

Bioethics has emerged for a number of reasons. The development of medical technology has created choices where once there was only chance. Also, there are real moral differences about what choices should or should not be made. Yet, there is a need to find ways for people with different moral views to work together in medical research and delivery. As one examines the agreement in the bioethical consensus one recognizes that the consensus may not be what people often hope that it is. Agreements in the field are not all the same. Nor are all disagreements the same. The more one understands the complexity of moral judgments, and the various types and degrees of agreement, the more one understands how limited the force of agreements often is and how important disagreements are often masked. Scrutiny of the bioethical consensus reveals more dissensus than first appeared. Bayertz's examination of European bioethics, in this volume provides a good example of the fragile, limited nature of consensus.

Boyle's insight about moral judgment, in his essay, helps make clear the limits of any notion of "global bioethics". A natural law method will yield general moral guidance but not specific judgments. An analysis of moral judgment leads to more modest views on the possibilities for a global bioethics. Solomon also raises important questions about the possibilities for global bioethics by posing the export problem. One can turn the problem around and see the essential dilemma in a different light. If there is really a global bioethics, can we *import* as well as export bioethics or is there a bioethics trade surplus? Even if there is "thick" agreement concerning a moral view of the world, the application of the view will vary in particular judgments. Some may argue that this criticism is unfair as it is a problem for every systematic moral view. This would be a fair objection except that many in the field of bioethics have portrayed the field as responding to very particular questions and moral controversies.

Even in the midst of moral pluralism and fragmentation Boyle raises an important point when he talks about finding some common moral ground.

In his essay Boyle points out that a natural law method has often rested on some sense of a *jus gentium*. But, in contemporary societies marked by moral pluralism one can ask to what extent a *jus gentium* exists. One could argue that what does bind people of different moral views together is the role of consent of free individuals. Such a view also limits government intervention and regulation in bioethical matters. This common ground allows others, outside a moral community, to raise questions about the moral practices of a community. I have argued elsewhere that the realm of procedural ethics, based on consent and agreement, provides our best hope of a common ground. This procedural ethics will not provide the rich, think ethic that many long for in a global ethics. But, it can provide a thin framework for limited, common moral conversation. One can understand the thin agreements of procedural ethics only if they are built on thicker, richer understandings of the moral life. Absent such overlapping values the procedures could not succeed ethically. Procedures need some form of moral justification if they are to be moral. If there are procedures that transcend moral communities then they may provide a way to identify the common ground of moral acquaintances. The agreement about procedures provides a way to articulate the overlapping agreements that exist for moral strangers and acquaintances.

In the end we are left with as many questions as answers. How might we explore, and respond, to the global questions that Boyle has raised about the ability to critique a particular moral community? How might we respond to the export problems raised by Solomon? If the domestic problems are as significant as he argues, can we even speak of a "regional" bioethics? These questions are not trivial. As bioethics continues to play a role in the development of health care policy, the way the field is conceived will have a direct bearing on the evolution of policy and the authority given to policy makers. The tension of global and local will continue to be an on going challenge in thinking about these issues. We may do well to learn from the emphasis in bioethics on "respect for persons" which has grounded our search for ways to acknowledge different moral views and still cooperate. Respect for persons, for example, is the foundation of procedures such as informed consent. The challenge for us now is to think of procedures that can help to protect the integrity of cultures in bioethics.

Notes

1. See, for example, Alastair Campbell (1999); Hyakudai Sakamoto (1999); Lori Knowles (2001); Tuija Takala (2001).
2. See, for example, Maura Ryan (2004).
3. David Solomon, "Domestic Disarray and Imperial Ambition: Contemporary Applied Ethics and the Prospects for Global Bioethics" and Joseph Boyle, "Natural Law and Global Bioethics" in this volume.
4. I use the term field consciously to distinguish bioethics from specific disciplines. While bioethics has been dominated by philosophical and legal thinking it is an

interdisciplinary field engaging medicine, law, philosophy, theology, and many other disciplines. See Albert Jonsen, (1998).

5. See Robert Veatch (1981).
6. See, for example, Callahan (1998).
7. See Cassell (1991).
8. See, K. Wildes (2003).
9. See Robert M. Veatch (1981).
10. See L. B. McCullough (1999).
11. One can argue that given the dilemmas of modern moral philosophy to speak about moral truth that philosophers have shifted claims away from truth towards consensus. In bioethics, for example, see, Jonathan D. Moreno (1995).
12. See, Kurt Bayertz, in this volume.
13. See, Jonathan Moreno (1991 & 1994).
14. See, James F. Childress (1994).
15. James Childress provides an interesting and instructive case study in the management of agreement and consensus in bioethics. Childress examines the deliberations of the Human Fetal Tissue Transplantation Research Panel (hereafter, HFTTR). In 1988 a moratorium was declared on the use of federal funds for HFTTR by Robert Windom, then Assistant Secretary for Health (U.S. Department of Health and Human Services). The National Institutes of Health appointed the HFTTR Panel in the fall of 1988 to respond to ten questions raised by Secretary Windom.

    Even before it began work, Secretary Windom and the NIH had given the HFTTR Panel significant help in its task since the framing of issues directs the ways in which any moral problem can be resolved. The framing process itself can make the moral pluralism of a committee more manageable. In the case of the HFTTR Panel, Assistant Secretary Windom had set the agenda in his ten questions. Childress notes that Windom's questions focused on the linkage between abortion and HFTTR practices. Indeed, Childress argues that Windom's questions constrained the Panel's deliberations. Childress himself makes the point that a different set of questions could have led to different outcomes. What is of interest here is that the process of deliberation and its outcome were helped and directed by the charge given to the Panel. As one looks to the agreements and consensus of panels, commissions, or hospital ethics committees, one needs to examine how the boundaries and agenda of deliberation were established.

    Childress also addresses the issue of dissent in the panel's work. He says that two of the eleven members had substantial dissent. The two dissenting Panel members produced a dissenting report, such that "panelists in the majority later expressed their concern that such a long and eloquent dissent would simply smother the report's brief responses." Childress notes that an additional meeting of the Panel was called to structure the form of the final report so that it would not be overwhelmed by the dissenting report.

    The discussion of dissent raises two important questions. First, how much agreement is necessary to a consensus? If a committee is unanimous, the consensus is obvious. However, absent unanimity, and when there is strong dissent, the degree of consensus is difficult to ascertain. Second, is the consensus based on the moral issues? A consensus report may play on certain ambiguities. Childress, for example, points out that the questions raised by the Assistant

Secretary were empirical, legal, medical, scientific, and moral. As one listens to claims of consensus it is important to determine whether the consensus is actually about the moral questions.

16. It is worth noting that Albert Jonsen and Stephen Toulmin offer a different account of consensus building. They argue that the National Commission reached consensus around cases (not principles) from which principles were articulated.
17. See National Bioethics Advisory Commission, *Ethical Issues In Stem Cell Research.* June 2000. For current documents by The Presidents Council on Bioethics go to http://www.bioethics.gov.

References

Blumenstyk, G. (2004). 'Two scientists from Bush's bioethics council say panel's reports favor ideology over facts,' *The Chronicle of Higher Education* [Online]. Available: http://chronicle.com/prm/daily/2004/03/2004030801n.htm

Callahan, D. (1993). 'Why America accepted bioethics,' *Hastings Center Report* (Special Supplement, November-December), 8-9.

Callahan, D. (1998). *False Hopes: Why America's Quest for Perfect Health is a Recipe for Failure.* New York: Simon & Schuster.

Campbell, A. (1999). 'Presidential address: global bioethics—dream or nightmare?,' *Bioethics,* 13(3/4), 183-190.

Caplan, A.L. (1993). 'What bioethics brought to the public,' *Hastings Center Report* (Special Supplement, November-December), 14-15.

Carrick, P.J. (2001). *Medical Ethics in the Ancient World.* Washington, D.C.: Georgetown University Press.

Cassell, E. (1991). *The Nature of Suffering and the Goals of Medicine.* New York: Oxford University Press.

Childress, J.F. (1994). 'Consensus in ethics and public policy: the deliberations of the U.S. human fetal tissue transplantation research panel,' in K. Bayertz (Ed.), *The Concept of Moral Consensus* (pp. 163-187). Dordrecht, The Netherlands: Kluwer Academic Publishers.

Daniels, N. (1994). 'The articulation of values and principles involved in health care reform.' *The Journal of Medicine and Philosophy,* 19(5), 425-434.

Engelhardt, H.T., Jr. (2000). Recent Developments in the Philosophy of Medicine: The Dialectic of Theory and Practice and the Moral-Political Authority of Bioethicists. Paper APA Eastern Meeting.

Fletcher, J. (1960). *Morals and Medicine.* Boston: Beacon Press.

Gustafson, J. (1975). *The Contributions of Theology in Medical Ethics.* Milwaukee: Marquette University Press.

Healy, E.F. (1956). *Medical Ethics.* Chicago: Loyola University Press.

Jakobvits, I. (1958). *Jewish Medical Ethics.* New York: Block.

Jonsen, A.R. (1998). *The Birth of Bioethics.* New York: Oxford University Press.

Knowles, L. (2001). 'The lingua franca of human rights and the rise of a global bioethics,' *Cambridge Quarterly of Healthcare Ethics,* 10(3), 253-263.

McCormick, R. (1984). *Health and Medicine in the Catholic Tradition.* New York: Crossroad Press.

McCullough, L.B. (1999). 'Laying medicine open: understanding major turning points in the history of medical ethics,' *Kennedy Institute of Ethics Journal*, 9 (1), 7-23

Moreno, J.D. (1994). 'Consensus, contracts, and committees,' *The Journal of Medicine and Philosophy*, 16(4), 393-408.

Moreno, J.D. (1994). 'Consensus by committee: philosophical and social the concept aspects of ethics committees,' in K. Bayertz (Ed.), *The Concept of Moral Consensus: The Case aof Technological Interventions into Human Reproduction* (pp. 145-162). Dordrecht: Kluwer Academic Publishers.

Moreno, J.D. (1995). *Deciding For Others.* New York: Oxford University Press.

National Bioethics Advisory Commission (June 2000). Ethical issues in stem cell research. [On-line]. Available: http://www.georgetown.edu/research/nrcbl/nbac/pubs.html

Ramsey, P. (1970). *Fabricated Man.* New Haven: Yale University Press.

Reich, W. (1994). 'The word 'bioethics': its birth and the legacies of those who shaped its meaning,' *Kennedy Institute of Ethics Journal*, 4(4), 319-336.

Rescher, N. (1993). *Pluralism: Against the Demand for Consensus.* New York: Oxford University Press.

Ryan, M. (2004). 'Beyond a western bioethics,' *Theological Studies*, 65(1), 158-177.

Sakamoto, H. (1999). 'Towards a new 'global bioethics',' *Bioethics*, 13(3/4), 191-197.

Smallwood, S. (2004). *Bush drops two supporters of embryo research from bioethics panel. The Chronicle of Higher Educations* [Online]. Available: http://chronicle.com/prm/daily/2004/03/2004030103n.htm

Stevens, M.L.T. (2000). *Bioethics in America: Origins and Cultural Politics.* Baltimore: Johns Hopkins University Press.

Stolberg, S.G. (2001, August 2). 'Bioethicists find themselves the ones being scrutinized,' *The New York Times*, p. A-1.

Takala, T. (2001). 'What is wrong with global bioethics? On the limitations of the four principles approach,' *Cambridge Quarterly of Healthcare Ethics*, 10(1), 72-77.

Veatch, R. M. (1981). *A Theory of Medical Ethics.* New York: Basic Books.

Veatch, R.M. (2000). 'Doctor does not know best: why in the new century physicians must stop trying to benefit patients,' *Journal of Medicine and Philosophy*, 25(6), 701-721.

Walter, J. & Klein, E. (Eds.). (2003). *The Story of Bioethics: From Seminal Works to Contemporary Explorations.* Washington: Georgetown University Press.

Wildes, K.S.J. (1997). 'Healthy skepticism: the emperor has very few clothes,' *Journal of Medicine and Philosophy*, 22(4), 365-371.

Wildes, K.S.J. (2000). *Moral Acquaintances: Methodology in Bioethics.* South Bend, IN: University of Notre Dame Press.

Wildes, K.S.J. (2003). 'Reshaping the human: technology, medicine, and bioethics,' in D. Hüber (Ed.), *Jahrbuch für Wissenschaft und Ethik*, (pp. 227-237). Berlin: Walter de Gruyter.

Contributors

Kurt Bayertz is a professor in the department of philosophy at the University of Münster in Germany. He was the head of the department of technology assessment at the Institute for the Systems and Technology Analyses in Biomedicine in Bad Oeynhausen.

Joseph Boyle is professor of philosophy at St Michael's College in the University of Toronto and he is also a Senior Scholar at the Canadian Catholic Bioethics Institute.

Nicholas Capaldi is the Legendre-Soulé Distinguished Chair in Business Ethics at Loyola University New Orleans.

Mark Cherry is the Dr. Patricia A. Hayes Endowed Professor of Applied Ethics and Associate Professor of Philosophy at St. Edward's University in Austin, Texas. He is the senior associate editor of *The Journal of Medicine and Philosophy,* senior associate editor of *Christian Bioethics,* and editor-in-chief of *HealthCare Ethics Committee Forum.*

Corinna Delkeskamp-Hayes is the director of International Studies in Philosophy and Medicine European Programs and is co-editor of Christian Bioethics and sits on the editorial board of *The Journal of Medicine and Philosophy.*

H. Tristram Engelhardt, Jr., is a professor in the department of philosophy at Rice University and is professor emeritus in the department of medicine at Baylor College of Medicine.

Stephen Erickson is the E. Wilson Lyon Professor of the Humanities and professor of philosophy at Pomona College.

Ruiping Fan is assistant professor in the department of public and social administration at City University of Hong Kong.

Angelo Petroni is the director of Advanced School of Public Administration of the Prime Minister's Office in Italy. He is a professor of logic and philosophy of science and the epistemology of the human sciences at the University of Bologna.

Julia Tao Lai, Po-wah is professor in the department of public and social administration at the City University of Hong Kong. She is currently a member of the Ethics Committee of the Hong Kong Medical Council. She is also a member of the editorial advisory board of the *International Journal of Medicine and Philosophy.*

Kurt W. Schmidt is the director of the Center for Medical Ethics at the Markus-Hospital in Frankfurt, Germany.

David Solomon is the W.P. and H.B. White Director of the Notre Dame Center for Ethics and Culture and is associate professor in the department of philosophy at the University of Notre Dame.

Kevin Wildes, S.J., is the president of Loyola University, New Orleans and he was a member of the department of philosophy and a Senior Research Scholar in the Kennedy Institute of Ethics at Georgetown University where he also held a secondary appointment in the department of medicine at the Georgetown University School of Medicine.

Index